METROPOLITAN COLLEGE OF NY
LIBRARY, 12TH FLOOR
431 CANAL STREET
NEW YORK, NY 10013

HEALTH IN THE CITY

CULTURE, LABOR, HISTORY SERIES
General Editors: Daniel Bender and Kimberley L. Phillips

The Forests Gave Way before Them: The Impact of African Workers on the Anglo-American World, 1650–1850
Frederick C. Knight

Unknown Class: Undercover Investigations of American Work and Poverty from the Progressive Era to the Present
Mark Pittenger

Steel Barrio: The Great Mexican Migration to South Chicago, 1915–1940
Michael D. Innis-Jiménez

Ordering Coal: Railroads, Miners, and Disorder in the Gilded Age, 1870–1900
Andrew B. Arnold

A Great Conspiracy Against Our Race: Italian Immigrant Newspapers and the Construction of Whiteness in the Early 20th Century
Peter G. Vellon

Reframing Randolph: A Reassessment of A. Philip Randolph's Legacies to Labor and Black Freedom
Edited by Andrew E. Kersten and Clarence Lang

Working the Empire
Edited by Daniel Bender and Jana K. Lipman

Whose Harlem Is It Anyway? Community and Working-Class Family Politics during the New Negro Era
Shannon King

Health in the City: Race, Poverty, and the Negotiation of Women's Health in New York City, 1915–1930
Tanya Hart

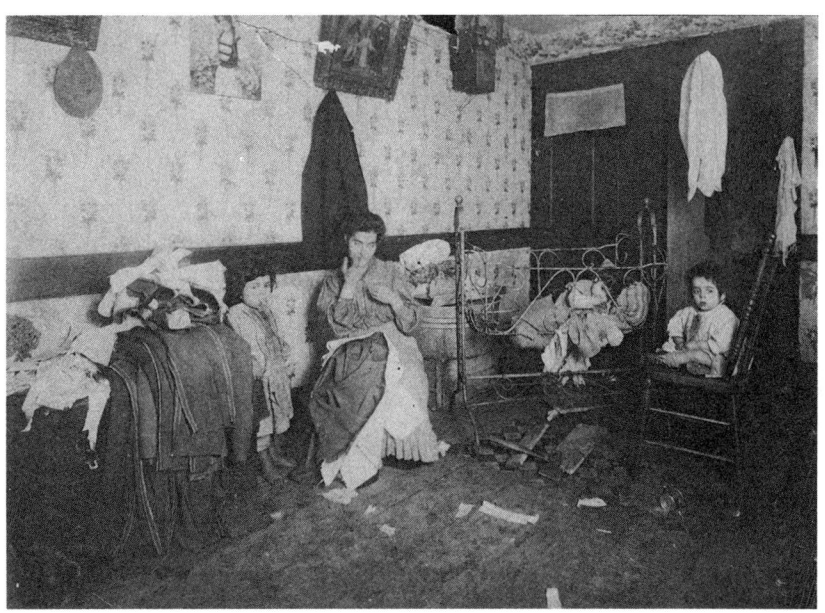

"Mrs. Guadina, living in a dirty, poverty-stricken home. On the trunk is the work of four days. She was struggling along, actually weak for want of food, trying to finish this batch so she could get the pay. There seemed to be no food in the house. The father is out of work. Three small children and another expected soon." Department of Commerce and Labor. Children's Bureau. (1912–1913) New York City. Digital ID: (color digital file from black and white original print) nclc 04144 http://hdl.loc.gov/loc.pnp/nclc.04144 (accessed March 10, 2014).

Health in the City

Race, Poverty, and the Negotiation of Women's Health in New York City, 1915–1930

Tanya Hart

NEW YORK UNIVERSITY PRESS
New York and London

NEW YORK UNIVERSITY PRESS
New York and London
www.nyupress.org

© 2015 by New York University
All rights reserved

References to Internet websites (URLs) were accurate at the time of writing. Neither the author nor New York University Press is responsible for URLs that may have expired or changed since the manuscript was prepared.

Library of Congress Cataloging-in-Publication Data
Hart, Tanya, 1956– , author.
Health in the city : race, poverty, and the negotiation of women's health in New York City, 1915–1930 / Tanya Hart.
p. ; cm. — (Culture, labor, history series)
Includes bibliographical references and index.
ISBN 978-1-4798-6799-8 (cl : alk. paper)
I. Title. II. Series: Culture, labor, history.
[DNLM: 1. Urban Health—history—New York City. 2. Women's Health—history—New York City. 3. African Americans—history—New York City. 4. History, 20th Century—New York City. 5. Maternal Health Services—history—New York City. 6. Minority Health—history—New York City. 7. Poverty—history—New York City. WA 11 AN7]
RA566.4.I3
362.1'042097471—dc23   2015000476

New York University Press books are printed on acid-free paper, and their binding materials are chosen for strength and durability. We strive to use environmentally responsible suppliers and materials to the greatest extent possible in publishing our books.

Manufactured in the United States of America

10 9 8 7 6 5 4 3 2 1

Also available as an ebook

To impoverished mothers all over the world, who carry their dreams and customs embodied in their hopes for the unborn and newly born, and to those professionals who work tirelessly to improve their health and the health of their children, I dedicate this book.

METROPOLITAN COLLEGE OF NY
LIBRARY, 12TH FLOOR
431 CANAL STREET
NEW YORK, NY 10013

CONTENTS

Acknowledgments	xi
Introduction	1
1. Migration and the City	15
2. Professionalization in the City	64
3. Work in the City	85
4. Culture in the City	108
5. Birthing in the City: Columbus Hill	138
6. Health in Columbus Hill	162
7. Birthing in the City: The Mulberry District	188
8. Health in the Mulberry District	218
Notes	245
Bibliography	291
Index	315
About the Author	329

ACKNOWLEDGMENTS

First and always, I want to give praise and thanks to God and His son, Jesus Christ. Without them, I would have nothing. They are my all in all.

I want to thank the faculty at Yale University and Harvard University for their undying support and encouragement throughout the graduate research that provided the foundation for this work: Nancy Cott, Glenda Gilmore, Matthew Jacobson, Naomi Rogers; David Brion Davis, David Blight, and Hazel Carby.

Archivists are invaluable to any historical work—they can really save your bacon. I wish to thank the archivists, curators and staff at the Columbia University Rare Book and Manuscript Library, especially Thai Jones and Devon Nevola; the archivists and staff at the New York-Presbyterian Hospital / Weill Cornell Medical Center, New York Presbyterian Hospital / Columbia University Medical Center, New York Public Library, Schomburg Center for Research in Black Culture, Beinecke Library at Yale University, Yale Medical Library, and the New York City Municipal Archives. I also want to thank Alia Winters, Judith Whiting, and the staff at the Community Service Society of New York for granting me access to its archives at the Columbia University Rare Book and Manuscript Library.

At the University of Kansas, I give my heartfelt gratitude to colleagues who encouraged me to press on, even as I encountered numerous obstacles over the years: Jennifer Hamer, Clarence Lang, Sherrie Tucker, Martha Jerrim, Christina Lux, Randal Jelks, David Katzman, Maryemma Graham, John Edgar Tidwell, Omofolabo Ajayi-Soyinka, Marta Vicente, and Hannah Britton. I also extend humble thanks to other colleagues and friends who have given critical support at strategic times: Troy Duster, Darlene Clark Hine, David Holmes, Judith Gordon, and Rhonda Lehman-Davenport.

My brothers and sisters in Christ have been amazingly supportive and encouraging over the years. My greatest thanks and blessings to everyone at the Whitney Avenue Church of Christ in North Haven, Connecticut, the Dover Church of Christ in Dover, New Hampshire (special thanks to Tom and Dorothy Olbricht), and the Southside Church of Christ in Lawrence, Kansas. I particularly want to extend much love and gratitude to the members of the Tuesday night small group Bible study where I was a member for seven years: thanks to David and Mary Beth Petr, Larry and Elaine McCullough, Victor and Marla Braden, Emily Braden, Chris and Krista Howard, the late Ione Sells, Adrian Lewis, Leatrice Smith, and Southside's minister and his wife, Chris and Beth Newton, for enduring all the tears and frustrations, and for always remaining loving, patient, and supportive. You all have helped me stay sane—no small feat.

Finally, I owe more than I can say to family members who have passed on before me. My grandparents, Alfred and Cecile Bell; great-grandmother, Lena Evans; and mother, Mona Blakeley, instilled within me an appreciation for the past, a sense of humor, and the ability to see the importance of everyday people. I love you, miss you terribly, and look forward to heaven.

Introduction

Shortly after the dawning of the twentieth century, the New York City Department of Health proclaimed its mission to protect public health in the motto "Public health is purchasable. Within natural limitations a community can determine its own death rate."[1] To test its credo, the Department of Health conducted its first citywide mortality study in 1915.[2] Starting with the results of the study, the programs and action that would occur over the next fifteen years reflected the city's power and promise to make public health a reality, the actions and reactions of its subject clientele, and the often resultant cultural clash between these competing groups.

Health in the City explores infant and maternal health care created for impoverished women in turn-of-the-twentieth-century New York City, and their responses. In particular, I compare the health outcomes of three different groups of poor and working-class women whose stories of infant and maternal health care are linked by New York City's first citywide mortality study in 1915, and trace their experiences through 1930. Poor and working-class African American, British West Indian, and southern Italian women received some of the nation's best health care, albeit shrouded in racially gendered and classed misconceptions and stereotypes of their supposed inferiority. As impoverished women, their responses to health worker's expectations—whether accommodation, manipulation, or resistance—revealed their agency and "work" as they carved out their own health care, while living in an era when the meanings of "woman" and resistance began in the womb.

Numerous historians of public health have shown that socioeconomic factors and cultural traditions have influenced how client communities have responded to the health care they received.[3] In a different vein, migration historians have argued that socioeconomic factors and cultural traditions influenced the ways in which migrating populations created new post-migration identities. Building upon both strains of scholarship, the socioeconomic status and cultural traditions of post-migration women of African and Southern Italian descent—and how public health and medical workers treated them—influenced their agency. In turn, the agency exhibited by these women also reflected newly forged identities, developed as they accepted or rejected tenets of the health systems that were being created around them.

To track what it perceived as the racial nature of health, the New York City Department of Health created sanitary districts defined by race in the late 1890s, then conducted its first citywide mortality study in 1915. After compiling the data, in 1916 it selected the New York City Association for Improving the Condition of the Poor (AICP) to create and conduct a health demonstration aimed at decreasing infant and maternal deaths among poverty-stricken African Americans and British West Indians in Columbus Hill, a midtown Manhattan neighborhood and the city's worst mortality "sore spot."[4] At first, the AICP focused its efforts on respiratory diseases. However, it quickly shifted its lens to syphilis among black women and congenital syphilis in their infants to explain high mortality rates, taking a page from southern white physicians who viewed all blacks as syphilitic—especially black women. To continue this mind-set, the AICP mandated that parturient black women undergo syphilis testing and treatment as a condition of receiving prenatal care, then in its infancy.

In 1917, after declaring its first year of health work in Columbus Hill a success when the infant death rate was cut in half, the AICP found and chose what it termed a more "racially distinct" area for expansion of its infant/maternal health care experiment: Lower Manhattan's Little Italy, or the Mulberry District. Here, the New York City Department of Health and the AICP ignored issues of syphilis among childbearing, impoverished Southern Italian women, and instead focused on tuberculosis-related illnesses and deaths among adult women, and pneumonia and enteritis among their infants. By 1924, this health program expanded to cover preschool and school-age children, and an area health care clinic was built. These successes aside, the Italian maternal acceptance of Anglo American prenatal care and physician deliveries never approached the enthusiasm held by African American and British West Indian women for similar programs: they rejected the AICP's top-down approach and rejected most native-born white pressures to trade midwives for non-Italian physicians. By the late 1920s, the AICP realized that other agencies were duplicating its work in the Mulberry District; its infant and maternal demonstration came to an end as the area contracted and Italian families moved to East Harlem and other neighborhoods. Farther uptown, in Columbus Hill, poverty and the mixed-use nature of the neighborhood worked to change its landscape forever. A tiny health care center—created specifically for blacks—could do little to accommodate even the dwindling numbers of inhabitants still living in the area. In the 1940s, most of Columbus Hill was razed for what would become the Lincoln Center complex. Blacks who had lived in the neighborhood moved northward to Harlem, or to other boroughs.

I am challenging traditional ideas of early twentieth century urban black health care by showing a program that was simultaneously racialized *and* cutting-edge. Moreover, Columbus Hill's health demonstration became the model for a European immigrant neighborhood, which contradicts the normal separation of black and nonblack urban health care and encourages scholars to take another look at race, health, and the evolution of health care programs across groups. Certainly, there may have been other European immigrant health care efforts built on foundations of black health care.

The AICP's health demonstrations in both Columbus Hill and the Mulberry District were framed and hampered by issues of race and class, and fractured by conflicts between mothers and health care workers over "correct" and "modern" birthing and child-rearing methods. In addition, when pressured to show the efficacy of its work, the AICP produced pamphlets distributed among the public health and medical communities that stretched results favorably: in the case of both neighborhoods, the agency claimed successes that an exploration of its own internal data call into question.

By examining health demonstrations and client responses from almost a century ago I am not only detailing a history of health work but also offering a cautionary tale for contemporary health officials and health care workers. When developing and carrying out health care programs for minority and poor communities, one should always consider and factor in the agency of women, their concerns, their importance within their communities, and their attachments to valued cultural traditions. As a comparative health study, *Health in the City* engages and crosses the fields of women's studies, the histories of public health and medicine, transnational migration and urban studies, and ethnic and African American studies. It reveals that even the most well meaning public health officials and medical workers may inadvertently reinforce perceptions of inherited or learned inferiority as a determinant of health that their programs are created to fix. Today, when biogenetic engineering promises much but remains linked to the very notions of "race" and racialized difference that the mapping of the human genome has disproved, we need to look back at a time when workers in public health and medicine could have used new technologies to question the immutability of race—but didn't—so that we may have a chance to challenge deterministic notions of "race" and dismantle racism in the future.

Methodology and Sources

Many have questioned the origins of my obsession with the lives and health of black and Southern Italian women and their children. I admit my positionality as a "boomer" kid, an only child who watched way too many old movies when I should have been outside playing in the yard. It seemed that every other film was set in New York City, and the "dead end" female or male protagonist always climbed to success by hard work. I also noted the absence of African American women from the silver screen. Most who were on screen were unattractive and overweight, and they were always subservient. As a child, I found the "dead end"–to–Park Avenue immigrant and the smiling, verbally challenged "Mammy" tropes deeply disturbing.

Sociologist Stanley Lieberson's *A Piece of the Pie: Blacks and White Immigrants Since 1880* shaped my scholarly interests in the late nineteenth and early twentieth century black and Southern Italian women who lived in New York City. Lieberson successfully quantified the reasons behind black/European immigrant economic differentials that developed from 1880 to 1930. However, I questioned the absence of women's socioeconomic roles in Lieberson's book and determined that a comparative examination of these women's lives should be done.

In *A Piece of the Pie*, Lieberson questioned past sociological studies that privileged either racial discrimination against poor and working-class African Americans or perceptions of their inferior cultural mores as the sole impediments that barred them from attaining the same higher economic levels as those achieved by southern, central, and eastern Europeans immigrants (or, using his abbreviation, SCE) of similar economic stature and job skills during the twentieth century. While retaining the salience of racism as a barrier to black status achievement, Lieberson went further, employing empirical data and socioeconomic theories of racial stratification to argue that other measurable obstacles explained the black/European immigrant status gap that appeared between 1880 and 1950. He revealed that although racism has always been an impediment to nonwhite success, other measurable factors, such as educational differentials, occupational niches, and residential segregation, must be evaluated to determine why African Americans have historically lagged behind other nonwhite groups and SCE immigrants.[5]

Lieberson's work laid an important methodological foundation for my research and thinking. As he states early on, one should not compare "apples to oranges" when analyzing why so many people of African descent found it difficult to match the socioeconomic upward movement of the first SCEs and their descendants. In other words, using assumptions of the cultural superiority of SCE immigrants and their children to explain their economic successes while stating that the slowness of African American economic gains can be explained by cultural inferiority can be an attempt to mask scholarly prejudices, feed into common historic misperceptions, and hide the difficulties that SCEs had had while "making it." The effect of cultural traditions alone on social mobility is difficult to quantify. Thus Lieberson sought quantifiable data that could better explain black/European socioeconomic differences over time. He eschewed culture, only employing it to show that African Americans were equally or more concerned with education than many SCE immigrant groups. In addition, even with the absence of women's perspectives and contributions to their family's economic, social, and emotional welfare, he successfully illustrated that, if one constructed a solid socioeconomic structure based on empirical data, one could incorporate culture and thus competently compare racialized migrant's lives without relying upon "culture" or "race" alone.[6]

Over time, some public health reformers between the 1880s and 1930s acknowledged that environmental factors, shaped by socioeconomic inequalities, were significant causal agents in determining infant and maternal health, while arguing among themselves about how much heredity or the à la carte subjectivities found in definitions of "race" could also influence individual and group health. I weigh these environmental, socioeconomic, and assumed heredity factors in explaining why I think African American, British West Indian, and Southern Italian women behaved differently with regard to the public health care they received. My research unearthed the tensions between racialists and environmentalists at the time, and their ability to accept and inhabit the varying shades of racialism and environment in between. Correspondingly, internal communications reflected not only the personal perspectives of social workers, physicians, and nurses but also acts of agency from their clientele.[7]

Although some of my primary source data comes from medical journals and health records as part of my attempt to chronicle black and Southern Italian women's responses to the health work created for them, I must confess that my interest in public health and medical history happened quite unexpectedly. I knew when considering graduate school that I would research black and Italian women in early twentieth century New York City. In 1996, while conducting initial research at UCLA on an Urban Studies seminar paper on black and Southern Italian women for the late Eric Monkkonen, I happened upon a 1923 *Opportunity* magazine article that reviewed how blacks had fared in New York City since the start of the 1910s Great Migration of African Americans out of the South. The author had briefly mentioned an unnamed black neighborhood where, in 1915, almost one-third of the infants had died within their first year of life.[8] Because of the arbitrary racialization that had been incorporated in the establishment of sanitary districts, neither the author nor the City had considered calculating the black infant mortality of an adjoining district that also contained Irish, German, Italian, and native-born white inhabitants. However, when I later incorporated the black infant mortality rate for this district, the death rate for the black area on West 61st, 62nd, and 63rd Streets soared even higher, to 46 percent.[9] Mesmerized by the enormity of human suffering that corresponded even with the lower statistic, my task became one of excavating the information surrounding the incredible numbers—namely, recovering the steps taken in the 1915 Department of Health citywide mortality survey, and what had transpired afterward. In the process, my earlier interests in women's identity became more focused on issues of maternal and infant health as I conducted a never-before-attempted health client study.

Many historians of medicine and public health have investigated how social inequalities influenced and thus complicated perceptions of science and medicine as empirical and objective, seen in the past as somehow set apart from the biases of practitioners and researchers.[10] For example, in *Silent Travelers: Germs and the Immigrant Menace*, Alan Kraut revealed the symbiotic relationship between U.S. politics, economics, Anglo American culture and identity, medicine, and public health in the period between 1880 and 1924. Immigration officials, armed with newly minted scientific knowledge about bacteria and the etiologies of diseases, inflamed nativist concerns over cheap immigrant labor by stigmatizing migrants from southern and eastern Europe as disease carriers whose presence threatened native-born white American health. In particular, as state agencies increased their ability to identify, classify, and quantify diseases, and as notions of intelligence testing and the hierarchy of supposedly superior and inferior races increased, the numbers of immigrants whom they deemed "fit" to become naturalized citizens decreased. Although most immigrants gained admittance, they found themselves under the constant scrutiny of public health officials and reformers who blamed immigrants for any signs of poor health and justified their views by citing the impoverishment, strange customs, and perceived racial inferiority of each group.[11]

Europeans experienced the links between "disease and difference" in contacts with native American populations, who later succumbed to European-borne diseases.[12] Explorers and colonists had also learned valuable lessons while dealing with their own "virgin soil" epidemics, such as malaria and yellow fever, which felled the vulnerable and unseasoned.[13] Pre-bacterial-era explanations of epidemic diseases centered on airborne miasmas, or foul air, that carried effluvia, or microscopic particles. Humoralists and anti-contagionists usually argued that disease required decaying filth as a growth medium for disease. Morality and religious beliefs also played a hand in understanding health and disease. This mode of thought and belief shifted slightly into the foreground during the 1800s. For example, between the cholera epidemics of 1832, 1848, and 1866, Anglo Americans' perspectives altered from viewing illness as God's will or wrath to exploring how poverty and filth exacerbated the spread of disease. Yet the rise of sanitarianism, and concerns over environmental factors as the cause of disease coexisted with the stigmatization or "othering" of nonwhites. Pro-slavery apologists such as doctors Samuel Cartwright and Josiah Nott led the fight against abolitionism by racializing African American health and disease, thus also racializing health differentials between blacks and whites and providing further scientific justifications for enslavement. This foundation of hereditary difference also influenced the treatment of Irish immigrants, whom reformers linked to the cholera epidemics due to their poverty, "drunkenness," and dirty surroundings.[14]

Of the immigrants that Kraut surveyed, the *contadini*, or townsfolk of southern Italy, felt the weight of white nativism with a disturbing frequency through the encroachments of public health officials and visiting nurses. Despite proof from "spokesmen" of the Italian community, such as Dr. Antonio Stella, and data compiled by Ellis Island officials that revealed low levels of premigration disease, U.S. health reformers continued to argue that Italian migrants fell ill to diseases they brought with them, not those they encountered through impoverished lives spent in overcrowded tenements, workplaces that lacked adequate ventilation, or malnutrition.[15]

The growth of their numbers frightened even the most tolerant Americans: between 1880 and 1921, more than 4.5 million Italians, mostly rural unskilled peasants from the south, moved to the United States. Most gained entry through the port of Ellis Island, and many settled in the New York City area. A vast cultural gulf existed between Anglo and Italian customs and responses to health and illness. The Italians became the focus of public health reformers as a result of their "strangeness" and recalcitrant attitudes toward authority figures—they brought with them a mistrust of uniformed "officials" that had been cultivated in Italy. Thus, with mistrust and cultural differences on both sides, public health officials castigated them for retaining their cultural perspectives on health care ("magic and superstition" to Anglos), and Italians resisted many incursions of health workers.[16]

Kraut's work is vastly important because he correlates the edicts of health officials, nativists' fears about the onslaught of racial inferiors, industrialists' need for cheap immigrant labor, the cultural clash over disease and its spread that occurred between native-born whites and immigrants, and the ways in which immigrant groups resisted or accommodated the desires of public health officials. Missing, of course, are people of African descent who either lived in New York City during the time of massive immigration from southern and central European immigration or migrated from the Caribbean, West Indies, and South America. Regardless of geographic origins, their numbers increased as Anglo nativists placed a firmer legal damper on non–northern European immigration. Moreover, some white northern reformers tagged blacks as socially dangerous because of the belief that they carried the same diseases as SCE migrants, a token from southern white physicians who warned their northern counterparts of diseased black women as domestics and their closeness to white families.

Therefore, the movement of blacks out of the South during the first Great Migration should be studied in concert with the era of massive European migration, because the two movements fed upon and supported the other. Since historians of science and public health have grounded Anglo American notions of racial differentials in health and disease within the legacy of slavery and Emancipation, a comparison of the health care received by groups of African and southern European ancestries and their responses is long overdue.[17]

Lastly, when public health reformers targeted women's reproduction, childbirth, and child rearing as objects of public health concerns, they commingled notions of women's bodies and bodily integrity, the home, and cultural traditions. James Scott's theory of "public transcripts" and "hidden transcripts" is invaluable in unearthing how seemingly powerless subgroups (such as my impoverished black and Italian women) always possess some measure of agency and may hide collective actions and words of resistance from the public sphere. There, representatives of the dominant culture (such as the public health workers and officials who served these female immigrant clients) wear a public mask that also may hide hidden private words and actions that belie their dominant position. According to Scott, "[by] assessing the discrepancy *between* [emphasis his] the hidden transcript and the public transcript we may begin to judge the impact of domination on public discourse."[18]

I raise several questions where a scrutiny of public and hidden transcripts provides alternate answers that explicate the complexity of these women's lives. For example, when AICP nurses questioned Columbus Hill's black women to find their marital status, they overwhelming replied "married." Historian Herbert Gutman revealed a marked difference in the Columbus Hill black male-to-female ratio, which did not become equal until 1925. He maintained that most black women were not single heads of households.[19] Studies done in the 1910s and 1920s by Frances Blascoer and Abram Harris—respectively, a white female and a black male social worker who were both sympathetic to the women of Columbus Hill—revealed difficulties in collecting critical data, or much lower rates of marriage for these women than the 96 percent marriage rate reported by the AICP.[20]

Who was right—the AICP and Gutman, or Blascoer and Harris? Or, better yet, should one instead look at the power held by these women to map the terrain, see what was expected and at stake, and reveal just so much to authority figures? At the turn of the twentieth century, much of white American society stigmatized women of African ancestry as wanton or hypersexual. One can easily surmise that these women told public health nurses they were married in order to receive better prenatal care, or to receive care at all, because they felt that monogamous (though extralegal) relations equated with marriage. In addition, I believe they may have lied to counter prevalent white stereotypes of black female sexuality. They may have been motivated by both reasons, including stretching the truth to keep whites out of their personal business. Were black female statements of marriage public transcripts that masked the reality of their private lives?

Regarding the Southern Italian Mulberry population, the City of New York instituted its first anti-tuberculosis campaigns in 1900. Part of the new public behavior that officials demanded was an end to public spitting, where air circulated from common instances of walking or wind could become a vector for the inhalation of dried tuberculosis sputum particles. Moreover, tuberculosis pamphlets disseminated by public health officials stressed that in order to avoid ingesting contaminated sputum, individuals should not drink or eat from the same cups, plates, or eating utensils. These public health warnings ran head on into cultural differences. For example, Alan Kraut has shown that spitting was an integral part of Italian culture. According to Kraut, Southern Italian mothers believed that their spit, used on an infant's eyes, would protect it from conjunctivitis, or treat impetigo. Italian women undergoing a difficult delivery also asked neighbor women to spit out the window to ward off evil spirits. They also used spittle as a purgative or to protect against the evil eye.[21] Did they hold on to these traditional methods at home? Were these actions hidden from those in public authority—especially since most Italian women continued to use midwives? Inquiries into and answers for these and other questions help reveal how, from seemingly powerless positions of racial, cultural, socioeconomic, and political subjugation, African American, British West Indian, and Southern Italian women may have successfully hidden their private lives from public view at a time when public health officials felt that their private lives demanded public scrutiny.

Chapter Outline

Chapter 1, "Migration and the City," charts the worlds that African American, British West Indian, and Southern Italian women encountered and created after coming to New York City, juxtaposed against the spaces, attitudes, and expectations of their homelands. Here I reorient the narrative around excerpts from social work files that reveal the lives of individual women and migration theories, inserting African Americans and British West Indians into standing European migration literature that has excluded them. While there were some differences, black and Southern Italian women often had parallel and overlapping reasons for their migrations and competed for housing, services, and even prospective sexual mates. This chapter also includes sociological, literary and cultural aspects of their lives, imperative in postulating how they felt about themselves, their expectations, and the demands of their pre- and post-migration communities. I also briefly explore what life was like for impoverished women and children who lived in Columbus Hill and the Mulberry District. Using census and sociological data from the 1910s and 1920s and Community Organization Society social work interviews of women living within the areas, I reconstruct how these poor and working-class women dealt with the vagaries of daily urban living: abandonment, poor health, caring for their children, work, and abandonment.

Chapter 2, "Professionalization in the City," examines the historical tenets of "maternalist" movements as loci to investigate how the professionalization of medicine and nursing combined in New York City to transform it into apex of "modern" municipal medicine at the dawn of the twentieth century. Here I argue that it is important to interrogate these constructions as contradictory, yet complementary, conceptions of racially gendered and classed identities in the United States that were firmly rooted in the perception and existence of racial and gendered differences, yet undergoing contestations at the same time.

Chapter 3, "Work in the City," charts the professionalization of public health and social work and its effects on Columbus Hill, the chapter's focus. In this chapter, I look at the amalgamation of top-down efforts to aid and analyze the poor, starting with Dr. S. Josephine Baker, head of the Division of Child Hygiene and the first woman to lead a municipal city department in the U.S., and continuing to the legendary Dr. W. E. B. DuBois who, in 1900, studied black life in San Juan Hill (the earlier name for Columbus Hill). I then discuss a more "middle-up" perspective from social worker Frances Blascoer, who worked in Columbus Hill, and Mary White Ovington, the activist and "mother" of the National Association for the Advancement of Colored People, who actually lived among blacks in Columbus Hill.

Chapter 4, "Culture in the City," begins with an 1892 Frances Ellen Watkins Harper speech to Brooklyn women on black mothering, and then incorporates popular cultural artifacts—work and blues songs, poetry, folklore, and short stories—to elicit cross-class perspectives of black womanhood from African American and British West Indian men and women in each particular group. I use this dialog to interrogate how women and men within these cultures responded to debates surrounding issues of privacy that were withheld from women, especially women of color: their bodies, female sexuality, being a "good mother," and the meaning of motherhood.

Chapter 5, "Birthing in the City: Columbus Hill," starts with the 1915 citywide health study, the Health Department's decision to start health work in the black section of Columbus Hill, which it saw as a "hot zone," and its devolution of power to the AICP, which decided to ignore the effects of tuberculosis, pneumonia, enteritis, and other respiratory diseases for infant and maternal syphilis. I posit that health officials ignored respiratory diseases for syphilis because of their acceptance of age-old stereotypes. Moreover, while changes in the diagnosis and treatment of syphilis infections were still dependent on the determinations of physicians and the efficacy of laboratories, the existence of multiple sites of maternal health care within the neighborhood—and of the Vanderbilt Clinic, which was staffed by medical students and syphilologists from Columbia University—made it prime territory for a public health demonstration *and* the subject of multiple articles on syphilis treatments, which were published in medical journals.

Chapter 6, "Health in Columbus Hill," continues by critiquing the actual health work done in Columbus Hill, and the pernicious effects of tuberculosis—the widespread disease that the AICP chose to ignore. While the neighborhood experienced a small yet significant decrease in infant deaths from syphilitic infections, this cannot explain the enormous decline in infant and maternal deaths that occurred in the AICP's first year of research. More to the point was the agency of African American and British West Indian women, who went out of their way to seek prenatal and postnatal care, even while dealing with mandatory syphilis testing and treatment.

Chapter 7, "Birthing in the City: The Mulberry District," tracks why—then how—the AICP in 1918 expanded its Columbus Hill-model of public/private infant and maternal health care into Lower Manhattan's Little Italy, the Mulberry District, which the agency deemed a more "racially pure" neighborhood in its own internal documents. Here, the AICP chose to forego the mandatory syphilis testing and treatments for parturient women to receive prenatal care that they were mandating for black women in Columbus Hill. Instead, in an effort to introduce prenatal care, the agency took the Italian preference for Italian midwives in its crosshairs and, viewing itself as an "entering wedge" into the community's health care and cultural traditions, implemented Anglo American physician deliveries in lieu of Italian midwife deliveries. To answer "why," I engage the broader anti-midwifery movement in this chapter, and its racial and classed foundations, to help explain why Columbus Hill's African American and British West Indian women had eschewed midwives and overwhelmingly accepted physician deliveries in Columbus Hill, while Southern Italian women doggedly clung to midwives throughout the 1920s.

Chapter 8, "Health in the Mulberry District," contrasts the actual health work done by the AICP and the Department of Health in the Mulberry District, from the perspectives of officials, the efforts of works, and the reactions of clients. The AICP's designation of the "midwife problem" became an enduring "line in the sand" between the district's Italian women, the larger community, and health care workers. This is clearly reflected in the agency's 1924 pamphlet *Protecting the Mother and Child*; however, despite maternal resistance, the AICP again lauds it efforts, much as it does in *Health Work for Mothers and Children in a Colored Community*. The internal data from which the AICP constructed *Protecting the Mother and Child* reveals that the agency may have "helped" its public image by inflating some of its reported data on maternal/infant health outcomes. This may have been done so that Italian maternal and community acceptance of Anglo preschool public health and medical programs made more sense. Regardless, the basis of the AICP's medical work in the Mulberry District was racially gendered and classed. The AICP mistakenly believed that, like Columbus Hill's African American and British West Indian women, Southern Italian women would similarly adopt Anglo birthing and prenatal programs. Instead, the women resisted, leading the AICP to blame them for their ignorance when, in fact, it was the AICP's ignorance of Italian culture and mores that had thwarted some of the outcomes it had wanted to achieve. By 1930, the AICP reviewed its efficacy in the Mulberry District and realized that its efforts had been limited by resistance from the neighborhood's Southern Italian women—even though it had publically trumpeted its successes only six years earlier.

1

Migration and the City

The New York City Department of Health conducted its first citywide health survey in 1915. The racially segregated African American and British West Indian section of Columbus Hill, an impoverished midtown Manhattan neighborhood, had exhibited inordinately high rates of infant and maternal mortality. The Department of Health termed it a "sore spot" in its 1916 report, a place warranting immediate help.[1]

So, beginning in 1917, with powers devolved from the Department of Health, the New York Association for Improving the Condition of the Poor (AICP) coordinated public and private efforts to stem the tide of black infant and maternal deaths within this area, targeting syphilis among black women and congenital syphilis among their young as the culprits. All the while, the Department of Health and the AICP closely monitored and measured the progress and results of their Columbus Hill work because they wanted to further test their methods and hypotheses in an additional area: one they believed was purer, more racially distinct. To meet this need, in 1918, they selected Lower Manhattan's "Little Italy," or the Mulberry District—even though the neighborhood's infant and maternal mortality rates were vastly eclipsed by other "sore spots," areas with health problems nearly as problematic as those of Columbus Hill. Nevertheless, the AICP focused on tuberculosis-related morbidity and mortality among childbearing Southern Italian women, and pneumonia and enteritis among their infants.

Mothers and children in both neighborhoods received modern, cutting-edge health care—at the time, New York City stood at the apex of maternal care in the United States—but the care they received was often shrouded in racially gendered and classed misconceptions and stereotypes of their supposed inferiority. Health care efforts in both neighborhoods were framed and hampered by issues of race and fractured by conflicts between mothers and health care workers over "correct" and "modern" birthing and child-rearing methods. In addition, when pressured to show that its methods worked, the AICP produced pamphlets that it distributed among the public health and medical communities. These reflected the biases and positions of the agency, even as it labored to improve the health of women and children. Physicians who treated Columbus Hill's black women and children for syphilis may have used their clients to further their own research agendas. And in the Southern Italian Mulberry District, where the AICP was surprised by maternal resistance to its prenatal work, it may have "encouraged" its results when the publication of its infant and maternal health work is compared to internal documents.

Years of health demonstrations—experimentations—in both areas passed, and, despite its racialized foundations and questions regarding the efficacy of its programs and validity of its data, the AICP coordinated and oversaw modern infant and maternal health care for black and Southern Italian women. These initial programs—their purpose, structure, and outcomes—and how the African American, British West Indian, and Southern Italian female clientele of Columbus Hill and the Mulberry District responded, are the basis of this book. Officials and the general populace alike targeted poor migrating populations as carriers of contagions; more narrowly, they targeted impoverished migrating women as potential carriers of contagions, through their bodies and the bodies of their unborn children. Seeing them as more than bearers of disease—seeing the cultural and social systems of identity and agency that they bore—means analyzing migration historiographies created by scholars as well as creatively mining other nontraditional methods of cultural and social transmission—stories, plays, and poetry. All are equally important in creating a comparative study of African American, British West Indian, and southern Italian women's responses to infant and maternal health care—basically, creating multiple client-based studies that never before existed.

But for now: Who were the women of Columbus Hill and the Mulberry District? Where did they come from, why did they migrate, and what cultural and social systems of identity and agency did they bring to New York City?

Immigration and Migration History and Historiography

Migration scholars have traditionally conceptualized the reasons behind group movement from one land to another in terms of "push and pull"; in other words, concretized and/or ideological agents (better jobs; the notion of freedom) *pulled* persons to a perceived, hoped-for better land, while other concrete and/or ideological agents (poverty and the lack of jobs; oppression from those in domination) *pushed* populations from their homelands. In the case of migration into the United States, primary emphases on the modes and types of migrations have also been bounded by historical era and origin. Many migrationists, with a culturalist perspective, accept the premise that this is a "land of immigrants" without questioning what "immigrant" means and, even more significant, without a recognition of the native populations who inhabited (and whose descendants still inhabit) the land. These "First Peoples" do not fit into the "immigrant" trope, nor does their forced or willing movement within the Americas. Furthermore, the tens of millions of West and Central Africans, also trans-Atlantic migrants, who came to the Americas by force, or whose descendants have moved forcibly or willingly throughout the Americas, have been considered outside the pale of trans-Atlantic (read: European) migration history. Often, these disparate but linked groups of peoples brushed elbows on a daily basis, intermarried and had children, competed for jobs and housing, were used to define how they and other groups would be conceptualized within the social, cultural, and legal fabric of the country, and how the United States conceived of itself and how it also would (and should) be reconceived as a land containing heterogeneous immigrants within its own seemingly homogeneous, collective identity.[2]

To criticize the creation of subfields in history at large, and in immigration and migration history in general, is not my purpose here: to refresh, challenge, or even subvert the telling of history by questioning, rethinking, and reworking popularly accepted notions of the past is part and parcel of how humans create history. Often, the perspectives and voices of the subordinated and disenfranchised provide a more nuanced depiction of an era than those who fear dragging out any other perspectives and voices that would question accepted narratives of the status quo. I am purposefully questioning the status quo by asking why the immigrations and migrations of those of African descent are still kept outside the boundaries of trans-Atlantic European migration history, particularly when the movements occurred simultaneously, often to the same areas and, while seeming different on the surface, often occurring for similar reasons. For a time, racial difference needed to flex its muscles to demand its place in the sun of migration scholarship. Gendered perspectives on migration have had to perform the same task.

Currently, however, a major flaw that continues in migration history has been the continued separation of so-called racial groups as if their perceived identities have made their movements—and reasons for moving—different, to the point of conflating differences of histories as salient divisions to justify differences of scholarship. As Russell Menard has stated, both the American colonies and the United States resulted from outer migrations, usually conceptualized as European and heterogeneous in origin. America's imagined homogeneity was thus achieved not by constructing a cross-cultural and transnational identity based upon "Old World Origins" but upon race, since the "'re-peopling' of North America . . . resulted in a holocaust for the Indians and in slavery for the transported Africans."[3] Simultaneous events with different origins and reasons, but simultaneous outcomes: after the creation of the new republic, membership for aliens became racialized because, always at the bottom, were "inferior" groups who, even if indigenous to the land or having had several generations born on the land, were not recognized as citizenship material. In fact, migrating Europeans, whether apprised of the situation in the United States beforehand or not, were usually the only group to hold the "whiteness" key to naturalization between 1790 and the 1870s.[4] It is for this reason that Menard advocates the inclusion of the migrations of African peoples in the literature of normally European trans-Atlantic migration history, which has been stifled by a "profound Eurocentrism" in the past.[5]

Therefore, the effect of separating group migrations by race, while necessary at times and enlightening in monographs, has created scholarship based upon separate "racialized" and also "gendered" and "classed" group differences. To look at comparative migrations at their fullest, I will examine the movement of African Americans, Southern Italians, and British West Indians to New York City from 1880 to 1930s in relation to one another and, later, in relation to their interactions with the New York City public health care and medical systems.

African Americans and British West Indians in Columbus Hill

What type of environment did African Americans and British West Indians encounter upon arriving in New York City? In the case of Columbus Hill, blacks encountered a community unique in its incongruities of ethnic diversity and racial segregation, picturesque surroundings and intense poverty, and a "cultured" past buried in a discordant, tenuous present. In short, Columbus Hill both enervated and exasperated. Its inhabitants were a diverse mixture of native- and foreign-born blacks, native-born whites, and Irish, Jewish, and Italian immigrants.[6] The earlier race riots that occurred between blacks and whites when the area had been known as San Juan Hill were but a distant memory by the 1915 census.[7] Unfortunately, the détente merely reinforced Northern de facto segregation: by 1922, the bulk of Columbus Hill's black community resided on West 61st Street, where 1,641 people lived in two and a half acres of squalid tenements.[8]

Columbus Hill proper was an elevated area that covered fifty-five city blocks and extended northward from 54th Street to the south, 70th Street to the north, and between Central Park West and Eighth Avenue

TABLE 1.1. Population by Race, 1910 and 1920

Racial group	Columbus Hill and vicinity		Areas 147 and 151	
	1910	1920	1910	1920
Native whites	13,150	14,383	873	1,065
Whites (foreign descent)	20,991	19,857	2,442	1,773
Foreign-born whites	19,169	18,115	2,222	1,348
Negroes*	9,825	8,180	7,291	6,248
Other colored	113	175	23	5
Total	63,248	60,170	12,851	10,471

* The black population of Columbus Hill proper (Sanitary Areas 147 and 151) was 15.5 percent of the total Columbus Hill population in 1910, and 13.5 percent in 1920. Part of Sanitary Area 147 (created in 1920) corresponds to Areas 113 and 115 (created in 1915); Area 151 (created in 1920) corresponds with Area 119 (created in 1915). Also, the black population in the area had increased to 8,928 in 1922. Data are taken from Holmes, "Sociological Survey," 2.

on the east to the Hudson River on the west. While the total neighborhood reflected its multinational basis, most of the area's native-born blacks and those from the West Indies lived segregated lives, crammed into tenements on 61st through 63rd Streets, from Amsterdam Avenue to the Hudson River.[9]

Referred to by one social worker as the "first stopping place for the newcomers from the British West Indies, the Virgin Islands, and the Southern [United] States," Columbus Hill's black community included newly arrived persons from various Central and South American countries as well.[10] As primarily native-born American rural and urban migrants and nonnative immigrants to the largest urban center in the nation, Columbus Hill's black men and women constituted a marginalized workforce, exploited by employers who placed a higher value on southern and eastern European migrant labor.

Despite the neighborhood's poverty, the areas outside of Columbus Hill's boundaries possessed an urban ambience. The urban wonders of Central Part and the Hudson River—one manmade and the other natural—created an atmosphere that provided its citizens with those "periods of refreshment" so immensely important to an area heavily congested with tenements and businesses. The neighborhood was also steeped in early New York City history. Columbus Hill was part of what had been the Bloomingdale (from the Dutch *Bloemendael*, or "vale of flowers") section of Dutch Manhattan in the seventeenth century. DeWitt Clinton Park now occupied the area that had been the eighteenth-century homes of General Garrit Hopper Stryker and the Mott family, and the Bloomingdale Academy, first opened in 1815, was located at West 74th Street.[11]

By the 1910s, Columbus Hill underwent rapid changes, shifting from a heavily residential district to a business area. Newspaper magnate William Randolph Hearst and Arthur Brisbane, another wealthy New Yorker, owned the lion's share of residential and business properties in the district.[12] Blacks owned few residences. The housing situation was deplorable. Overcrowding became the primary problem in older tenements and houses: 7.2 people per apartment on average resided in dilapidated, pre-1901 dwellings (see figure 1.1). Older housing was cheaper than the new model apartments (on average, the

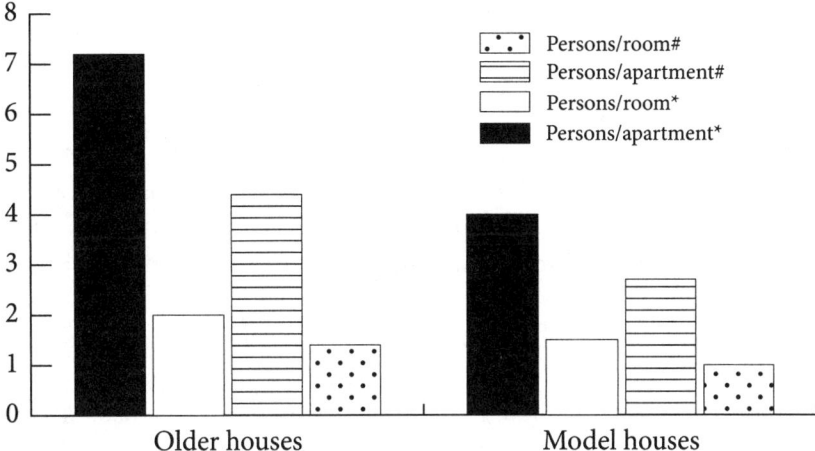

Figure 1.1. Comparison of overcrowded conditions between older and model houses. The data are taken from Norman A. Holmes, "Sociological Survey of the Negro Population of Columbus Hill of New York City," photocopy (New York: Lincoln House Committee of the Henry Street Settlement, 1922), 5.

* Observation 1: A sampling of 100 apartments in older houses and 100 apartments in model houses containing the largest families.

\# Observation 2: A sampling of 100 apartments in older houses and 100 apartments in model houses, with no consideration of family size.

rents for older apartments were $1.20 per week, versus $1.85 in modernized tenement "homes"), yet the differences were financially and aesthetically significant.[13]

Although they were few, model apartments such as the "513 desirable apartments" called the Phipps Houses and the City and Suburban Homes were located on 62nd, 63rd, and 64th Streets, just north of Columbus Hill's heavily black 61st Street. Built after 1901 and constructed to comply with New York City's newer housing laws, they possessed considerably more frontage space than older tenements (approximately 45′6″, compared to the general 25′ of older houses) and were built with interior courts and fireproof halls. Out of one hundred model apartments randomly sampled in Norman Holmes's "Sociological Study" of Columbus Hill, each had at least its own private toilet, and eleven four-room apartments had full baths. Understandably, in a city where poverty and poor housing had more than a casual acquaintance, the waiting list was long for such dwellings. If one were lucky enough to afford and procure a model apartment, the aesthetic and social benefits were tremendous.

"Too much cannot be said of the benefits of good housing in a colored neighborhood," declared social activist Mary White Ovington, the only white resident of the model Phipps House apartments on 63rd Street. "Church[es] and philanthropy had done and are doing excellent work on these blocks, but a sudden and marked improvement came from good housing, from the building of clean, healthful homes for law-abiding people."[14]

Those who could not afford newer housing suffered in every sense. Only 732 of Columbus Hill's older apartments, or 21 percent of its total residences, were considered "passable," and Lincoln House's social workers argued that although some had modern amenities, the dimly lit buildings with narrow airshafts were prime candidates for demolition and replacement. Even worse were the remaining 2,132 apartments that made up 63 percent of the area's available (and affordable) housing. Termed by social workers as "absolutely undesirable as habituous [sic] for human beings," their conditions were abysmal. Unsanitary and unsafe, the older houses were incommodiously separated into twenty apartments of three to four cramped rooms each, lacked heat and proper ventilation, and were vermin-infested hovels of "disease, crime, and filth." Norman Holmes, author of the Lincoln House study, recalled visiting one such tenement: "On entering the hall, the most nauseating odors poured forth from a dark, dismal room into a dark, dismal, filthy hall of a house which had seen better days. The appalling fact is that this can be duplicated many times." The "duplication" Holmes spoke of was no exaggeration, but a chilling reality for most of Columbus Hill's black poor, and a depressing reminder of class inequality and racial segregation for the white social workers and nurses who tried to serve the community's health needs.[15] The AICP itself believed that at the core of the inferior housing was commercial "progress." As more businesses moved into the area, fewer landlords than usual wanted to face the prospect of expensive renovations if the buildings could later be sold and torn down for new office space.[16]

Public health officials believed that tenement filth, disease-carrying flies, roaches, and other vermin, and the noxious odors trapped by poor ventilation directly affected health, particularly that of infants and small children. Nevertheless, although Columbus Hill's older tenement houses were substandard and virtually uninhabitable, they provided badly needed housing to impoverished, newly arrived southerners and nonnative black immigrants. Their condition may have justified a wrecking ball, but at $1.20 for a week's rent, they were "very reasonable" in price, considering the exorbitant rents paid by Harlem blacks. Still, coming up with the rent each week could be a daunting task. Therefore, the blacks who remained in Columbus Hill were those who could not afford to move uptown to the more expensive, newly created "Negro mecca" of Harlem.[17]

The AICP weighed the needs of Columbus Hill's African American and British West Indian residents; staff members were keenly aware of the causal relationship between poverty and poor health, but they considered that "the health approach to the colored problem is in our judgment the wisest and safest approach." In the words of AICP's director, Bailey B. Burritt, providing financial assistance "from the relief side rather than from the health side would be a waste of good money resulting in a breaking down of the fine spirit" of Columbus Hill's black residents. As a result, the AICP believed that funding one nurse in the initial 1917–1918 period of the health work in Columbus Hill proved to be far more effective than relief work alone.[18] This stance reflects the weak side of Progressive Era public health reform. Municipal authorities and private reformers could assemble funding for visiting nurse services and health education. Yet, because the public largely opposed the eradication of the environmental factors associated with poverty, much of the infrastructure that exacerbated ill health among the poor remained.[19] Impoverished, newly arriving black migrants from the American South and from the British West Indies thus moved into an area that, despite their hopes and dreams for a better life, may have provided fewer opportunities than they wished or imagined.

"She was told that we expect her to start in to work very soon": Private Lives and African American Migration Historiography

Ellen was almost eighteen years old when she married her husband, Thomas Simms, in 1908. She had been born and raised in Montgomery County, Maryland; Thomas, fifteen years her senior, came from

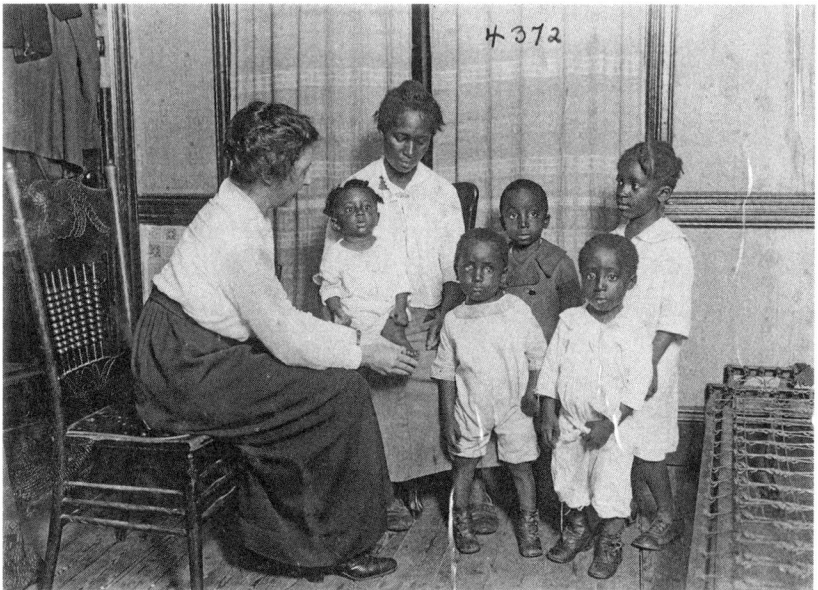

Figure 1.2. Creator unknown, "Columbus Hill Health Center Album, Woman and Four Children with Nurse," between 1879 and 1950, Rare Book and Manuscript Library, Columbia University, Community Service Society Collection, http://css.cul.columbia.edu/catalog/rbml_css_0553 (accessed March 2, 2014).

Charlotte, North Carolina.[20] What we know of Ellen and Thomas comes from a surviving COS casework file, notes made by white female social workers outlining home visits and information gleaned from letters and court documents that became the public part of Ellen's private life, all contained within a single file.

The file tells of illness and hardship, joy and hope, of an impoverished, illiterate woman struggling to care for herself and four children while her husband was imprisoned in New Jersey for sexually assaulting her eldest child, an eight-year-old girl named Sara. Ellen states that she had always fended for herself and the children: that Thomas had never worked to support them during their marriage. A letter from a white employer in Maryland supports her allegation: Ellen had worked for them for several years prior to marriage, and they had "[a]lways found her honest and trustworthy." Going further, they state that things started going wrong for her when she had "married a stranger in the neighborhood; he had a bad name and proved to be a bad man in his family particularly when drinking."²¹ Hope followed through movement, but uncertainty and deprivation intervened. The couple first migrated to New York, to be near Thomas's mother, and where Ellen quit working after having the first child, then to Washington, D.C., then to New Jersey, where physical abuse and the sexual assault and Thomas's imprisonment occurred. Ellen and the children then moved back to New York City, to again be near Thomas's mother, a live-in maid for a white family; Thomas's mother helped with rent and food whenever possible.²²

Ellen never contacted COS for assistance—this happened through a letter from the Urban League, which informed COS that the family desperately needed food.²³ After the initial visit, however, she never shrank from exposing her private life to gain assistance for her children. Ellen literally put everything on the table: illiteracy; her inability to do mathematics; that sometimes the house was dirty because she was ill from rheumatism, tuberculosis, and a "cold" that never seemed to go away; that, despite the fact that she fed her year-old child table scraps while also breastfeeding, she feared taking her off the breast and refused to work until she was fully weaned; that she had no idea where her three older brothers lived and was estranged from family members; that her husband had infected her with syphilis and may have also infected her daughter.²⁴

Without this record, Ellen and millions of African Americans like her remain invisible, their private lives hidden, their existence reflected only in raw data which charted their movements, hopes and dreams. The final entry in the Simms family case file is revealing:

Closing Entry
Case opened 07-30-17, referred by Urban League for general assistance. Family consisting of man, who is serving a long prison term for assaulting his daughter; woman and four little girls under age eight. Home is dirty and children badly cared for. Man's mother, a cook, supports family, except when out of city. Assistance given for a few months in groceries and clothing supplied during winter. Later, the baby was killed by falling from the fire escape. Woman placed the older children in a day nursery and now works in a cherry factory in the neighborhood, supplying food. Man's mother still pays rent. Family now self-supporting. Case closed.²⁵

Case closed. The now-public end of black private lives forms the basis of African American migration historiography.

Multiple archival sites and research methods offer glimpses into the private lives and agency of women like Ellen; they are necessary to put flesh on the bones of statistical data that, by itself, forms the necessary but sometimes limited scaffolding available for migration historiographers. The bustle of New York City—its promise in the imagination and reputation as the mode of entry for the world's "huddled masses yearning to be free"—pulled Europeans, British West Indians and Afro-Caribbeans, and peoples of other nations to its gate of entry, as well as African Americans like Ellen and other internal groups from areas around the nation.[26] Unfortunately, little has survived of their individual stories. Historian Nell Painter wisely argues that, although few historians have accorded the term "immigrant" to blacks who moved out of the U.S. South, especially during the Great Migration of the early twentieth century, these migrating populations deserve the label. Painter points out that "the women and men who made the break from their bad 'Old Country'—the rural South—sought their fortune (with all the meanings of the word in folklore) in the same manner as other immigrants who came to the United States."[27] For southern black immigrants, and females especially, the act of seeking their fortunes outside the South revolved about the interconnected spokes of economic betterment, escaping the ongoing, unchallenged threats of violence to their bodies and bodily integrity, and an expansion of roles as full civic actors.[28]

Southern African Americans who migrated out of the South after Reconstruction ended in 1876 left with a vigor that mirrored many of their religious sentiments. With promises of equality and freedom appearing for many as elusive as the wind, and as recalcitrant "Bourbon" Democrats and other whites who had been too poor to own slaves but now had to compete economically, politically, and, God forbid, socially with supposed racial inferiors, blacks were forced into debt peonage and increased physical violence. Frustrated blacks moved northward and westward with hope of better futures.[29] The earlier "trickle" of a black southern tide became a flood between 1916 and 1921, when 500,000 blacks (or 5 percent of the entire black population in the South) migrated northward. By 1920, fully one-quarter of northern blacks resided in New York City, Philadelphia, or Chicago. As Jacqueline Jones eloquently states, black migrants believed their exodus from "Pharaoh's Egypt" was an escape into a northern "Promised Land."[30]

However, an earlier Emancipation and Reconstruction-era generation of black women had also claimed those years as ones of promise that could elevate them from past racial, gendered, and class constraints and indignities. With their ancestors having forcibly arrived to the New World enslaved, and with African females becoming "beast[s] of burden," newly freed southern black women had acknowledged that their expected position in American society had always been that of workers.[31] Thus, for most, Emancipation and Reconstruction had not meant an opportunity to escape from working outside the home. Although the white dominant culture throughout the United States had stressed the ideal of women staying within the home as the only fitting place for respectable white women of the middle and upper classes, poor white and minority women had not fit into this paradigm. They were expected to work for white families, supervised by white married women, and then they were expected to return home and care for their own families. As the perfected embodiment of "double-shift" women, during their enslavement and in freedom, African American women had always been relegated to servile spaces, far outside the accepted boundaries of female respectability.[32]

Although many Reconstruction-era black women had preferred not to work outside the home, this luxury had not been an option. Instead, they had reveled in the choice that freedom had given them: the chance to choose the type of work they would perform. Having equated field labor to slavery, they removed themselves from the field in order to work at a more unsupervised pace, far from the prying eyes of white overseers. Because of the persistence of economic discrimination and the low wages paid to black men, most black families needed two wages to survive. Black women had risen to the challenge, augmenting their husband's salaries as cooks, laundresses, and domestic servants, or had tended gardens and sold the excess crops. However, as the economic, social, and political noose of Jim Crow segregation constricted the necks of African American men at the end of the nineteenth century and in the infancy of the twentieth century, a trickle of male and female "Exodusters" who had initially moved West in the 1870s and 1880s now metamorphosed into a steady stream northward and into the Midwest that would become known as the first "Great Migration."[33]

But the glitter of the North soon proved vulnerable to tarnish: the glossy attraction of higher wages and a "freer life" shrouded a peculiarly northern brand of racism, prejudice, and discrimination. Northern employers increasingly preferred immigrant laborers to southern black workers, even though African Americans were not hindered by language barriers and were usually better educated than their immigrant counterparts, especially those from southern Europe. Black males were relegated to domestic labor that paid far less than factory work. Black women initially fared better, with some finding work in factories. But most soon found "whiteness," used by native-born white women to forcibly segregate their workspaces from southern and eastern European women whom they considered racially inferior, was also used by women in these groups to force employers to segregate workplaces from each other and from African American women. Many black men who had moved North with wives did so purposefully, not only because they perceived economic, political, and social chances for masculine dignity and betterment, but also to protect their women from onerous fieldwork, white male sexual harassment, and the overall "degraded status of their womenfolk."[34] Shut out from clerical work or retail sales jobs, many black women quickly discovered that they had "gone from the fire into the frying pan," back into positions of closely supervised, low-paid servile work.[35]

Prior to 1900, working women, black or white, had commonly labored as domestics. An appreciable shift occurred after 1900, however, when native-born white women moved from domestic service into factory and white-collar clerical work, leaving behind black women who became synonymous with the term "domestic."[36] The work done by African American men had usually determined the economic and social status of their daughters or wives. But northern black men, displaced by immigrant laborers and lacking occupational "niches," found themselves mired in marginalized, low-paying, menial work that was often seasonal or part-time in nature. Plagued by both "chronic underemployment and sporadic unemployment," they were aided by the labor of other family members, particularly that of their wives. Whether single or married, black women again took up the mantle of out-of-the-home workers: they were five times as likely as white women to work. In New York City alone, 46.4 percent of black women were employed in 1920.[37]

Thus, for African American women, the promises sought with northern migration came with strong doses of reality. Historian Joe William Trotter Jr. isolates three historiographic models within African American migration studies. Through the "race relations" model (used from the 1900s through the 1950s, but peaking in the 1930s), sociologists such as W. E. B. Du Bois employed the "push/pull" method to explain what had motivated contemporary black migration. While arguing that northern white hiring and housing discrimination thwarted most African American gains, Du Bois simultaneously pathologized southern blacks as rural migrants ill-prepared for northern living. From World War I through the early 1930s, sociologists and social anthropologists, such as Robert Park and E. Franklin Frazier of the famed Chicago School at the University of Chicago, continued in Du Bois's vein, further emphasizing the entrance of black rural migrants as a strain on already tense northern urban race relations. However, these scholars placed more emphasis on economic and social push/pull factors and downplayed issues of black urban pathology—and African American migration gained a positive spin as a necessary corollary to expanding northern labor needs. However, in general, the race relations model left little room for black agency, kinship, or culture as reasons for their "push" from the South. Instead, external forces beyond their control propelled them from the South, *then* pathologized them in a North where their existing cultural capital, gleaned from the South, prepared them little for urban living and upholding standards of existing black self-definition outside the South.

During the 1960s and 1970s, black migration scholars attempted to complicate earlier push/pull analyses through what Trotter refers to as the "ghetto model." Within this construct, historians combined the push/pull model with interdisciplinary methods to create historical analyses of black urban ghetto formation that also looked at "social disorganization." Unfortunately, these methodologies largely failed to account for the social reasons within southern black culture that led to migration, and again ignored African American agency. Fortunately, however, as the ghetto model gained adherents, historians such as Florette Henry and William Tuttle began critiquing the decisions and actions of working-class black migrants of aspects of agency. Spurred by these efforts, and beginning in the 1980s and continuing in the decades that followed, dissertations and monographs increasingly used this "proletarian" model of subaltern agency to investigate black migration from the perspectives of southern rural and northern urban working-class lives.[38]

Since the mid-1990s, African American migration historiography has seen the value of subaltern positionality and interdisciplinary approaches. It combines economic, social, political, and environmental forces—a faltering sharecropping system, Jim Crow segregation, increased levels of gendered racial and intra-racial violence, and boll weevil attacks on the cotton market—along with southern black culture and community, and the agency found in kinship and family ties, to explain the first Great Migration. And, in the fields of literature and artwork, Farah Jasmine Griffin chronicles how African American migration history has gone through specific changes, reflecting the problems, consciousness, and hopes of each prominent historiographic era.[39] It is the exposure of the human quality of history that historians "get" at different levels: we know the often invisible hands behind the backdrop that manipulate what audiences see; we also know and admit (again, to differing levels) how society influences what we write and the debates that go on over who gets to tell history and how it is told, sometimes subtly, sometimes vociferously. The public is aware and unaware; those who are aware realize that the "history" they were told in school does not mesh with that passed on orally; those who are unaware also know there is a dislocation between "histories": the history they were taught, and the new history wars that threaten to rewrite the "truth." In this vein, the more "real," organic approach to African American migration informs the sticky and seemingly impassable gulf between diverging history camps by first blasting apart past methodologies (not all of them were wrong), including new methods, questions, and sources, bemoaning at the resulting mess, seeing links, and then putting them back together. This process transfers easily into the immigration and migration histories of other groups and the historiographic debates within each era that may have shaped perceptions of migration history.[40]

Returning to African American migration in the literary and popular mind, those affected by the first Great Migration—for example, novelist and literary critic Richard Wright and his cohort—configured black flight from the South as a direct response to white threats to the black male body. In other words, black men could not be black *men* in the South and exercise all the rights and responsibilities of manhood as long as patriarchal power, configured as citizenship—with all its white-male defined rights and obligations—remained transfixed and stratified along a one-drop color line. Once one left the South, return was not optional; it was only for visits or for "show," where African American southern émigrés would physically and rhetorically show why *anywhere* outside the South was better. Often hidden behind flashy clothes, cars, money, and the cultural currency of high-toned or fast-talking, urbanized speech—or, perhaps deftly understood within a larger knowledge of what it meant to live permanently on the wrong side of the veil—was the sliding scale meant in the term "better."[41]

For Wright's generation, and generations of black men since Reconstruction, the violent specter of lynching as a solution to white fears and preoccupations with black male success, white male unfettered access to black female bodies, and threats to white male supremacy—whether within the southern economy, its political structure, or in the bedroom—was real and omnipresent. To be a black man in the South meant exercising resistance in all its grayed manifestations, and resulting acts of agency within the critical unspoken and unwritten bounds of discernment. Perceived as and appearing to have little or no control over one's reputation and body,[42] or being unable to protect the bodies of one's wife or children left wide space for actions that often reflected acceptance, ambivalence, adherence, resistance (subtle or overt), and nihilism.[43] Furthermore, attempts at economic uplift could be thwarted or ended at any time by any white man or woman of any class, fully justified and protected under white-controlled law. At times, black men even castigated black women for lacking respectability when approached or sexually attacked by white men; black male responses ranged from physical confrontation to passivity and patriarchal impotence, all read within the ever-present standard of lynching for those African American men or women who questioned white supremacy and stepped out of their "place."[44]

This early literary black migration focus on violence and the black male body always begged the question: If black male bodies were under constant threat, what about those of black women and their children? What about women like Ellen and her daughters? To pose this question and further enrich this early mode of migration examination, historians such as Darlene Clark Hine have reconfigured black migration history from a male-gendered perspective that also considers southern violence against African American women's bodies and those of their children as a salient determinant in the questions of push, pull, and subaltern agency in southern migration. Again, the vulnerability of these black bodies to violence reflected the reality of bodily threats perpetrated by white men. Just as cogent to Hine, however, are acts of the heretofore unspeakable violence hidden in her theory of black female "dissemblance": bodily threats perpetrated against black females and their children by males, both in the home and in the larger community. These revelations, as well as issues of sexuality and sexual reproduction, maternal and infant health, and civic mobility, often recognized but unsaid in the work of black club women to "uplift" their benighted sisters, have all become significant lenses for current and future migration studies.

African American Migration
John F. Matheus's 'Cruiter

In his 1931 play, 'Cruiter, John F. Matheus incorporates some of the crucial aspects of black migration from the South that have been previously examined: the hope of economic prosperity, the quest for an end of violence and bodily integrity, and the desire to become actors in the civic sphere. He pits two weighty African American tropes against each other: the character Granny, an elderly former slave who is described by Matheus as "a typical Negro 'Mammy,'" and the power and salience of long-deceased southern Negro ancestors, ultimately embodied as the family dog. As Farah Griffin has argued, black ancestors—ranging from real, departed family members to the sights, sounds, tastes, and smells that evoke emotional, spiritual, and mental images of "down home" for migrating African Americans, the better side of an imagined South—played special roles in the third-phase twentieth-century black migration narrative, particularly in the works of African American female novelists like Toni Morrison. In this vein, Matheus was before his time in acknowledging the power of this psychological magnet; at the time, novelists centered their narratives on "leaving Dodge" for good. Yet, for good, ill, or spaces in between, ancestors could drive migrants northward or encourage them to return home. Time and gender also influenced the force of ancestors, as in the case of the main characters Sonny, Sissy, and Granny. Here, African American ancestors become a powerful tool that ties Granny to Georgia, but drives Sonny, her young grandson, and his wife, to the North.

The short play takes place in 1918, in a small cabin in rural Georgia. Sonny and his wife Sissy work as sharecroppers for Mistah Bob, a white landowner. Granny, age seventy-seven and still working in the fields, lives with them. The first scene opens with a breakfast discussion between the three. World War I has increased the need for corn and other foodstuffs—something not lost to Sonny or Mistah Bob, who feared that the draft was "raisin' hell wid his business, takin' all de niggahs fum de plantation." Sonny believes that Mistah Bob had somehow used his influence with the Georgia Draft Board to keep Sonny from being drafted, so that he could remain on the farm. He also believes that, given the chance, the powerful white landowner would block the efforts of a northern white labor recruiter who was combing the countryside in search of black male laborers who want to leave the South for work in northern munitions factories.[45]

As the narrative unfolds, a conflict arises between Granny, who evokes ancestors, fear of the unknown, Christian faith, and a solid distrust of whites—southern or northern—as reasons why Sonny and Sissy should stay in Georgia. Sonny counters, arguing that the recruiter is valid in depicting "[u]p No'th" as a place "wha' we kin be treated lak fo'ks." Even the first steps of the passage—gathering them up in the dark and taking them to a place unpatrolled by the white sheriff, where they can safely board the train out of the South—does not discourage him. The only thing they would gain by staying is a lifetime of hard work, being treated like animals for their labor, and with no freedoms to speak of.

When the white recruiter shows up on their doorstep to confirm that he will return later that night for them, the stage is set in the conventional "push/pull" economic migration format of the era, as he further kindles their hopes of freedom and advancement against strict boundaries between black life, southern or northern. He tells Granny that he is "giving this boy a chance to get out, to be a man, like anybody else, make plenty money and have time to enjoy it," and draws Sissy into the conversation by asking, "Don't you want to live like a lady and wear fine clothes?" "Yas, sir," she responds. He leaves and, despite his belief in the white recruiter's promises and his own desire to flee from the South, Sonny remains torn and confused, mired in a quandary. He and Sissy want to leave but fear making a wrong decision. Neither wants to leave Granny behind. Sonny warns Granny that only she will be left to endure Mistah Bob's wrath after Sonny and Sissy's departure; while Granny has lived in the cabin for fifty years, the shack is on the white man's land.

In the end, Sonny and Sissy decide to leave—but Granny stays because she refuses to leave without Berry, the family dog, who cannot be found when the recruiter calls. Granny later releases Berry, the missing hound, from a crate where he had been hidden. Matheus leaves it to his audience to figure out who had hidden Berry away. Sissy first mentions the need to find and take the dog, but only as they were leaving. Had Sissy purposefully hidden the dog in the crate in order to give Granny an "out," or way to concretize her decision to not leave? Had Granny been the culprit? Or Sonny? Regardless, for Granny, the dog embodies everything she would miss about Georgia: love, heritage, culture, and home. If ancestors propel Sonny and Sissy northward, they tie Granny to the South. Matheus's depiction of the classed, gendered, and generational struggle surrounding African American migration from the South may have reflected his own movements. Matheus was a migrant himself or the son of migrants. His roots sprang from Keyser, West Virginia—far from the environs of Columbia University and the Sorbonne, where he later studied. But, unlike Sonny, the traveler returned home as a professor of romance languages at West Virginia State College.[46] For Matheus, class and education became tangibles that might allure former southerners back home.

In moving to New York City, the African American women who lived in Columbus Hill had completed the first critical step of the journey; like Sonny and Sissy, they had weighed their options and, like other immigrants from foreign shores, had made the crucial decision to leave their "vale of tears" for what they hoped would be a better land. Encompassed in this movement were also considerations faced by Sonny, Sissy, and Granny: private desires for economic betterment, the end to violent reprisals against their bodies, and for civic stature in society. Moreover, like Sonny and Sissy, they became the "uppity Negroes" who moved from the South because they hoped for, and expected, better lives for themselves and their offspring. This better treatment included access to cutting-edge medicine and health care, something that they could only dream about as southern African American women. By moving North, they put their dreams into action and brought with them modes of decision making and agency from the South; some customs and beliefs would be retained, others discarded. But the actions of Columbus Hill's native-born black women were predicated upon decisions made in the South: as human agents, movement became a means toward the realization of a new, and hoped-for better, status. Sometimes things turned out well; sometimes, they did not. But privately held hopes for a better life undergirded their public decisions.

"She was most desirous to return to her native home": Private Lives, and British West Indian Migration Historiography and Literature

Things must have seemed to have been going so well at first. Before marriage, Katie Owens had been employed as a domestic in Kingston, Jamaica, where her mother had later described her behavior as "healthy and hardworking." Retrospectively, in a 1921 letter to the City Magistrates' Courts in New York City, COS echoed this sentiment, stating that when Katie's family had "first [come] under our care" in 1918, their initial research revealed a commendable work record, that she had been given "excellent references from places where she was employed at domestic service."[47] Katie had left Jamaica in 1909 for New York when she was twenty-four or twenty-five. She later met and in 1914 married her husband, Lester Calhoun, who was about ten years her senior and also from Jamaica. She had continued domestic work until giving birth to their son, Martin, in 1916. Lester had been employed as a porter, making sixty dollars a month, until ill health and a hospitalization ended his employment in March 1917. Both were literate, and listed as Protestants in their case file. Katie's parents still lived in Jamaica, but she had three sisters living in New York.[48] Publicly, both Katie and Lester are numbers, part of the initial British West Indian migration that occurred in the early twentieth century. As their private lives unfolded, they appeared to have been acclimating to New York, with employment and relatives in the area. Along the way, something happened.

From the file alone, it is difficult to tell exactly how and when their troubles began, but social workers, the courts, Katie's mother and, apparently, her other siblings believed that she had somehow gone insane and needed to be forcibly institutionalized. According to letters in the COS file, Katie's mental health seemed fine until after her marriage to Lester in 1914. In 1915, Katie became pregnant with the couple's first child but denied the pregnancy until the child's birth. After delivery, her physical appearance declined and she became increasingly angry and difficult to deal with. Soon after, the child died, and a social worker accused her of having "neglected her child, failing to give him necessary medical care and often going out leaving him locked alone in the room."[49] Katie attempted suicide by jumping from a window after the child's death. As her mental health deteriorated, she became angrier. Estranged from a husband who could no longer work due to ambulatory problems, left to raise Martin on her own, and, according to one letter in the file, pregnant again in 1918, all Katie wanted to do was return to Jamaica.

> The husband and relatives were willing to have her placed in a proper institution by commitment, but she absolutely declined to go voluntary[il]y, and forced commitment in this city in such a case was not possible. She was most desirous to return to her native home and make a home with her mother but this plan, while approved by her husband, was disapproved by other relatives. On communicating with our correspondent in the West Indies, we learned that it was not felt advisable for any action to be taken in the way of carrying out the woman's plan. Her parents had no means of supporting her and it was thought there would be great difficulty of her having proper treatment if returned.[50]

The file falls silent after 1925: we know nothing more of her private struggles, of whether she received care in the United States or returned to Jamaica, or what happened to Lester and the children. The self-determination that Katie had once exhibited in her successful work life and decision to migrate to New York City had run head-on into familial and legal barriers.

Decisions to stay or leave, to navigate post-migration waters or return to those of home, complicate the single-direction assumptions we may entertain when talking about early twentieth century British West Indian migration to the United States. At first glance, the reasons for Afro-Caribbean and British West Indian migrations to the United States parallel many of those that historians have cited in the push-pull of southern African American movement to the North, or southern Italian movement to the United States.[51] However, like Katie, British West Indian migrants felt they *could* return home—however hard that existence might be—while African Americans might *visit* the South by choice, but not choose to return permanently. Experiences of race and racism, of identity and how one was identified, troubled issues of blackness and African heritage between migrating blacks from the U.S. South and migrating blacks from the West Indies. Afro-Caribbean and West Indian accounts of the United States—and particularly New York City—as a place of opportunity, advancement, and freedom constituted a major "pull" for blacks, especially overly embellished letters stating that "New Yorkers did not have to work if they did not care to, for money was abundantly available for all."[52] Many who migrated to the United States, especially to New York City, believed themselves better than African Americans. In *The West Indian Americans*, Mirian Klevan notes that, in the 1930s, an animosity brewed in West Indian / African American relations: "West Indian immigrants were generally status conscious and often looked down on American blacks for their lack of education." On the other hand, she states that African Americans ridiculed West Indians, referring to them as "'monkey chasers,' 'Jewmaicans,' 'Garveyites,' and 'cockneys.'"[53] It was only after arriving and settling that black West Indians truly found out what living in New York City and in the United States was all about.

Still, as a push factor and more important than their social status mind-set or quest for upward mobility and education, were the harsh socioeconomic factors in the West Indies. Most West Indians and Afro-Caribbeans wanted to emigrate from the poverty, unemployment, malnutrition, overcrowded housing, and high rates of infant mortality they witnessed, and that could imperil their standard of living. In addition, as the sugar industry faced an overall decline in the decades between 1900 and 1940, devastating earthquakes and hurricanes roared through the Caribbean. In Jamaica alone, hurricanes hit with a vengeance four times between 1912 and 1917. Yet, although third-class steerage rates were relatively inexpensive, most unskilled laborers and their families never escaped. As with African Americans, it was usually the more educated and striving West Indians who left in search of bettering themselves.[54]

The West Indians who immigrated to New York City included persons from the unskilled, skilled, and professional classes whose overall literacy rate did exceed that of the U.S. average, regardless of race. Oscar Handlin has remarked that between the decades of 1900–1910, the British West Indian presence swelled to 40,000.[55] Official immigration data reveal that for the period between 1900 and 1917 (and prior to the institution of the 1917 U.S. Literacy Act), while 54 percent of arriving Afro-Caribbean migrants listed themselves as unskilled, 83 percent were literate. In subsequent years, the numbers of unskilled workers declined—and their literacy rates soared even higher to qualify for entrance into the U.S. through the new literacy law. Along with the money for steerage and a new start, West Indian migrants needed to be literate in order to transcend the innumerable bureaucratic barriers they faced in securing visas or passports. Unskilled, skilled, or professional adults came not from the rural or urban impoverished classes; rather, they had been artisans, civil servants with little chance of advancement, or small farmers. Upon arrival in New York City, they became laborers and domestics—but retained many of their petit bourgeois sentimentalities. Members of the professional class had been teachers, preachers, middle-level civil servants, writers, and engineers.

In his seminal work on black migration to the United States, *The Negro Immigrant: His Background, Characteristics, and Social Adjustment, 1899–1937*, sociologist Ira De Augustine Reid maintains that immigration—particularly the migration of so-called racial groups—should be the purview of sociologists. However, during Reid's era, other than the work done by the Chicago School, few sociologists had taken immigration seriously, except for applying a few choice statistics and thereby creating a history, or economics, of migration. Reid wanted to change that by creating a history of Negro immigration to the United States that maintained exacting sociological standards and methodologies used in other areas of research.

There were distinct problems with the project, however, mainly stemming from the source materials and the categorizations employed at the time. First, Reid admits that "race," even in the 1930s, was a troublesome term when used to study international migration, but nonetheless employed lavishly by the United States government and the popular masses to measure and categorize the character of the racial mixture coming to its shores. Therefore, to Reid, the U.S. immigration category of "Africans, black" became a dumping ground or, in his terms, a "conjure word that metamorphoses persons who, prior to embarking for the United States, may have been known as 'colored,' 'mulatto,' or 'black,' or who had not been grouped by race or color."[56] Welcome to the United States. From this undesirable polyglot of racial construction, Reid asked a few main questions. First, he demystified a dirty little secret created to bring in Europeans who were "white" enough for acculturation and naturalization but, according to eugenic theory, nativist fears, and the ideologies spouted by advocates of ending U.S. "race suicide," not white enough for exogamous mating with Anglo-Saxon whites: How did the United States, famous for its "melting pot" rhetoric, propose to assimilate or accommodate groups of people of African descent (whom, in reality, they deemed completely unassimilable because of their African ancestry)? If true assimilation occurred, what would it look like, and how would (could) it occur? And what affect would this process have on the larger social, political, economic, and racial big picture? Basically, if native-born American whites were not ready to assimilate immigrants of southern, central, and eastern European background, could they ever truly consider assimilating non-African American immigrants of African background?[57]

De jure and de facto barriers to exogamy in whiteness were not new in the late nineteenth and early twentieth centuries; they can be traced back to antimiscegenation laws that began cropping up in the early colonial era in the Chesapeake which forbade intermarriage between African males and English women.[58] In addition, the widening of what Andrew Hacker has described as the "umbrella of whiteness" that occurred after World War II remains the major feat that restructured the American identity and imagination with regard to what constituted "race," and what made the new term "ethnicity" a viable catchall for the European "races" previously conceived as racially inferior.[59] The notions of white nativism and legal immigration restrictions by race began in 1790 but were tempered in a congressional act in 1875 that extended citizenship to naturalized migrants of African ancestry. But the opened door began closing for non-Europeans and non-Africans with the Chinese Exclusion Act of 1882. By the early 1900s, in an effort to keep them from competing with native-born white workers and driving wages downward, Japanese and Chinese workers were deprived of entry into the United States and, for those who were already in the country, naturalized status. In 1917, U.S. immigration restrictions grew even tighter as new literacy requirements denied entry to anyone illiterate in English or any other language.[60]

Fueled by general American acceptance of the tenets of eugenic science and increased racial tensions, immigration levels were pared back again in 1921 law, this time by country, to 3 percent of their 1910 levels. This downward trend continued in a revised 1924 law, when yearly immigration totals declined to 2 percent of 1890 totals.[61] Thus, within three years, U.S. immigration officials had stemmed the tide of southern, and central and eastern European immigration without ever mentioning the word "race." Moreover, by keeping their numbers at lower levels that were based on pre-1890 totals, when migration from these parts of Europe to the United States had been significantly less, U.S. immigration officials had given in to nativist and eugenicist demands to end the flood of European racial inferiors whose unrelenting fecundity threatened to overpopulate the white nation. Nonetheless, the focus on Asian and SCE European immigration left the door open for other groups. From 1917 onward, the numbers of immigrants to the United States from North and South America increased, as did the numbers of blacks from the British West Indies.[62]

Yet, in keeping with its battle to keep those deemed racially inferior outside U.S. boundaries, far beyond its golden door, and even further from citizen status, between 1908 and 1937 the United States barred Afro-Caribbean and British West Indian immigrants from entering the country at a higher rate than their percentage as aliens on the grounds of the narrowed 1924 immigration law (5,000 persons of African ancestry were barred between 1921 and 1932; the time period reflects changes in U.S. immigration law that, while not openly racializing admittance to the United States, rolled back immigration levels to pre-1890 numbers, when the majority of U.S. immigrants had originated from northern European racial stock). For example, almost 3 percent of Afro-Caribbeans and British West Indians were denied entry into the United States from 1908 to 1937; their percentage of all immigrants allowed access never numbered over 2 percent, however.[63] In terms of female-to-male sexual ratios among West Indian immigrants, four things become clear from the available statistics compiled by Reid. First, young marriageable blacks (age sixteen and over) formed the core of the migration group. Second, British West Indian males outnumbered females. Third, age and sex would later become important factors in West Indian "adjustment" to U.S. culture; and fourth, more than 90 percent of West Indian immigrants stayed on the East Coast of the United States, where many had disembarked.[64] Most nonnative migrating Negroes were between the ages of 14 and 44 (considered prime working ages); the percentage increased from about 70 percent in 1899 to between 80 and 86 percent prior to World War I.[65]

In general, black males immigrated in larger numbers than black females, especially during the period 1917–1934, when the greatest pre–World War II migration of West Indian blacks occurred. A female-to-male gender imbalance occurred after 1924, when all-around Afro-Caribbean migration quickly slowed. However, men usually outnumbered female migrants (51–59 percent). In many cases, after men settled, they soon sent for relatives or spouses, since travel between the United States and the Caribbean remained inexpensive and speedy. Reid also points to West Indian male "clandestine arrival[s]" as another reason for the black female-to-male disparity. Black men simply found it easier to enter the country surreptitiously as sailors, unannounced and beneath the radar of U.S. customs officials. Eventually they would surface in census data. Reid supports his theory with the fact that, per the 1920 census, black nonnative-born women were naturalized at a far higher rate than their black male counterparts. In addition, some 2,600 Afro-Caribbean men brought to work in the U.S. as laborers in South Carolina eventually disappeared without a trace.[66] The disparity between the native-born black / nonnative-born black sex ratio also reflects Reid's hypothesis. Native-born black women continued to outnumber their male counterparts; by 1930, there were only 91 native-born African American men for every 100 black women. Afro-Caribbean sex ratios reversed this trend, however; in 1930, nonnative black men outnumbered nonnative black women, 143/100. Nonnative-born black men outnumbered their women at a higher rate than that of "Nordic" European immigrants, but at a lower rate than that of southern and eastern European immigrants.[67]

While Reid defines Afro-Caribbean immigrants as "future male industrial workers and female domestics," skilled workers (former middle-class professionals such as bankers, lawyers, shopkeepers, and artisans) comprised 25–33% of Negro immigrants after 1923. The majority of non-native born blacks who emigrated back to the West Indies or Caribbean were categorized as laborers or servants—few if any formerly migrant middle-class blacks left the United States. Thus, migrating West Indian blacks—many from successful professional backgrounds—brought education, experience, and sensibilities to the United States that were not expected from African Americans, males or females, in the North or South. This racialized culture shock undoubtedly made adjustment harder for some nonnative blacks.[68]

While immigrating blacks may have had more educational or business advantages than many of their southern African American counterparts (who, in terms of this study, were also, in general, better educated than blacks who remained in the South and better educated than southern Italian migrants), the passage of the 1917 immigration statute made literacy (in the language of choice of the proposed immigrant) mandatory for admission into the United States. West Indian black immigrants had higher rates of literacy than their African American counterparts (98 percent in 1923; 99 percent in 1930 out of immigrants age 16 and over). Between 1910 and 1930, only 2 percent of the blacks who immigrated to the United States spoke no English (Afro-Caribbeans originating from French, Spanish, or Portuguese-speaking countries).[69] While non-English-speaking black immigrants may have passed literacy tests in their native tongues, West Indians competed for jobs with the benefit of knowing the English language. Most, however, bore the additional burden of having darker skin than southern Italians. Whatever educational capital West Indians brought with them may have been more slowly put into play after admission into the United States.

Most of the foreign-born immigrants of African descent who disembarked and were allowed to stay in the U.S. not only tended to remain on the East Coast at but lived in the northern states of New York and Massachusetts, or in Florida. Although 37 percent had lived in the South in 1900, by 1930, 65 percent of Afro-Caribbeans and British West Indians lived in New York City alone; correspondingly, by 1930 the number of southern-born African Americans living in New York City decreased to less than 15 percent of the city's African American total. Jim Crow segregation, racial violence, discrimination, and prejudice wedged West Indian blacks into an uncomfortable and powerless position in a southern binary system of black/white power relations. Black, but not native-born African American, foreign-born blacks found themselves cast as outsiders in a region that cared little for immigrants in general. Reid maintains that "[i]n such communities, where the number of foreign-born Negroes was sufficiently large to make them highly visible, the foreign-born Negro workers ranked even lower [on] the occupational scale than the 'black devils'—the native Negroes."[70] Afro-Caribbeans also preferred urban life; with the exception of Cubanos, 80 percent had originated from cities and, upon arriving in the United States, doggedly clung to ethnic enclaves in large metropolitan areas. In this regard, while the movement of West Indian blacks to the United States paralleled the initial onslaught of southern black migration into the North, foreign-born blacks tended to prefer urban areas more than did their native-born counterparts.[71] As one Trinidadian remarked, after "day-dream[ing] in the semi-tropics" and having tasted life in the big city, few West Indians wanted to return to the country. Statistics seemed to confirm popular knowledge: by 1930, 93 percent of all foreign-born blacks lived in large northern cities on the Eastern Seaboard. In New York City alone, the number of West Indians grew to more than 50,000 by 1940. By then, only a smattering of black migrants lived in Miami and Tampa.[72]

In short, regardless of former class or status, many West Indian migrants came to New York City armed with survival tools in their cultural capital that some of their migrating African American counterparts may have lacked. Both groups came searching for better lives; one group simply started off with better tools.[73] Since West Indian migrants made up one-half of Columbus Hill's black population, intraracial frictions could have occurred during competitions over housing, jobs, sexual partners, and social status. Outside sources—such as visiting nurses and physicians—may have also inadvertently added to this tension by preferring one group over the other.

In addition, single-head-of-household status for black women in urban centers after the turn of the twentieth century still fuels many historiographic and sociological debates. For decades, since the ponderous works of sociologist E. Franklin Frazier in the 1930s and 1940s, scholars accepted as fact the stereotypical paradigm of the strong-willed black matriarch, forced to fend for her family in the face of a deserting male.[74] In the 1970s, historian Herbert Gutman used data from New York City to persuasively argue for the resilience of the black-male-headed family.[75]

The statistics regarding the percentages of African American women to African American men could be misleading, however, since, on a nationwide scale, black women took control of their lives and departed from older traditions, such as early marriage and large families. Out-of-wedlock births still occurred among African American women. Even though the AICP health care workers remarked that almost all of the black women they saw were married, some of Columbus Hill's black women may have lied to receive prenatal care and lower the chances of judgment. Many Jamaican women birthed children out of wedlock, or outside state- or church-sanctioned marriages, because black Jamaican society recognized these unions as stable and legitimate. Church marriage increased a couple's social position, but its absence placed little stigma on the resulting children.[76] Historian Deborah Grey White has examined this acceptance of out-of-wedlock births during U.S. slavery, and traced it back to western and central African gendered cultural expectations, where more status was accorded births if they occurred before marriage than the other way around. This cultural retention, coupled with the paucity of marriageable men and the prospect of husbands or boyfriends leaving mothers-to-be in the lurch may have left marriage desirable as an ideal, while difficult as a reality.[77] Moreover, W. E. B. Du Bois remarked that while their mothers and grandmothers "had married at twelve and fifteen," by 1910, 27 percent of the black women over the age of fifteen were still single.[78] Still, even using Du Bois's 1910 statistics, a full 73 percent of black women would have been married, and married at some time after the age of fifteen. Therefore, African American women, in search of husbands or trying to keep the ones they had, may have found themselves in direct competition with West Indian women for the dwindling numbers of available black men. The New York City black male-to-female population did not reach parity until 1925.[79]

Paule Marshall, *Brown Girl, Brownstones*

Novelist Paule Marshall discusses the lives of post-migration Barbadian women who lived in Brooklyn in the 1930s in *Brown Girl, Brownstones*. Marshall adroitly refers to Ralph Ellison's *Invisible Man*, published in 1952, for his depiction of African American men as "invisible" in the white psyche. She builds upon this by arguing that "if the Black foreigner has been treated to a double invisibility, then the West Indian immigrant woman might be said to suffer from a triple invisibility as a Black, a foreigner, and a woman." These women's experiences, at the time of Marshall's publication of *Brown Girls, Brownstones*, had been absent from what she refers to as "social science literature." By correcting this omission Marshall, whose parents had migrated from Barbados to the United States during World War I, gives voice to her mother's generation and her own as well.[80]

Describing a generation that arrived in a migration that coincided with the first Great Migration of blacks from the South, Marshall agrees with Reid and others that, although they came from a single-economy sugar island and dire poverty, Barbadian women believed they were better than African American women: more militant and assertive in their relations with whites, harder working, and firmly wedded to achieving higher social positions for themselves and their children. Marshall reveals that her mother once admitted that she could never live in the South because her words would have gotten her killed. At the outset, Barbadian women seemed the rural antithesis of their Jamaican counterparts: less educated, from a congested, rural area. However, upon arrival and regardless of their occupations in their homelands, like African American and other British West Indian women, they worked as live-in domestics with every second Thursday off. If less lucky or more independent, they weathered the vagaries of "day's work," standing on corners as white women looked them over and decided whether to employ them for the day.

Whites helped reinforce the attitudinal divide between native-born and immigrant blacks, touting the hard work and ease at which West Indian women accepted their lot as domestics without complaint. "She was that kind of person," one white woman stated. "I've always told my friends there's something different, something special about Negroes from the West Indies. Some of the others are . . . well . . . just impossible!" Marshall writes that they were able to endure such indignities because, starting work straight off the boat, they endured whatever manual labor and indignities that followed with the goal of homeownership, nice clothing, college educations for their children, and yearly trips back to Barbados. Yet, while embracing the commercialism and materialism of the white United States, they remained distant, spending time after work each day with friends discussing "home" and never feeling accepted in what Marshall's character calls "this man's country." Unable and unwilling to seek commonality with African Americans and invisible to whites as foreign-born black women, they clung to their cultural identities. "They were," Marshall argues, "for all their insularity, fears and misguided materialism, women of impressive strength, authority, and style. Unfortunately," she laments, "because they were women—and Black women at that—this country never saw fit to acknowledge their presence or their worth, or to make full use of their tremendous human resource they represented." Try as they might, while achieving a measure of material success and status achievement, West Indian women were closer to African American women than they admitted or dared realize. Most women in both groups found the color, gender, and class boundaries set too high to successfully scale.[81]

The women in *Brown Girl, Brownstones* create an informal mutual support group based upon their common homeland and culture, their aspirations for better lives for themselves and their families, and their conjoined strength which they share and take in times of need. Silla, a primary character, is the strong-willed, hardworking, and wise matriarch of her family, headed by her husband, the "beautiful-ugly" Deighton, as termed by a close friend; an eldest daughter entering womanhood; a younger daughter who sees and analyzes everything within the family dynamic; and the strong, painful memory of the boy child who would have been her eldest had he not died from a heart condition in infancy.[82] Selina, the ten-year-old, categorizes her mother and all the other Barbadian mothers in the same manner.

> It was always the mother and the others, for they were alike—those watchful, wrathful women whose eyes seared and searched and laid bare, whose tongues lashed the world in unremitting distrust. Each morning they took the train to Flatbush and Sheepshead Bay to scrub floors. The lucky ones had their steady madams while the others wandered those neat blocks or waited on corners—each with her apron and working shoes in a bag under her arm until someone offered her a day's work. Sometimes the white children on their way to school laughed at their blackness and shouted "nigger," but the Barbadian women sucked their teeth, dismissing them. Their only thought was of the "few raw-mout' pennies" at the end of the day which would eventually "buy house."[83]

The pressure to get ahead and "buy house" comes to a boil early in the novel, when Deighton discovers that his recently deceased sister has left him two choice acres in Barbados where he wants to relocate the family, grow crops, and build a house "just like the white people own. A house to end all house." He reveals this to Selina, his release valve who, of course, immediately asks if he will tell her mother. "His smile faltered and failed; his eyes closed in a kind of weariness," Marshall writes. Deighton's actions reveal the tensions underlying the relationship between him and Silla: she is, as Selina has stated, the hardworking, cautious woman who sees everything and endures every slight so that their family will soon have enough saved to buy a house. Deighton, on the other hand, is the dreamer (or lazy, drifting womanizer who has no goals, according to Silla). It was he who was raised in a large city in Barbados and fantasizes an idyllic rural existence as a landed planter who "was always dressing up like white people."[84] Silla is a child of the sugar plantations: she understands hard work for little money and no future. Later that evening, when Deighton tells Silla about the land, she is at first dismissive, unbelieving. When he shows her the paperwork, she rejoices and asks what he thinks it is worth. "What I care—I ain selling," he retorts. Then, giving her a bone, he responds "Eight hundred, I guess." Silla is overwhelmed with their good fortune. Eight hundred dollars puts them in the running for a home, along with the money she has saved. (Silla had minutes earlier growled at him for not saving any money that week toward the house or for the family, instead claiming that "You mean it all gone on fancy silk shirt and shoes and caterwauling with your concubine").[85]

Then the battle of wills and desires begins: Silla demands he sell the land; Deighton wants to emigrate back to Barbados and live on the land. Marshall paints a raw portrait of pre-, post-, and possible future migration life for Silla and her family. A tough, disciplined, and goal-oriented woman, Silla came from nothing to the United States in the 1920s with dreams that are still unfulfilled. As she stands on the brink of partial fulfillment, Deighton, her husband, has other plans. It is interesting that Silla knows about and tolerates his philandering; other comments suggest that the latest "concubine" may have competitors and has had many progenitors in the past. But Silla's primary focus is material: after bearing three children and losing a beloved son, after bearing the indignities of domestic work and racial epithets from children, after working long, tedious hours to make a few dollars and set aside a portion for her dream, she wants the American Dream, their own house. Here Marshall shows how female Barbadian cultural expectations and group identity have changed after migration: women may have dreamed of better lives while working in sugar fields. But now they have the chance to make dreams come true. No one will stop them—not even loved ones.

In keeping with the ideas of ethnic and cultural capital differences, both African American and West Indian women shared a key similarity: both groups worked outside the home in large numbers: 52 percent of the black adults surveyed in the Lincoln House study of Columbus Hill were black female laborers. Their male counterparts fared no better: the top occupations for Columbus Hill's black males were laborers, porters, longshoremen, and elevator operators. Low pay and hard labor were not their only problems; many men and women could only find part-time employment. This was particularly true for black males employed as longshoremen, whose jobs were seasonal. Thus black women like Silla and Sissy, her migrating Georgia counterpart, had to work outside the home at twice the rate of native white or European women in order to augment their husband's meager earnings, or to support their families as single heads of households. Performing the double duties of workers and mothers, Columbus Hill's black women composed the largest segment of working African American and West Indian women in New York City at the time of the 1915 health survey, and as a result of the rampant poverty and overcrowding in their neighborhood, they often experienced poor maternal health.[86] The increased physical and emotional stress faced by black women who worked outside the home and then returned home to perform the duties of homemaker, wife, and mother created an additional component of their physical well-being that directly affected their health and that of their unborn children. Katie Calhoun may be the tip of a larger, unseen iceberg, a critical example of how the pressures of migration, work, and motherhood could undermine the mental health of an otherwise strong woman.

"She was too ill to care for her children": Private Lives and Southern Italian Migration Historiography and Literature

Social workers' comments found in surviving Community Organization Society (COS) files about southern Italians living in the Mulberry District are sparse; instead of perceptions of the people interviewed, we see names, dates, addresses, and times/dates of hospitalizations or clinic attendance. Maria Massini's file breaks the silence. She was born in Naples in 1881 and had married her husband, Guiseppi, while still living in Italy. Like many southern Italian male workers, he had arrived first in the United States in 1908, and Maria had arrived one year later, traveling with a four-year-old and an infant. While living in an undisclosed place, Maria had three other children, with the latest born less than one month before Guiseppi's death in 1914. In 1915, she and the children moved into a crowded three-room apartment with her married sister and brother-in-law, their three children, and Maria's brother.[87] Sometime between this move and the opening of the COS file on Maria, she was diagnosed with a "neurasthenic" defect, a catchall phrase that reveals little, and her five children were placed in "city institutions." We do know that in November 1917 she had been "persuaded" to undergo a health-restoring operation and that COS believed she could return to work and care for at least one single child.

Maria's life—that of an impoverished, widowed mother of five in poor health—was influenced by traditions and modernity, by family and the city. Like many Italian women who migrated to the United States, Maria and the children arrived after Guiseppi, presumably after he had obtained a job and the means to pay for their transport and living space. Neither she nor Guiseppi had lived alone—even after his death, she had lived on Houston Street with extended family in a crowded, but familial, setting. She had had to negotiate larger social structures, however, when she dealt with the health care system for herself, and with social service agencies after becoming ill and unable to care for her children. Even the letter from COS to the supervisor of the Lower Manhattan District Department of Charities makes it clear that whether Maria was ready to work again and care for her children would not be up to her alone, or her family. They would have their say.

> From our knowledge of the situation, we believe that Mrs. Massini is not now well enough to resume responsibility for all her children and we should not feel justified in undertaking the burden of the allowance which would be necessary to permit her to do so. We do believe, however, that she is able, both financially and physically, to care for at least one child. The purpose of this letter is merely to bring that possibility to your attention, in case you care to take up the question of discharge or of her making a small payment to the city for the support of one child.[88]

The decisions and actions of social workers and public health workers regarding southern Italian women and their children who were living in the Mulberry District reveal the complex actions of formerly rural women encountering a modern city filled with new expectations that challenged older, racially gendered traditions, versus the actions of workers tasked with providing care for them. Sociologist Kathie Friedman-Kasaba has analyzed the pre- and post-migration experiences of Italian women and Russian Jewish women in global and localized structures of patriarchy. Central to her analysis is how these women, in relation to each other, struggled against patriarchal constraints to redefine and remake their identities during the massive European migrations to the United States during the late nineteenth and early twentieth centuries. Friedman-Kasaba argues that, for these women, U.S. migration created a paradox: it emancipated women as easily as it reinforced their adherence to existing systems of domination. In general, massive migrations threatened the preexisting identities of groups and individuals. Migration itself, and its timing in a modern world system, was shaped by the dynamics of race, class, and gender inequalities. But migration also tended to offer individuals and groups the opportunity to challenge or subvert categories of inequality previously considered immutable, natural, or God-ordained.

Issues of family, work, and community relations make gender an integral part of migration, as migrating women constructed identities apart from their communities, evoking their own sense of emancipation. Viewing European migration from a gendered perspective—like viewing international immigration from the perspectives of African American migration or Afro-Caribbean and British West Indian migrations—has been a fairly recent phenomena and an uphill battle.[89] The overlaps and parallels between the histories of oppressed groups on either side of the Atlantic, how the dominant cultures in their homelands and in their receiving countries viewed them, and how they had fit and were expected to fit within the economic, political, sociocultural, and sexual frameworks of their homelands and receiving countries should have tipped off migration scholars to think "out of the box," more integrally, and in new comparative ways.

When Friedman-Kasaba created her own migration theory to view immigration to the United States from the comparative positionalities of Russian Jewish and southern Italian women, she did so out of necessity. Earlier scholars of European migration—even those who had written extensively on eastern European Jews and southern Italians—had done so from a male perspective, configuring migration in "push-pull" terms of workers and their motivations to leave home. Of course, these workers had been male; until the end of colonialism, the U.S. civil rights movement, and various national and worldwide empowerment movements of the 1950s through the 1970s, few scholars had questioned gendered aspects of European immigration. Moreover, the "worker" perspective of transmigration literature was primarily of a Marxist or (in the 1960s and 1970s) a neo-Marxist tilt that usually subsumed gender or race as resulting from class conflicts. In addition, the sources normally used for migration studies were statistical; in much the same manner that Ira Reid had decried racial statistics and the American misuse of "race" as an ambiguous term to malign or assess racial status to immigrants, statistics employed by migration scholars reflected the idea that "worker" was a male-defined term—women, as workers within the home, or even outside the home, found their work and therefore their worth often excluded from statistics. Even worse, the invaluable unpaid and unnoticed work done by women (accepted even by them as culturally validated via traditional sex-segregated roles), such as child rearing, housekeeping, the acculturation of children, and the passing down of traditions, did not only fall beneath the radar of non-gendered immigration studies: they did not exist.[90]

Friedman-Kasaba compensated for these past historiographic oversights by restructuring world-systems migration theory to analyze women's cultural adaptations to migration, thus revealing their agency within international and local frameworks. This new theoretical formulation broadened the concept of economics to include changes in women's paid and unpaid labor and expanded indicators of education, literacy, and skill to include the culturally defined training given to girls by female kin. Political structures also underwent redefinition by showing how the changing world system influenced social relations; race, class, and gender inequalities influenced who could stay behind or leave. Also, the position of the sending or receiving states within the world system influenced human movement, governmental policies, and income production. Lastly, kinship and community ties influenced women's migration through the material and moral support given to or withheld from women. By creating a model that embraces gender, class, and racial differences and how they impact international migrations, Friedman-Kasaba has inserted racially gendered women—all women, if the concept of race is carried to its logical end—within a labor framework that does not battle over their race or gender.[91]

Feminist scholars added to what had been lacking in the scholarly tradition of immigration history by adding women; unfortunately, many got lost in neo-Marxist feminist debates over how to quantify the importance of gender bias over class, or of lumping all women together into one "gender class," which considers all males their oppressors and all their oppression the same. Friedman-Kasaba broke the mold by tearing everything apart and rebuilding from the ground up. Borrowing from feminist scholar Sandra Harding, Friedman-Kasaba argues that within hierarchical societies stratified by race and gender, gender becomes racialized and race takes on a gendered component, as reflected in institutions, social relations, economics, and politics. She places herself firmly in the whiteness studies camp by categorizing Europeans who migrated to the United States from the 1870s through the 1920s as racialized groups, through the blurring of culture, nationhood, and biology that occurred in U.S. scientific, political, and popular culture at the time.[92] By looking at how stratifications between migrating European groups shaped their individual and group identity constructions, she agrees with historian Matthew Frye Jacobson and distinguishes the nineteenth and early twentieth centuries as times when Anglo-Saxon or "white" Americans did not consider southern, central, or eastern Europeans "totally white," but marginally white and racially inferior.

Decades before the official dawnings of the "[N[egro question[s]" or the "woman question[s]" that would preoccupy U.S. society from the late nineteenth through the twentieth centuries, Italy, after its Risorgimento, or unification in 1860–1861, dealt with its own variant of racial inferiority and white supremacy: *la questione meridionale*, or the "southern" question.[93] Quickly after unification in 1860–1861, Italy's new leaders—members of a "whitened" northern Italian elite gleaned from the political, scholarly, economic, and scientific realms—realized that the newly formed nation had just inherited millions of literal unknowns whom they had no idea what to do with. Separated geopolitically, culturally, and economically from the more urbane and wealthier north, southern Italy—the area south of Naples—seemed a backward paradise of landless, inferior, illiterate rural peasants, ruled by absentee landowners in what could only be described as a remnant of feudalism.

The initial approach taken by officials confronting the *meridionalismo* problem was one of research; in an era when Darwinism and the fledgling field of anthropology promised scientific answers to social questions, researchers conducted innumerable studies on southern Italians, trying to discover why they were backward and how (or if) they could become transformed from rural regional (darker) identities to nationalized (whitened) citizens. Works written in the latter half of the nineteenth century and the early twentieth century by Italian intellectuals and scholars gave scientific legitimacy and justifications for centuries of discrimination and, thus, the further maligning of southern Italians by northerners. Giorgio Bertellini writes that

> Specifically, their work developed a racist, misogynist and misopedic perspective by derogatorily pairing Southerners with female subjects and children (*popolo-femmina* and *popolo-bambino*) and by opposing them to Northern, mature and rational subjects. As the most popular version of *Southernism*, this *vulgata* contended that Southerners, like women, children, and crowds (with the ultimate configuration being Southern female crowds) were weak, immature, and unreliable, unable to tame their primitive instinctual and emotional life. Described as sensual, vicious, frivolous, and superstitious creatures, Southerners, "like women and children," were thus regarded as intellectually inferior and morally inadequate to the burgeoning ideal of the Italian citizen, who was instead defined as adult, male, and Northern.[94]

The parallels between the attitudes describe here and how most U.S. whites viewed African Americans before and after Emancipation, and particularly after the end of Reconstruction and the advent of the "Negro problem" are staggering. The eighteenth- and nineteenth-century Atlantic was not only a site that migration scholars have used for studies; through the transmigration of intellectual thought surrounding abolitionism and pro-slavery, worker-versus-capital, and male-versus-female rhetoric, it also became a petri dish for inequality theories and practices. The similarities between how racialized superiors viewed racially inferior peoples of African and of southern Italian descent (viewed as remnants of northern African and Italian miscegenation), and then gendered their races as feminine and immature should not be surprising.[95]

Similarly, much northern Italian writing about southern Italians during the late nineteenth century reads like a U.S. southern white blueprint for explaining the "Negro problem" to northern whites: ignorant of black innate inferiority, after black migration out of the South began, southern whites believed their northern counterparts needed to be told why blacks must still occupy the bottom rungs of society as a perpetual working class after arriving in the North, and not be entrusted with the rights and responsibilities of civic status. Northern Italians had also characterized southern Italians as vicious criminals and biologically

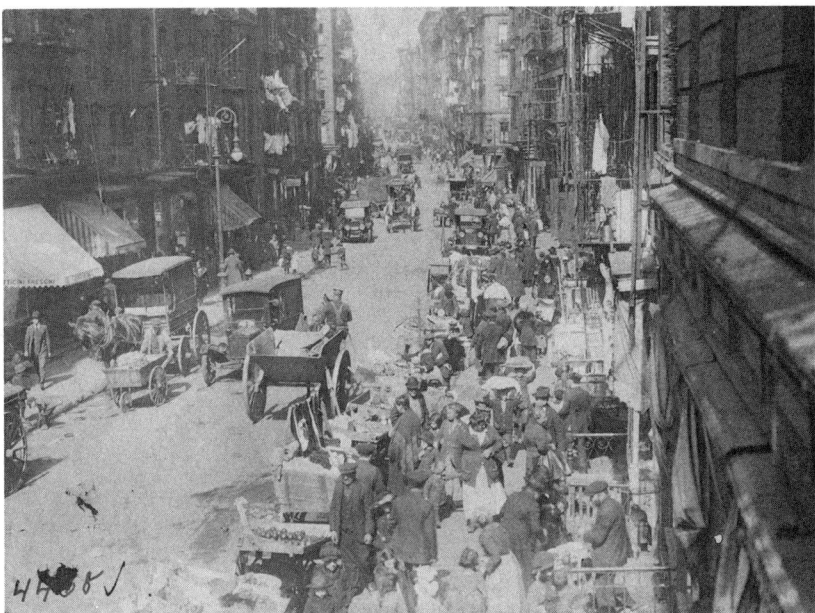

Figure 1.3. Manhattan's "Little Italy." Creator unknown, "Looking North on Mott Street from Hester," circa 1908, Rare Book and Manuscript Library, Columbia University, Community Service Society Collection. http://css.cul.columbia.edu/catalog/rbml_css_0573 (accessed March 10, 2014).

inferior to themselves. Southern Italian men were viewed as violent, emotional, and prone to enacting vendettas to retain their positions and respect. These negative stereotypes were passed on to American white public health officials and physicians; southern whites also schooled northern whites on how to handle blacks. Many native-born white maternalists accepted that southern Italian men imposed their will upon their wives through violence and physical force. Considering the apparent power wielded by southern Italian women in the home, compared to the need for external respect in the larger (read: male) Italian community, one may surmise that, as with black male violence against black women, some of these assertions were true. Still, to portray any migrating groups in one-dimensional stereotypes masks why dominant groups may have tried to contain them within marginalized spaces in their sending lands, and why dominant groups may have tried to contain them within marginalized spaces in their receiving lands.[96]

Zoe Norris: *The East Side*

Some within the white dominant culture of United States were more sensitive to the plight of southern Italian men and women. Would their depictions of Italians differ from those promulgated by maternalist social workers, visiting nurses, and the white masses in general? Mrs. Zoe Anderson Norris was a well-known twice-married, twice-divorced writer from Harrodsburg, Kentucky, who had made Manhattan her home. In 1909 she began her own magazine, called *The East Side*. In the first issue she reveals that she is of English and French descent ("And can I help it if a few centuries of English Vicars willed me their tendency to live among the poor, while a French grandmother on my mother's side left me as her only legacy to her inclination to dance?").[97] She created the magazine to reflect her own concerns for the poor and disenfranchised who inhabited the tenements, alleys, and docks of New York City's Lower East Side; in essence, like many other Progressives of the era, she championed the lives of immigrants and the poor and saw herself as their loudspeaker.[98] While refusing to wear the title of suffragette, Norris definitely sided with poor women who worked—as single heads of household whose husbands or boyfriends had abandoned their families, or as women who worked hard inside and outside the home just to keep their men. Many southern Italian women worked in the needle trades; Italian women gravitated to the needle trades because they saw them in concert with homemaking and, according to an interviewer of one young woman, "most Italian girls went into dressmaking and the sewing trades because they believed they would be useful to them after marriage."[99] Norris tells of the other side of women like this whose expectations were colored by men who flitted in and out of their lives.

> You have seen the little lace-sellers sitting flat on the pavements of the East side, smilingly offering you their laces, have you not? Well, nearly all these little lace-sellers have husbands and children at home whom they support. Nearly all of them have known what it is to be left alone to shift for themselves upon the advent of the Stork when they are no longer able to shift for their Husbands. For that is a common occurrence on the East Side, the flitting of the Husband upon the advent of the stork.[100]

Norris the bohemian frequently and openly stated that she preferred male companionship to that of females as long as she and other women did not take them seriously: "They must be treated as a Joke." She took the Joke metaphor gravely, branding men a "sad Joke" in a world where if "there are only seven original jokes in the world," then "one of these is Man." Keeping men in their places and warning women about them (and men about themselves) was Norris's self-proclaimed duty, as a non-suffragette but proto-feminist.[101] Here she revolves the positionality of a poor working woman around inequalities of sexuality, gender, and class: the lace seller probably works because she has to help support her family, and, when she becomes pregnant, there is a good chance that her husband may become a "bird of passage" and at least temporarily abandon the nest. This "bird of passage" term had been given to Italian men who, like Guilio Massini decades before Italian women began migrating with their families to the United States in larger numbers, made the trans-Atlantic trip multiple times, never intending to stay in the United States, and returning to Italy with money. It also invokes the experiences of Italian women left behind as *vedove bianche,* or "white widows," who fended for themselves and their families as their husbands sought the family fortune abroad, returning occasionally or sending money home.[102]

Norris's take on the southern Italian family structure and gender role expectations plunges into the depths of family violence in another writing. In "The Song of the Tubs," Norris writes about the closeness of the tenements, her open access to a line of windows and the inhabitants inside from her seventh-story kitchen window, and the closeness she feels to the elderly lady across the way. One morning, Norris discovers the lady is gone—she never speculates about her death—but says that, as the older woman had been Italian, "in the kaleidoscopic way of the East Side, came these other people to inhabit the flat" who were also Italian. The family consisted of a husband, pregnant wife, her sister, and "a brood of big eyed children." Norris was impressed by the wife's beauty and cheerful attitude: "This girl was a beauty, black hair, big eyed and curly lashed as [her son]" and because of the ten-foot space between the tenements, she was able to spend time observing her as she washed clothing in a tub, cared for the children, cooked meals, and cleaned.

Norris states that, particularly while washing, the wife would sing "a very cheery little song, much more cheery that I should have sung under the circumstances," and that once she looked across and smiled at Norris "in a pretty way, pretty as her sister, except that the children had faded her, as children will." Norris does nothing to hide her compassion for this woman and her children; she keeps her sympathies with impoverished, overburdened women constant in her writings, and chides those who cannot read men and hand over their power to them.[103]

The father—also darkly handsome, but possessing "a fiendish temper," soon turns the direction of the story from the everyday to "tragic," but Norris grounds this shift by stating that what was to occur could only happen on the East Side, where "life is very simple, simple and tragic," and where its inhabitants "act as they feel." One evening during their dinner, she watches from her window as the Italian husband first slaps, then begins to beat his sister-in-law. His wife watched in horror, crying into her hands but saying nothing and not interfering. Although she could not understand Italian, Norris says she ran to the window crying, "Let the girl alone! I won't stand it! Quit!" Suddenly, aware that their private lives are under public observation by an outsider, both the husband and wife pale, and the sister lowers the curtains. Afterward, the entire dynamic between Norris and the family changed. The son stopped visiting and passing on family secrets; the wife partly closed the curtain when cleaning or cooking but still sang the same happy song while washing. What amazed Norris was the action of the sister-in-law; when she closed the curtain, Norris writes, "She was independent then! It was impossible to refrain from admiring this spirit," but the wife's sister's actions had chilled her to the bone. Moreover, she now expected that if the husband beat his sister-in-law in front of his wife, he had also probably beaten his wife while Norris had been asleep. "How strangely her nature was that she could so easily recover," Norris remarked, as the young wife sang her familiar song the very morning after her sister's beating. "There mere sight of it [presumably, what had happened to the sister] had taken all the little tunes out of my heart."

When the boy finally talks to Norris again, it is to tell another family secret: he reveals from the window that his mother and the child she had carried had died. He quickly recovered though, according to Norris, as the sister-in-law now stepped in to take her sister's place in the home. Norris sized up the situation from her "man-as-a-Joke" perspective: "It appeared to be difficult to find another to take her place, for she remained and cared for them and cooked and washed and ironed, and life went on more evenly than when the wife was alive, for the girl, being necessary to the well being of the household and free to come or go, the father of the family dared not beat her. He was forced to treat her with respect."[104]

This life of nonviolent cohabitation continued until the day that the boy revealed that his new mother was his aunt. Norris notes the situation with ambiguity; while she does not condone the man marrying his wife's sister, there are the many children to consider. "I have often thought that I should come back and haunt a husband who had married my beautiful younger sister," she muses, "but not in this case." The new wife had inherited a mess, though a familiar one: total care and responsibility for the children, the running of the home, and a bad-tempered husband. Soon after their marriage, Norris' belief that the sister-in-law would only remain unharmed as long as she remained unlinked by marriage to her sister's husband came to fruition: the man lost his temper, struck one of the children, and, as the new wife attempted to serve him, began beating her. Norris had feared this would happen: "It is impossible to change the nature of a man without decapitating him." It seems it was impossible for Norris to change her nature as well. Again she interfered, screaming across the divide for the husband to stop. Again, frozen by the realization that their private lives had become public and an outsider was watching, he stopped. Again, his new young wife lowered the curtain as she sobbed. "It might have been expected," Norris writes. "She might have known. She married him with her eyes open." Still, Norris's contempt for weak women softens; she rethinks her stance, relents, and reminds herself that the first wife and baby had been spared further suffering: "A beaten woman suffers a thousand deaths in humiliation and despair." For Norris, such was life in the lower East Side of Manhattan, "where life is so primitive, where no attempt is made to conceal the emotions and the windows flare wide!"[105]

How does one read Norris's story of familial violence in an Italian family? The openness that gives her story resonance also provides the lens to see it as tainted and fictional, even jingoistic; patronizing, misanthropic, and misogynistic. Norris wears her politics on her sleeve throughout each issue of her magazine. Described in her 1914 *New York Times* obituary as a "Bohemian" writer and founder of the Ragged Edge Klub, a group composed of "writers of radical tendencies and their sympathizers," and a woman whose burial was attended by the wealthy as well as the poor, she never hid her disdain for men who were unfaithful or cruel to their wives, or who abandoned their families and paid no alimony. Norris also revealed her disdain (tempered by empathy, however) for young women who too quickly relinquished themselves for marriage and childbearing, without the slightest concept of a Plan B—education, work, training, money of any kind—if the marriage collapsed and the ex-husband acted like a stinker. She herself had been married twice and divorced twice; to hypothesize that she carried over bitterness from these relationships is to not stretch an idea to improbability. Moreover, Norris wrote from a position of a woman who had once been better off; though educated and intelligent, she had experienced poverty and described a time when, huddled in fur coats, she had suffered through the cold because a landlord had refused to turn on the heat in the tenement. Little wonder that she paints such a dire portrait of Italian women and children under the thrall of an overbearing, violent husband.

Norris does paint a plausible picture that could illustrate a post-migration story not only for southern Italian women but for those of any descent. The pressures of acclimating to a new environment, the strictures of sex-role traditions and expectations, the pressures placed on breadwinners, and child rearers and housekeepers, and the weight of poverty, overcrowded conditions, too many children and another on the way—this could have been anyone's story, without regard for private dreams and place of origin. It certainly fits for Ellen Simms, Katie Calhoun, and Maria Massini. Norris touches on the important aspects that I highlight in the post-migration issues that many women encountered in Columbus Hill and in the Mulberry District.

In addition, Norris did not have to stretch the truth of Italian culture or prevaricate to illuminate the power behind the private, as carried in cultural traditions. That the wife works in the home is usual; Norris's panoptic gaze cannot monitor the actions of the wife all day, however. Since her sister lived with them, both may have also worked outside the home, varying hours to accommodate child care, or could have done the cottage-industry work common among Italian women of that time and place: sewing, needlework, or assembling clothing, or making artificial flowers. Or they could have taken in a boarder to increase the family coffers. The husband could have been a menial laborer, or even unemployed. Any of the above could have triggered his anger; youth, expectations of submissiveness to the male head of the household, and the absence of female kin—especially older cousins, aunts, or grandmothers—could have provided a breeding ground for female resignation. Not to say that other Italian women in similar conditions always bowed to threats or acts of violence; Norris tells of one wife who sits before the window all day, hitting her husband on the head with a flat iron any time he becomes irritating. But the bonds of culture and the fact that most southern Italian women traveled with their families, and not alone, did help to reinforce cultural norms. The eminent late sociologist Rose Laub Coser has written that Italian families tended to be centripetal during this era; the force of the center tended to draw everyone inward, shutting out others.[106] In this case, instead of defending one another, both sisters became their own centers of accepted oppression.

In the final stage, sexuality and culture inform female private lives. In rural villages, familial control of female sexuality was directly tied to familial power and status: in a society where male honor was a reflection of female virtue, a family with women of exceptional, virtuous provenance wielded more power in land and in marriage negotiations. This was a woman's public face in southern peasant societies: to bring honor to the family and, thus, to the community. Neither Norris nor her readers know why the husband hit his sister-in-law in the first place; perhaps he felt she had brought shame upon him and thus upon the family. Perhaps she had not handed him his plate quickly enough. No one knows if he beat his first wife (perhaps causing physical problems that may have led to the deaths of his wife and baby), or why he beat the second. Norris does tell us, however, that she performed what she considered her civic, public duty as an American woman: "For we have some rights as citizens. We are not obliged to stand by and see a woman beaten. But you should have seen the consternation," she writes. "The husband turned pale, then glared at me when he found that I was not an officer of the Law." This, he understood—the disdain and fear of Italian authorities who might have traversed the Atlantic and may have been staring into his window. When he saw that they were not there, he stopped—for the time being. The specter of the law, in the public form of a native-born Anglo woman, also affected the wife and sister. The wife stopped crying, then, when she realized no police was watching, she covered her face, which had become pale from Norris's shouting. The sister showed her reaction to the potential public power of the law, and also her imagined public role. After realizing no police officer would intervene (or could not officially interfere; the power of culture and tradition, as we have seen, could cut both ways), she closed the curtain.[107]

In this scenario, all four actors—the three Italians and Norris—had made decisions and committed acts of agency that belied their private and public lives. While southern Italian men, and southern Italian women to an even greater extent, may have arrived on these shores with cultural capital and social control that seemed out of sync with contemporary American society, they would exercise their power as immigrants to a land of freedom by deciding which traditions to keep, which to alter, and which to exchange for better tools.

Conclusion

Ellen, Katie, and Maria are just three of the tens of thousands of African American, British West Indian, and southern Italian women who migrated to the United States in the early twentieth century and, at some time, made New York City their home. How they lived and what their daily lives were like are often lost to our knowledge. People died; if they were literate, many of their writings have not survived; if their private lives became public through interactions with representatives of the public sector, their perspectives and opinions were lost if their comments were not recorded or have not survived. Even if their comments and opinions were recorded and survived, they were often written by authority figures who were working out their own professionalization at the same time and whose opinions may have clouded what they wrote. We know their numbers only because federal, state, city, and private agencies felt that their movement, for whatever private reasons, necessitated public knowledge and scrutiny. Migration, as measured by numbers alone, is more than movement, and it mandates the use of alternate, creative artifacts to reconstruct why people moved and how they negotiated their post-migration lives. At the core are people who decided to leave the familiar behind and relocate for a better future. They entered the United States at the same time that workers in the fields of public health, medicine, and social work were in the process of professionalizing, of elevating scientific methods as tools to analyze and treat modern urban ills. The clash between private desires and public demands will be discussed in the following chapters.

2

Professionalization in the City

In 1913, Frances Blascoer discovered the case of Mrs. R., a young woman of African descent, in Urban League referral records.[1] A white social worker who was studying the lives of black schoolchildren and their families in the San Juan Hill / Columbus Hill area, Blascoer was investigating cases of truancy and neglect, and how black social institutions were responding to the needs of the neighborhood. Mrs. R. was struggling to raise two daughters, ages nine and ten, and a two-month-old baby. Her husband had abandoned the family prior to the baby's birth, and the Charity Organization Society had provided aid until the baby reached the age of one month. When school officials noticed the malnourished condition of the two older children and their irregular school attendance, a social worker found the family living in a colored mission's boardinghouse. There, Mrs. R. and her older daughters cleaned and cooked for $2.50 per week, then paid $2.00 for room and board.

The case was referred to a black women's organization, which gave the children clothing and found another job for the mother. One month later, an Urban League investigator found the family living in a dank, cramped basement, with the older daughters alternately missing school to care for their infant sibling while their mother worked. Weeks later, however, the oldest daughter told the investigator that the younger sister was in St. Joseph's hospital with tuberculosis, and that the infant had died. The oldest daughter and her mother still lived in the basement. Blascoer comments, "The Urban League's visitor stated that the mother had failed to take advantage of the place secured in the Nursery, that she considered the woman to be slovenly and neglectful of her children, and the case was apparently dropped there."[2]

I do not believe that Frances Blascoer revealed this tragic story in her report merely to elicit false hopelessness or to romanticize the suffering and poverty of blacks in the San Juan Hill / Columbus Hill area. She tells other stories that are equally, or even more, disturbing. Nor should the tale be taken as the norm, if one considers the perspective shown in Dr. W. E. B. Du Bois' 1900 study of black Manhattan, which I will discuss later in this chapter. Or should it be taken as the norm? I will show later how Du Bois struggled to show that, at a certain level of poverty and degradation, it was hard to tell whether such conditions were the fault of the mother, as the Urban League visitor had judged, or of the larger economic system. He did, however, issue a caveat to readers at the end of his study: "[T]he morality and education [of] this black world is naturally below that of the white world." Was the Brahmin showing his stripes?[3] What had he meant by *this black world*? Only black New York? Was the missing husband another of Du Bois's criminal class who were giving "respectable" black New Yorkers a bad name? Had this couple even been married? Or had they simply been part of the migrating mass of rural southern African Americans or British West Indians whose backward "heritages" had left them unprepared for urban life?[4]

Women and their children were central figures in a Progressive Era drama in which the private became public as denizens of the worlds of medicine, public heath, and social science tried to manipulate the lives of women and children while professionalizing their own. Karla FC Holloway has forcefully argued that legal and medical notions of individual privacy and bodily integrity were not constructed for women, regardless of color, and African Americans, regardless of gender, because, historically and socially, their bodies have not been accorded the privileges of privacy. Regardless of how individual women and blacks have defined themselves, the larger American society, normalized as white and male and usually embodying privilege and power, has demanded the power to make its private bodies into public spectacles, to be used for the marketplace, for science, for medicine. Women have lacked legal and ethical power over their personal reproduction—black women and women of color, even more so. The idea that workers in the legal system, medical ethicists, and medicine are somehow magically devoid of the sociocultural baggage of racism and gender prejudice is unacceptable, because the very foundations and scaffoldings of the law, medical ethics, and medicine are built on the acceptance of difference. From the start, therefore, some bodies were deemed worthy of status and privacy; others were judged far beyond the pale, invalid, and unworthy of protected personhood.⁵ The legitimacy of applying science to social ills—issues of morality, depravity, poverty, and disease—was at stake.

The Culture of "Maternalism"

The rise of science as a world view and source of meaning, identity, and reason in the West, and particularly in the United States, was not a nineteenth-century phenomenon. Some have argued that in the post-Darwinian world, science and reason supplanted emotionalism and religion. In fact, the commingling of science and religion in the United States traces back to the colonial era, when botanists, physicians, and scientists looked to new discoveries and technologies as proofs of the existence of God and His powers. This belief extended into the late nineteenth century. To avoid either-or binaries, Charles Rosenberg suggests that we see science and religions resting comfortably together, with the "lack of conflict" the most surprising factor. The physical laws of science increasingly provided moral explanations for social concerns and individual actions. The discovery of nervous impulses, for example, provided rich metaphors for balance and moderation in life that mirrored those of the nervous system. At the time, scientists thought that each body was endowed with a limited amount of nervous energy. Use too much and become too excited and immoderation would sap vital energy; be female and lack the social freedom to release pent-up nervous energy and become hysterical. This thinking helped explain modernity. A society falling into intemperance risks losing its powers of control, yet there must be a means for tapping into the uncivilized to harness social energies. Progressive Era reformers were keen on understanding the need for a serious, empirical explanation of social ills, and they also believed that science and technology would provide the harnesses to control the savageries of human lust and greed that were necessary to continue along the path of modernity to world supremacy. Problems merely needed a good dose of science and religious fervor for solutions. And sometimes science came with an emotional fervor of its own.⁶

As urban problems increased, women reformers needed ideas steeped in scientific authority to protect women and children. Assaults on the family threatened to rupture the moral efficiency of society.

What were these assaults, however, who should be protected, and how? Reformers disagreed over these questions. But, contrary to the tenets of biological determinism, they agreed in some measure that science gave hope that the quality of children and their homes could improve, that they could be molded into future productive citizens, that their mothers could be taught modern methods of birthing, feeding, and child rearing, and that any differences among mothers in their "cultural and individual" values were not immutable.[7] Historians have been prompted to call these varied groups, who focused on the well-being of women and children, "maternalists." They placed more emphasis on environmental factors and the need to educate and acculturate migrating, formerly rural peoples than on capitulating to scientific racialisms. Yet the programs they created and studies they conducted to inculcate women and children with proper American cultural and citizenship status cut two ways, having both liberating and stigmatizing effects on group cultures, group perceptions, and group traditions.

From 1900 through 1930, three questions were key to how reformers and their female clients framed, challenged, acquiesced, and remapped female responsibilities in the home, community, and the state: the "woman" question, the "negro" question, and *la questione meridionale*. All three revolved around questions of heredity versus environment. The answers lay in the shadows between, as socially constructed explanations for human differences were typically defined by many as manifestations of inferiority or superiority. Moreover, it was not uncommon for some to view persons in these groups, whose identities often overlapped, as racially gendered individuals with problematic, even pathological, cultural traditions that did not fit into the modernizing world of the middle class and elites in their sending and receiving locales. But, as Robert Park and Herbert Miller pointed out, immigrating cultures also looked at U.S. customs and often viewed them as strange and unsettling, even inferior. Different degrees of moral worth were at stake across the board.[8] Although the board was stacked on the side of reformers and medical and health workers who were going through their own "scientification" as science influenced the professionalization of their pastimes, they found worthy contestants in the female clientele they served. First, what was maternalism? How did the culture of maternalism affect the lives of women who migrated to New York City, and their children?

Maternalism and Its Permutations

Seth Koven and Sonya Michel, scholars of the infant/maternal movement and the origins of child welfare, argue that the late nineteenth and early twentieth century maternalist discourse reflected the diverse and often competing sociopolitical concerns in industrializing nations as they dealt with declining birthrates and elite perceptions of social moral degeneracy. Although "Progressive" and "progressivism" were terms of their time, "maternalism" is an historical construct, a product of the 1990s, used to explicate the positionalities and actions of Progressive Era reformers and their preoccupations with maternal and children's issues. But as fluid and ambiguous as "Progressive" and "Progressivism" had been by definition and motivation,[9] "maternalism" has proven even harder to define because the concept embraces the contradictory ideals and movements of the Progressive Era.

For example, some scholars have used maternalism to explain the thoughts and actions of paternalists who supported children's issues as they vociferously fought against women's rights. Simultaneously, historians have used maternalism to explain why women's rights advocates lauded women's and children's issues as cultural panaceas for gender inequities, seeing the inequities as threats to women that directly impacted their children, the home, and the nation. By targeting women and children as fair objects for private and especially public financial support, maternalists could accomplish through women what they could not accomplish any other way: help poor and working men, expected to be self-sufficient and independent, by providing the foundation of what would become welfare support by providing health initiatives for their wives and children. Moreover, by placing an emphasis on the need to help the helpless, racial integrationists demanded equal rights for minority women and their offspring, while bringing the effects of job and housing discrimination against racialized men and their families to the fore. In essence, if maternalism could work to voice working men's concerns without specifically speaking about them, maternalism could express the needs of all working men, women, and children.[10]

Gwendolyn Mink has highlighted three points that were critical to the success of Progressive maternalism. First, the reformers themselves had to create a new public role for women that tied their reproductive bodies to their new political status as valued citizens with the rights and obligations tied to motherhood. Second, maternalists wanted cultural stability and homogeneity. To achieve this, they encouraged impoverished women to exchange social acceptance for dominant cultural conformity. And third, they successfully marketed the belief that they could acculturate those considered incapable of acculturation.[11] In *White Women's Rights*, Louise Newman adds one significant additional process: Progressive maternalist reformers still had to be able to encourage an acceptance of conformity by touting the benefits of eventual assimilation, even as they pushed actual assimilation farther into the future. Newman maintains that in the case of women of African descent, some native-born white women took acculturation, and certainly assimilation, completely off the board by emphasizing that there were too many unknown racialized variables. These women used evolutionary theory to balance the precarious divides between their own worlds of feminine and masculine ideals. White female reformers employed "race" to equate themselves with white males and thus place themselves at the pinnacle of womanhood. They then used their racial positionality as proof of their civilized status. This racially gendered identity qualified and justified their entrance into the public world as they carried a gospel of cultural uplift aimed at women and children on the lower rungs of humanity. The cultural reeducation and reidentification of mothers and infants was central to their work.[12]

Reformers concerned with maternal and infant health care needed to embrace the potentialities that the culture of maternalism could bring. They were faced with an indifferent American public that needed to be enlightened to the scientific possibilities of controlling life-threatening diseases. Even prior to the turn of the twentieth century, health officials stated that the stability and future of the United States depended on public protection of infants and their mothers. Health care and social reformers in the United States were not alone in their concerns; work to reduce infant mortality had been proceeding on an international scale, involving most of the world's industrialized countries. Key to these movements was the belief that "it was in the interest of the state to make an investment in the lives of its citizens." Possibly nowhere was the threat of decreased population due to infant and maternal deaths greater than in Europe. On the brink of World War I, many Europeans realized a crucial link existed between the welfare of the state and the care of its children and mothers. Faced with the specter of war with Germany, France led the way in infant mortality research as a result of its declining birthrate: future generations of soldiers would be needed to safeguard the country from external military threats. Throughout the continent, the connection between a growing maternalistic ethos on bearing and rearing healthy children as female civic identity—a "patriotic" duty and "public service"—vaulted the private into the public, the sexual into the cultural, as the need for civic infant and maternal health care programs took center stage.[13]

The connection between lifesaving programs for infants and mothers and protection of the United States' vital interests caused even prominent politicians to get into the act. Speaking before the National Congress of Mothers in 1908, Theodore Roosevelt asserted that the country "could not get along as a nation without the right kind of home life; the woman who shirked her duty as mother should be condemned as heartily as a soldier who fled from battle." Hidden in the statement was the inference that these female civic obligations applied only to native-born Anglo American women. Roosevelt also believed that less prolific native Anglo-American middle- and upper-class families were committing "race suicide."[14]

The implementation of infant and maternal health care programs faced serious societal and political barriers. Some Progressive Era reformers were alarmed at the dramatic influx of "racially inferior" southern, central, and eastern European immigrants and imagined the destabilizing effect they would have on white middle-class society, its health, its culture, and its identity. The fear that the changing ethnic composition of society would contaminate the pure, superior Nordic stock permeated the psyches of many Progressive reformers. Physicians and scientists in prestigious journals such as the *American Journal of Public Health* took a strict Darwinian approach to racialized reproduction; they decried the use of public funds to increase the life potential of "feeble infants and weakling adults" who prior to health care reform would normally die. Instead, the degeneration of the native white race would begin as it lost its capacity to ward off "sickliness" while its ability to competitively out-reproduce new immigrants decreased. It was clear to many that public efforts to universalize infant and maternal care had profited the wrong class, while "racial decay" threatened to destroy the best of the "human race," much like diseases that strike trees at their top.¹⁵ Thus the growth of public welfare programs was hampered by both resistance to governmental intervention and racism: strict eugenic and racialist Progressives thought it inappropriate to waste public funding to protect the lives of racially inferior poor women and their offspring.¹⁶

Although the U. S. Children's Bureau, created under the auspices of the Department of Labor in 1912, contained its own share of eugenicists, it adopted a kinder, more maternal, and less utilitarian stance. This did not mean that its advocacy of the "rights of children and mothers" encompassed the entire women's infant health care movement—many retooled and expanded their notions of eugenics to include societal problems such as "temperance, moderation in food consumption, and sexual morality." Thus the U. S. infant mortality movement contained an amalgam of hereditarian and environmental understandings—contrary beliefs that cultural differences reflected inherited racial distinctions, while maintaining that environment could, in fact, trump heredity and race—that coexisted and coalesced to provide social reformers and scientists with an atmosphere that maximized "national power" while preserving its racial focus on "ethnic purity." In the end, they all agreed that it was wiser to spend public and private funding to create a healthier society than to burden future citizens with an unhealthy and unproductive workforce.

Looming on the horizon were the reproductive needs of millions of African American women who lived in the South, and hundreds of thousands who were migrating to the North. Black middle-class clubwomen formed a national coalition in 1896—the National Association of Club Women (NACW)—and promoted themselves as models for racial uplift. Placing their focus on black women they saw as lower classed, impoverished, and sometimes immoral, the NACW adopted the motto "Lifting as We Rise," and worked to uplift the moral, social, and economic lives of rural and urban black women. In their wake, while the discriminatory practices of white club women and reformers barred most of them from equal participation in the programs that would become the foundations of the U.S. social welfare system, the NACW and other black women's associations worked at the grassroots level in their respective communities and created institutions parallel to those that white female reformers instituted in European immigrant communities. These included day care centers and resettlement centers that taught Anglo ideas of mothering. Especially among black women in the North, notions of mothering had shifted during the nineteenth century within the larger white culture, from an appreciation for midwives and motherhood as a natural, sexual phenomenon to viewing childbirth as pathological and requiring physician deliveries and professional education in new methods of scientific mothering.[17]

To change from natural motherhood traditions rooted in folklore and common sense to a woman's inability to give birth or raise a child without scientific expertise reflected larger issues surrounding the ascendancy of science as an American "religion," and the professionalization of medicine, nursing, hospitals, and social work. At the core were white reformers' concerns over migrating populations, the urban squalor where most lived, and microbes—the spread of disease to the general public. The movement of professionalization and the subsequent creation of the modern health care system were to counter these fears, real or imagined.

Therefore, the tasks set before U. S. maternalists were the conflicting goals of a growing population: the need for publicly funded protection for all infants and mothers and the need to serve the clientele with "sliding" programs that reflected the expertise and money of the private sector, the racially gendered, classed identity of the clientele, and the racially motivated construction of a "quality" native-white population. Intrinsic to this seemingly impossible job was the geographic location of infant mortality hot spots: maternal and infant mortality rates were higher in urban areas where most arriving immigrants gathered than in rural communities. Moreover, black infants born in urban areas died at a rate twice that of whites. Combating these ills fit perfectly into maternalism.[18]

The maternalistic ethos dominating the United States and industrializing countries in Europe at the turn of the twentieth century focused its attentions on issues pertinent to women (particularly mothers) and their children. In New York City, which was the center and breeding ground for cutting-edge maternalist thought, as well as of new public health and medical programs, the spread of infectious disease and the inordinately high infant and maternal morbidity and mortality rates were the problems. Competition between the culture of maternalism and the cultural traditions of the women the maternalists strove to educate and acculturate made some sort of cultural clashes seem an inevitability. However, the reasons behind these clashes and their outcomes were never self-evident, despite the power of the state that maternalist reformers and health care professionals wielded.

The Professionalization of Health and Medicine in the United States

From the 1850s through the 1920s, the ascendancy of science as a social, economic, and cultural paean for the ills of an urbanizing, modernizing United States shaped the popular acceptance of public health departments, medicine, nursing, hospitals, and social work as empirically grounded professional occupations that brought order and hope out of chaos. Humans have always feared illnesses and diseases and been touched by suffering. As George Rosen has observed, however, it is only recently that one could overhear a conversation in which a person complained about suffering from a viral or bacterial infection. The acceptance of microbial agents as the cause of diseases—living organisms only seen by microscope that did not spontaneously generate or travel via ambiguous miasmas—only occurred during the latter half of the nineteenth century. Earlier scientists had theorized that tiny "worms" or "animalculae" probably accounted for diseases. Lacking proof until the laboratory discoveries of Louis Pasteur, and later Robert Koch, the theories foundered and humoralism retained it primacy.[19]

Germ theory will be discussed later in this chapter. For now, it is only important to note the revelations over time concerning germs as contagions, often spread by people, associated with the poor, and the swelling numbers of what Alan Kraut has termed the "immigrant menace" in overcrowded cities.[20] If germs had no barriers, and migrants in tenements bred germs, then nothing barred diseases from entering the larger society. Moreover, diseases could place an interminable weight on many of the poor, lessening their fitness for work, decimating their family structures, and creating children that could financially drain the future society. Public health departments, ran by medical professionals, were seen as an answer. In addition, the collaborative use of private and public funding to protect and educate society on proper hygienic and preventive health methods created the modern, scientific, professionalized health care systems of the Progressive Era.

The Professionalization of Public Health

Germ theory relies on two points: humans live in a world of "germs," which are distinctive organisms, and germs do not spontaneously generate from filth or other items, but reproduce themselves.[21] Proof to support this theory was generated between the 1870s and the early 1900s. The theory did not immediately replace sanitarianism, the older belief that filth generated miasmas or conditions that made people ill, and that sanitation systems that purified water, better drainage systems, modern plumbing, and removing rotting refuse from streets would decrease the rates of illness and disease, especially in the poorer, crowded portions of cities. These methods were successful, to a point, and later easily blended with germ theory. But the notion that microscopic entities could be borne by water, air, or human contact, and that poverty accelerated their spread, fed into sympathies with the poor for some, and fed the fears of others. The establishment of boards of health in major cities signaled a public response to calls for tighter controls over the spread of filth and disease, especially when epidemics threatened. Gradually, it also armed city health departments with the powers to create laws to protect society from the threat of contagious germs that bred disease.[22]

In New York City during the late 1890s, after decades of largely halfhearted methods, the board of health grew serious in response to increased migration, poverty, disease, and calls from the public for protection. It expanded from sanitary measures into pure milk campaigns and milk stations, well-baby programs, distributing preventive health care literature, opening neighborhood clinics, inspecting food vendors and producers for sanitary violations, and passing new tenement laws. Such growth in responsibility required trained personnel. For example, former concerned female volunteers who had once worked with the poor were gradually replaced by professionally trained social workers and visiting nurses. Proper food, and workplace and tenement safety inspections, required scientifically trained personnel. Scientific methods of public health care made what had been private public, and the professionalization of public health began.[23]

Germ theory held the promise—though unrealized—that science possessed the knowledge to unearth "magic bullets" that would eradicate disease. More importantly, germ theory led to the marriage with sanitary science and produced forms of prevention. Older sanitarian methods, which had moralized cleanliness within the home, mirrored scientific mandates for cleanliness within laboratories to insure accurate methods and outcomes. Both systems pathologized the home as an unclean, potentially dangerous place that only scientific methods of sanitation could protect. This also encouraged public measures to change individual and communal behavior, all in an effort to curb the spread of infectious disease.[24] Private companies focused on selling their sanitation systems to those who could afford purer homes, helping to foster a physical and moral divide between the wealthy clean and the dirty poor. With the exception of health education campaigns that attacked public behavior (like the anti-tuberculosis movement and its anti-spitting campaign), most public health departments focused their energies on educating society about proper home and bodily hygiene. Women, especially mothers, became the focus of reformers and public health officials as the primary agents of health in their families, to the benefit or detriment of society. Since cleansed households required healthy, cleansed bodies, women's reproductive systems, mothering techniques, and housekeeping came under the purview of the state. The professionalization of public health responded to growing concerns with the poor and migrants by entering the home through the bodies of women, and then extending its reach outward.[25]

The Professionalization of Medicine

In the latter half of the nineteenth century, American methods of therapeutics changed from individual specificity to universalism as physicians professionalized their craft and thereby uplifted their status from one of ill-trained generalists and quacks to one of highly skilled, scientifically trained medical specialists. This sea change was built on the concurrent changes that lifted nurses from the ranks of the unskilled to being seen as vital additions to hospital and clinic staffs, and necessary assistants to physicians. Hospitals underwent three changes from the colonial period through the first half of the twentieth century, shifting from almshouses to death houses for the poor to hygienic spaces of healing, medical training, and research. And social workers advanced from eager volunteers to settlement workers to college-educated professionals trained in the social sciences. All in all, science and professionalism defined the notion of "progress" in the Progressive Era, and defined the U.S. cultural identity.

In the early 1800s, Europeans questioned, and gradually abandoned, the humoralism that had defined the nexus of the human body, diseases, and illnesses for nosology—the classification of diseases as distinct entities—which instead emphasized the importance of the bedside observation of the modes of diseases, and used autopsies as laboratories for learning human physiology and the effects of disease. Physicians in the United States took a different route. Until the 1840s, they still believed in treating the whole body to achieve the individual's natural balance. The principle of specificity, or the rationalized therapeutics used in the United States that individualized therapies based on the idiosyncrasies of the weather, age, region, time of year, and other assorted factors, placed the medical community at odds with what was seen as scientific or "cutting edge." Specificity helped define American bodies as different and thus requiring different therapeutics, and also placed the United States behind Europe in the creation of new scientific discoveries until the 1920s.

Humoralism was the Hippocratic belief that human bodies were composed of four "humors": blood, phlegm, black bile, and yellow bile. Galen took the concept one step further, believing that all illnesses resulted in a humoral imbalance, and that morbid humors had to be removed by heroic, or interventionistic, means.[26] U.S. physicians were emphatic heroicists. To restore a body's balance, they would excite patients who lacked vigor, or calm the overwrought by using methods that drained the patient's overexcitement, such as emetics, purgatives, and venesection or bloodletting. These methods always seemed to work; clients whose veins or intestines had been depleted quickly calmed, and everyone concerned was relieved. This is not to say that blanket methods were used for everyone in every case. Quite the contrary: doctors relied on specificity, tailoring therapeutics to each individual depending on the locale, time of the year, and other assorted factors. This knowledge depended on localized wisdom and experience. The American medical educational system did little to energize traditional modes of traditional therapeutics.[27]

The general state of education in the United States, and the state of medical education in particular, did not equip doctors with an epistemological foundation comparable to that learned by their European peers. The United States lagged behind Europe in producing new scientific methods and inventions and did not overcome this deficit until the period of 1910 to 1920, where the ongoing war in Europe helped change the situation. American physicians thus looked upon their European counterparts with a combination of awe, envy, scorn, and embarrassment. Europe's medical schools were funded by governments, U.S. schools by students paying tuition. Europe's professors were trained to both teach and conduct research; U.S. professors only taught and trained too many ill-equipped practitioners. U.S. medical schools received students who were often barely literate, and not prepared for intensive study. Even one of its most prestigious medical schools, the University of Pennsylvania, required about half the time in attendance than that required by the medical schools at Edinburgh and Paris. Moreover, the U.S. curriculum gave cursory attention to laboratory science, with most attention being placed on anatomy classes until the end of the nineteenth century. Student fees led to inferior faculties and uninspired teaching; this, coupled with the American obsession to learn by "practice," placed limited importance on incorporating the sciences into medicine and medical therapeutics. In his pathbreaking 1910 report on the status of U.S. medical education, Abraham Flexner looked back on the poor state of medical training prior to the 1870s.

> Nothing was really essential but professors. The laboratory movement is comparatively recent; and Thomas Bond's wise words about clinical teaching were long since out of print. Little or no investment was therefore involved. A hall could be cheaply rented and rude benches were inexpensive. Janitor service was unknown and is even now relatively rare. Occasional dissertation in time supplied a skeleton—in whole or part—and a box of odd bones. Other equipment there was practically none. The teaching was, except for a little anatomy, wholly didactic. The schools

were essentially private ventures, moneymaking in spirit and object. A school that began in October would graduate a class the next spring; it mattered not that the course of study was two or three years, immigration recruited a senior class at the start . . . No applicant for instruction who could pay his fees or sign his note was turned down. State boards were not as yet in existence. The school diploma was itself a license to practice. The examinations, brief, oral, and secret, plucked almost none at all; even at Harvard, a student for whom a majority of nine professors "voted" was passed.[28]

This ragged, unscientific, and unprofessional approach to medicine left many U.S. physicians in an increasingly degraded status, and a frightened and disgusted public flocked to alternative methods such as homeopathists, hydropathists, and Thomsonianists in response.[29]

The American dependence on heroic, therapeutic rationalism, taught haphazardly in medical schools, flew in the face of cutting-edge scientific therapeutics taught by the Paris School and its "therapeutic empiricism," which stressed linking therapies to particular diseases and relying on bedside observations instead of matching therapies to the "[i]diosyncrasy, or the peculiarities of the individual." In the latter, surgical and dental therapies lagged behind the universalized standardization that had been occurring other medical fields. Even Europeans agreed that American doctors excelled at surgeries, and U.S. surgeons never let them forget that this supremacy, including the use of ether anesthesia starting in 1846, was due to "native mechanical ingenuity and frontier resourcefulness."[30] Specificity played an important part in giving American physicians status, at least in their own minds, that Europeans could not touch. For example, some American physicians eschewed French or German empiricism because, they theorized, what worked on European bodies in France or Berlin would not work for Americans in the United States: different people, different climates, different places. Moreover, the therapies that worked on immigrants and the poor would not necessarily meet the needs of native-born whites. This helps explain why, until the 1880s, most whites who were not poor had never seen the inside of a hospital: the status of hospitals had barely risen from almshouses (or death houses) for those who were too poor to afford a physician at home, or who had no one to care for them.

Gradually, even U.S. physicians began realizing that heroic therapeutics placed undue harm on patients and often did more damage than good; after increasing numbers of complaints, they began moderating their practices by using milder, more natural treatments, or getting closer themselves to the empiricist's camp. From the 1860s onward, U.S. physicians shifted toward dispelling the "gloom" of rationalized medicine. While doing little to heal patients, rationalized medicine had also placed their own practices and social standing in jeopardy. Therapeutics based on the "physiological method" seemed a step in the right direction. As laboratory scientists increased their abilities to isolate, define, and replicate diseases, the physiological method could clarify new therapies and remedies. By understanding the components and functions of the parts of the body, and by understanding the "normal" state of the body, compared to the "natural," attention shifted away from the ambiguities of natural imbalances to specifics that could be analyzed and treated. This gave an incredible boost to the medical profession and filled its members with hope, as well as placing physicians on the higher, more professional plane of empirical science. This boost was more psychological than actual, however; laboratory science was still in its infancy between 1860 and 1880, and contributed less to substantiate its real power than the hope that doctors had in its potential as a "powerful vehicle of professional uplift."[31]

The means of training medical students to be in a position to achieve this uplift only came after medical schools abandoned their reliance on student fees, sought philanthropic endowments, and aligned themselves with universities. This allowed teachers to actually teach and research without relying on their own medical practices to support themselves. As long as medical schools remained "businesses" and kept their status separate from universities, philanthropists gave lucrative grants to other sciences, and even more to theology schools. Students who had studied abroad came home with much information and skill, and little hope of expanding upon their learning. Dr. William H. Welch, a renowned pathologist who had studied medicine in Germany and complained to his sister in a letter that "I sometimes feel rather blue when I look ahead and see that I am not going to be able to realize my aspirations in life" of carrying on scientific research, upset the status quo in 1893 when he headed the newly created Johns Hopkins School of Medicine in Baltimore, Maryland. First, no student could be admitted without a bachelor's degree. Second, the Johns Hopkins endowment released it from any dependency on student fees and made it the premier medical research institution in the nation. Other changes occurred to raise the status of medical schools. State legislatures started licensing physicians and requiring them to take examinations in order to practice medicine. Following the Hopkins model, other medical schools began requiring more than freshman status as an entrance requirement. This, of course, decreased the numbers of students who could qualify, and the number of medical schools declined from a lack of fees. In the process, however, the quality of medical schools that survived Abraham Flexner's suggestions and that aligned themselves with universities and hospitals increased.[32]

The Professionalization of Nursing

The professionalization of the field of nursing developed in an American society that had ordered nurses—predominantly women—to care, and yet has undervalued the work of caring because nursing has historically been defined as "women's work," or something women perform naturally, or innately. Inextricably bound with the development of the modern medical profession and hospitals, economic, cultural, political, and ideological limitations curtailed nurses and their ability to care, with "caring" defined as both emotional and work-valued. In essence, nurses were crowded into a sex-segregated labor market, riven by social inequalities that made it difficult (and nearly impossible) for them to achieve the political unity necessary to fight against patriarchal constraints from without and fractures from within.[33]

Before the 1870s, all women at some time probably experienced the unpaid job of caring for family, friends, or neighbors. Hired specialists, such as midwives, might also be called to provide in-home medical care, such as bathing, feeding, changing bandages, and administering medicine from doctors or self-cures.[34] As stated earlier, hospitals were still marginal care providers at the time, more institutions for the poor, homeless, and destitute ill than places of medical care. The few nurses they employed used skills that ranged from none ("brute strength") to those honed from years of experience. The hospital/

nursing link came with the post–Civil War social reform movements; slowly, hospitals developed into business spaces that sold medical care *and* nursing education.[35]

During the 1870s, the creation of in-hospital nursing training centers drew "respectable" young white women who wanted careers in caring. They became part of a "secular" Christian-based ministry that allowed hospitals to expand as nursing trainees exchanged their labor for hospital education. They were expected to be "good women" who used their womanly duty to care for the sick while remaining subservient to instructors and physicians.[36] Problems arose when few nursing graduates were hired by hospitals as supervisors or instructors. Most entered an overcrowded, competitive, sex-segregated field of trained and untrained nurses who worked in private homes. The 1890s saw an oversupply of nurses. Until the 1930s, hospitals ran staffs of untrained attendants and nursing students to cut costs. Nursing students were thus exploited by hospitals because nursing schools were financially dependent on hospitals, which, in turn, depended on the unquestioned labor of nursing students. In return, the demands of cheap labor often took precedence over the administrative and technical training of nursing students.

The rise of professional nursing reforms began in the 1890s, as small groups of nursing administrators, like physicians and, increasingly, medical schools, demanded standardized, scientific training and education requirements to limit the numbers of practitioners in the profession. Gendered problems arose again, however; the idea of professional status within a caring profession went against popular notions and depictions of nurses as ladylike and natural caregivers. Demanding higher wages and education equaled commercialization, also seen as unwomanly and uncaring. Both hospitals and physicians used these gendered arguments to exploit nurses and resist reform; both feared that standardization and education would result in a demand for trained nurses, and thus having to pay higher wages. Moreover, separate nursing organizations did not want standardization or mandatory education, but simply higher wages. Nurse administrators alienated these women who lacked power and a voice—they were left in a void, needing more money and seeing no tension between higher wages and their duty to care.

Scientific management, coined as the "morality of efficiency," became the credo of early twentieth century nursing reformers. These used

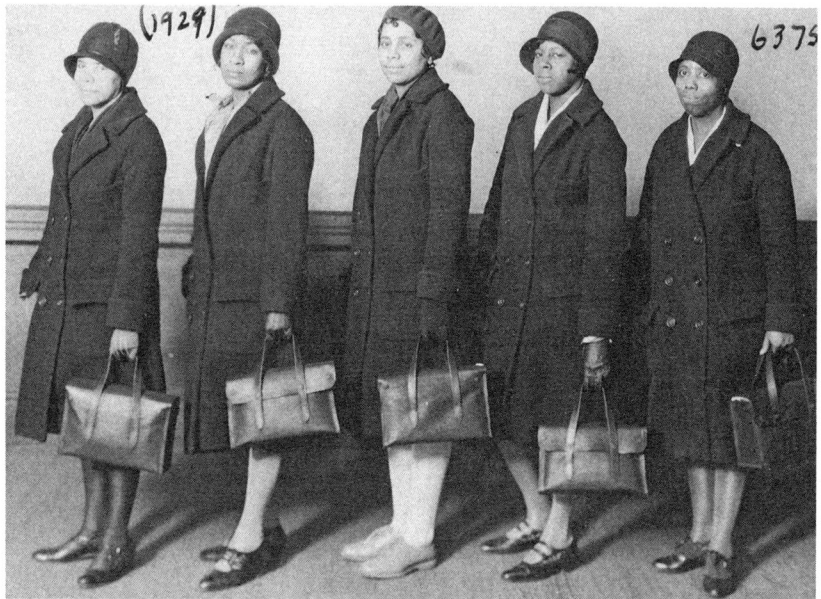

Figure 2.1. This 1929 photo of Columbus Hill black nurses underscores the importance that nursing held for black women and their communities. Creator unknown, "Columbus Hill Health Center Album—Columbus Hill Health Center Nurses," 1929, Rare Book and Manuscript Library, Columbia University, Community Service Society Collection, http://css.cul.columbia.edu/catalog/rbml_css_0624 (accessed March 2, 2014).

the growing complexities of acute care, medical and surgical care, the expanding numbers of paying patients, and the increased specialization of physicians as viable justifications for standardizing nursing and making education mandatory to practice nursing. But the science of efficiency meant the subdivision of nurses' jobs and increased their workload to the benefit of hospitals. In addition, the oppressive link between hospitals and nurse training still remained, bedeviling the multitude of women, trained and untrained, whose numbers glutted the field of nursing. The decade of the 1910s resulted in the overproduction of nurses due to the expansion of hospitals and the increased number of beds. And hospitals still resisted employing only accredited nurses because trainees were cheaper. By the 1930s, nursing leaders reassessed the profession and their collaborations with physicians and hospitals. Instead of trying to assist nurses who were already working in their fight for higher wages, nurse administrators sought to create a nursing elite by closing substandard hospital training programs, narrowing the definition of "nurse" to limit those who could work in the field, and by moving nurse training from hospitals into colleges and universities, thereby forcing hospitals to hire only properly trained nurses. The Depression hit the field extremely hard: less than 10 percent of the population hired private nurses, which resulted in massive unemployment. Those who were able to stay in the field who could not qualify to work in hospitals were older, improperly trained, and limped by on low wages. The professionalization of the field had worked out positively for very few nurses.[37]

Left on their own were African American women who were not accepted into most white nursing schools because of their race. In addition, some African American males at black medical schools blocked the admission of black women who wanted to receive training as physicians. This racially gendered discrimination was ironic and unfortunate. Nursing schools were competitive and, along with training women in exchange for cheap labor, many white women encountered problems entering nursing schools and, later, in achieving professionalized status. Many black men also found themselves excluded from white medical schools. Moreover, Abraham Flexner's 1910 report, which declared almost all black medical schools inferior in staffing, funding, equipment, and meeting state licensing standards, resulted in the closing of nearly all black medical schools, making medical or nursing educations even harder to achieve for African American men and women.[38]

This double bind did not keep some black women from overcoming tremendous odds and receiving training in medicine and nursing. By 1900, 115 black women had successfully completed medical training at the Meharry and Howard medical facilities. In contrast, 7,000 white women had become physicians during the same period. The Flexner report would hurt the chances of black women who wished to become physicians, however: only 65 African American women still practiced medicine by 1920, compared to almost 4,000 of their male counterparts.[39] The ideology of racial uplift in the 1890s and monies from white philanthropists did help black women past the racialized hurdles of entering nursing schools, however. During that decade, historian Darlene Clark Hine writes that as the numbers of nursing schools expanded at an extraordinary pace, nine out of the top ten black nursing schools were created. Black schools were affiliated with black hospitals, as white nursing schools were affiliated with white hospitals. As black communities created their own black-run, black-staffed hospitals, they also created a need for trained black nurses and physicians. Hospitals took on the role of providing internships and employment for black physicians, and training and jobs for black nurses. By 1928, more than 2,200 African American women were nurse professionals.[40] Despite the obstacles, nursing became a prestigious profession for black women, offering the persistent a way out of poverty and entrance into the black middle class.[41]

Conclusion

The professionalization of health and medicine in the United States was not a foregone conclusion, but one built on deep foundations of denying privacy to women, particularly women of color. Laying the bodies of women of color bare for the public to view, as problematic sites of reproductive excess, sexual immorality, and unhealthy living, became part of the process of professionalization as workers in the fields of public health and medicine separated themselves from the "volunteers" and poorly trained practitioners of the past and led the way to the highly educated professionals of the modern age.

3

Work in the City

In 1908, when Dr. Sara Josephine Baker became chief of what was then known as the Division of the Bureau of Child Hygiene in the New York City Department of Health, she was the first woman to head a municipal city department in the United States. Baker's focus on improving infant and child health employed an approach that was rather novel at the time but today would seem commonsense: instead of waiting until babies and children fell ill from contagions or substandard care, cities should invest in teaching new mothers preventive health care measures, and use visiting nurses as teachers and supervisors to monitor child care and re-instruct mothers, if necessary. Baker's initial interest in infant and child health and preventive education came from a medical school course given by Dr. Annie Sturgess Daniel that the young Baker had attended when she was a student at the Women's Medical College of the New York Infirmary in 1895. In a course titled "The Normal Child," Daniel argued that before physicians set out to find and analyze "abnormal" children, they should first become acquainted with "normal" children. This statement was rare and unusual for its day; Baker later wrote that "the intellectual soundness of that position left my callous young mind cold and disinterested."[1] After flunking the course and deciding that she would have to approach it with greater sincerity the next year, something clicked. She came away with the knowledge that approaching infant and child health from a pathologized perspective did not lend to preventive care or help tens of thousands of impoverished children survive.[2]

Her gradual acceptance of the efficacy of this approach came while working among the tenement poor in Boston, and later in New York's Lower East Side, Hell's Kitchen, and in San Juan (later Columbus) Hill. Whether working as a doctor on call to deliver babies, or as a medical inspector, meandering through side streets, alleyways, and up darkened stairs, Baker embodied the maternalist ethos: save the babies and teach the mothers. While in Boston, she found the work challenging and discouraging: challenging when what had been merely colored pictures of physical conditions became all too real in human flesh: discouraging because of the level of society she dealt with. "We were dealing with the dregs of Boston, ignorant, shiftless, settled irrevocably into surly degradation. Just to make sure they would be hopeless, many of them drank savagely. Having borne children and lived and fought and made love regardless, they took that method of dodging the consequences. Nothing admirable about it, but one could not honestly blame them for making use of alcohol as an anaesthetic [sic]."[3]

Here, Baker is speaking retrospectively, decades after her first encounter with social "dregs." Still, even if one could argue that her memoir embellished to make a point of how badly off her first patients had been, these words can also reflect an underlying disdain for poor or fallen mothers, seen again and again in her depictions. I am not attacking Baker for her judgmentalism, nor will I justify her positionality as a product of the times. I am placing her squarely within the gray areas of the maternalist culture. Some moralized, others did not; some swayed toward protecting children over mothers, others did not; some favored particular groups over others, some did not. Yet, as we will see in these New York City cases, many made their careers from exposing the private lives of poor women and the children, all in the name of saving lives.

Dr. S. Josephine Baker and the Ethos of Maternalism in New York City

Baker kept saving lives and, years later, after trying to establish a working practice with a friend from medical school, she became a medical inspector for New York City. Her thoroughness brought ire from fellow workers who suddenly looked bad when Baker reported numerous cases that needed attention while they apparently saw none. Her first assignment was Hell's Kitchen, the infamous violent Manhattan neighborhood with the name that bespoke its environment, and San Juan Hill, the area just above West 59th Street, and on the northern edge of Hell's Kitchen.

> This time I had let myself in for a really grueling ordeal. Summer anywhere in New York City is pretty bad. In my district, the heart of old

Hell's Kitchen on the west side, the heat, the smells, the squalor made it something not to be believed. Its residents were largely Irish, incredibly shiftless, altogether charming in their abject helplessness, wholly lacking in any ambition and dirty to an unbelievable degree. At the upper edge of Hell's Kitchen, just above Fifty-ninth Street, was the then largest colored district in town. Both races lived well below any decent level of subsistence. . . . I climbed stair after stair, knocked on door after door, met drunk after drunk, filthy mother after filthy mother and dying baby after dying baby. . . . The babies' mothers could not afford doctors and seemed too lackadaisical to carry their babies to the nearby clinics and too lazy or too indifferent to carry out the instructions you might give them. I do not mean that they were callous when their babies died. Then they cried like mothers, for a change. They were just horribly fatalistic about it while it was going on. Babies always died in summer and there was no point in trying to do anything about it.[4]

Baker was a working model of the best of maternalism at the time; despite her attitudes, she worked mightily to improve the lot of infants and children. Her work to provide mothers with purer milk helped lead to the creation of baby health stations. Her work with professionally trained visiting nurses helped lead to firmer crackdowns on homes harboring family members or boarders carrying contagious diseases and later to the first "supervisory" efforts of prenatal care. Overall, she worked to educate mothers, regardless of whether poverty had made them repugnant and worthless or if they purposefully lived in poverty because they were repugnant and worthless. Her motives within her work, however, are open to question.

As Katherine Kish Sklar said in a 1998 paper in which she reinserted the use of religious beliefs into maternalism, even among non-Protestant and secular reformers such as Jane Addams, Florence Kelley, and Lillian Wald, scholars investigating the prominence of maternalist thoughts and actions in Progressive Era culture should pay attention to the religious roots of its secularized, moral stance. While native-born white middle-class women did use the power of uplift to create their own professional niches, they also interrogated and brought to light class inequalities, and I would also add racially gendered inequalities as well.[5] Baker mentions little about her religious faith or upbringing in Poughkeepsie, New York, except that her elderly great-aunt on her father's side, who had been "one of a large family of old-fashioned Quakers," would trick her parents into believing that she constantly read the Holy Bible to them when Baker and her siblings visited when, instead, she pointed out that stories like Daniel in the Lion's Den were in fact "very silly" and contained nothing true. Although her sister Mary became "a religious devotee" of the high Episcopal Church, Baker had remained outside organized religion. "Perhaps my mind was fertile soil for that seed," she remarked, harking back to revealing the secret that they kept about Aunt Abby's "bible stories" until after her death at the age of 106. Baker could not see any harm that had been done to her or her sister. Instead, she felt that her aunt's irreligiousness regarding Old Testament stories had been "the beginning of my desire to question the right and wrong of all accepted doctrines."[6]

What Baker reveals as her moral center had more to do with a combination of wanting to make something great of herself, since she had not been the son that her father had wanted (this fact he had made plain to her since childhood), her family's interaction with students from Vassar, Yale, and Harvard, and the empathy she had felt toward African Americans. She begins her book by telling a story of how, at the age of six and all dolled up in beautiful new, lacy clothing, she saw an emaciated black girl of her age in a "ragged old dress the color of ashes." Her own egoism over how she looked immediately turned into pain. "Child that I was," she writes, "I could not stand it; it struck me to the heart." In response, she totally disrobed in the street down to the skin, giving everything to the black girl. She incurred no ire when she came home nude, because her parents had somehow understood why she had felt so moved to act.[7] Later, when commenting on the fairy-tale aspect of her growing years, filled with parties, outings, important upper-crust house guests, and leisure, she remarks that Frances, "our colored nurse of blessed memory," had been their "other mother and my love for and sympathy with and understanding of the colored race date back to her and all she meant to us children." Frances had not been alone; there had also been a cook, maid, and laundress of indeterminate heritage who had also been longstanding presences in the Baker home. However egalitarian on the surface, this bucolic setting is tempered when Baker decries the "changing servant problem of today" compared to that of her childhood. Frances,

Bridget, Mary, and a Mrs. Uniack had been "with them always." These women, undoubtedly, had represented hardworking, attentive, mothering influences in her life, far from the worthless mothers and the innocent infants and children that she would later encounter.[8]

Baker built on this moral foundation and carried out impressive organizational methods and moral reforms that helped wrench the New York City Department of Health from the dark ages into the most modern, influential, cutting-edge system of public health in the nation, looked upon as a beacon of health progress around the world until after the end of World War I. Historian John Duffy remarks that through solid drive, Baker did what Lillian Wald, the founder of the visiting nurse service and head of the Henry Street Settlement house, and Lina Rogers, who supervised the health of 4,500 people in one of the city's worst areas, could have never accomplished: she became the successful, respected female head of the nation's first and largest health department organization, created solely to care for mothers and their children. To do so, Baker rolled with the punches. Dressing in mannish suits to hide her femininity and savvy about city politics, she balanced her power between Tammany and anti-Tammany mayors who juggled political patronage and corruption against anti-corruption and radical reform every few years like bowling balls. In the process, Baker went from supervising a beginning division of slightly over 387 in 1908 to a bureau of 697 employees in 1914.[9]

When measured alongside the tactics that she and her workers used, her accomplishments come to the crux of maternalist culture during the Progressive Era: while creating public health systems that awakened politicians and the public to the need to pay attention to the health needs of children and their mothers, the means used reflected the notion that maternalist reformers deemed their own culture—that of the modern middle class, whether black or white—to be the height of achievement. In other words, while working to help the poor and downtrodden, they themselves, as workers, embodied the ethos of the progress that could be achieved during that time by concerned professionals and money. In response, they judged migrants, and particularly women, to be lacking what was necessary for modern living in New York City because of the cultural traditions they carried: they had nothing positive to teach moderns. This idea can also be seen with regard to notions of southern black cultural pathology in the early studies of Dr. W.E. B. Du Bois. He alternated between white prejudice and discrimination as reasons why rural black migrants struggled to acculturate into black middle-class models of respectability in the North and Midwest, while also feeling it necessary to distance respectable, *modern* blacks from the black underclass: always premodern, always criminal, always having just migrated from the South, always bringing a diseased, pathological culture with them.

Baker pathologized immigrant cultural traditions in much the same manner. Migrating women were ignorant and culturally ill equipped to mother modern children. They needed instruction from experts. Despite their cultural retardation (in terms of how to give birth properly and who should assist their birthing; how to feed, clothe, and care for babies and children; how to keep clean households), if they were compliant and willing to repent their shortcomings and learn, Baker praised and complimented them. For example, before she was selected to be the chief of the Division of Child Welfare, she proposed what she termed an "experiment" to test her theory that, with adequate education and supervision, visiting nurses could decrease the devastating infant death rate that occurred during the hottest months of each summer. Of course, to do so, she selected an Italian tenement neighborhood, the most "complicated, filthy, sunless and stifling nest of tenements on the lower east side of the city." To be successful against these odds would surely prove her point, she thought. Baker maintained that new immigrant women would be ready and willing to learn new methods of child care. "Mrs. Capozzi might be puzzled to find a perfect stranger dropping in to tell her how to take care of her perfectly well baby," she mused. But Baker theorized that learning modern infant care would be seen as just part of shedding the Italian language and culture that she had brought with her; "there was probably as much point in learning the American way of caring for babies as there was in learning the American way of talking."

But what happened when the Mrs. Capozzis of these tenements resisted, thinking instead that their culture was correct, and that the new methods proposed by these authoritarian figures were themselves pathologized? Like a nagging salesperson, Baker revealed that "if the mothers were sulky or apprehensive, the nurses went again and again, wearing down their resistance, establishing friendly contact, until they were ready and willing to cooperate." Acquiescence would lead to acculturation by sheer persistence—the more they resisted, the more the visiting nurses would try to gain entry into their homes and replace their habits with new, better ones. Baker maintains that once Italian mothers saw the benefit, they complied; during the summer experiment of 1908, they saved more than twelve hundred babies as about thirty nurses taught women how to combat infant diarrheal diseases.[10] Like Baker, one may argue that the ends justified the means. However, as later seen in the Mulberry District, the means used by health workers often blocked migrating women's access to the ends. They were expected to learn new techniques and leave old traditions behind because reformers saw themselves strictly on the teaching end. There was nothing important to learn from the cultures they encountered. And Baker got her job.

"Reading" Society: (Social) Work in New York City

The spirit of social work can be traced back through the reformist culture in the United States where, depending on the era and the condition, ministers and laypersons, teachers, businesspersons, workers, and housewives concerned over social conditions would, in the spirit of the Americans met by Alexis de Toqueville, join other like-minded citizens, form an association, volunteer their time, and take action for or against whatever cause united them.[11] Social work—a new, early twentieth century, science-based, female-gendered career path that replaced benevolent, volunteer-based philanthropy—gave white women the space to use their education to help society. But, as Daniel Walkowitz has demonstrated, the process of professionalizing social work as a middle-class occupation meant determining the boundaries between the deserving and undeserving poor, justifying their professional worth as "workers" doing jobs that had been previously done by Lady Bountiful–style wealthy volunteers, while making certain to distance themselves from both the poor and the wealthy, nonprofessional volunteers in the process. In particular, as they patrolled the borders between workers and the destitute who needed their services, they had to continually distance themselves, in terms of their speech, how they dispassionately analyzed and depicted the poor in case files. Though workers, striving to pull their ranks from semiprofessional to professional status and middle-class respectability, social workers walked an amorphous line between themselves and those they served.[12]

The scientific roots of social work rest in the field of sociology. W. E. B. Du Bois was the first sociologist to study the Negro population and its conditions in terms of the status of African Americans and British West Indians in New York City. As a man who walked among the early inhabitants of Columbus Hill (then San Juan Hill), his views of the neighborhood and its people in 1900 become an important early benchmark in describing the culture of the area's migrants. Mary White Ovington, a Du Bois contemporary, a colleague in the fight for racial equality, and the "mother" of the NAACP, provides the second voice. She lived in San Juan Hill for eight months in 1908. The third case is that of Frances Blascoer, a social worker and the first secretary of the NAACP, who studied the schoolchildren and families of Columbus Hill and Harlem in 1915, the year of the first citywide mortality study that undergirds this work. All three give valuable perspectives on life in Columbus Hill.

Dr. W. E. B. Du Bois and the New York City Sociological Study of 1900

In his study of African Americans who had migrated from the South and were living in northeastern and mid-Atlantic states, Du Bois announced that the "negro problem" had spread outside the South, where it was still most virulent. Many people, he declared, had wrongly assumed that, finally outside the deprivations and violence of the South, blacks had moved to areas where they could advance and experience equal access to what the U.S. had promised its citizens—*read*: native-born whites—or at least equal to that experienced by arriving Europeans. This was not the case, however. Du Bois explained that one must never forget that the North and South had both been spaces of enslavement, and that even after Emancipation, blacks lived in a "serfdom of poverty and rights" even though some improvements had occurred. Of the estimated 385,000 African Americans living in the North by 1900, one-third had been born in the North from free parents; the remainder had migrated from the urban and rural South. These differences in birthplace and parental status amounted to class stratifications in northern urban black communities, where most blacks lived, and had an influence on the status that they were able to attain.[13]

The African American population in New York City increased threefold from 1880 to 1900, rising from 20,000 to 60,660. Most lived in the borough of Manhattan in a rectangular swath that spread westward from Fourth to Seventh Avenues to the Hudson River, and north from 16th Street to 65th Street. Twenty thousand blacks inhabited this space and, following the historic march of blacks on the island, were continually being moved northward with the arrival of each new European immigrant group. Du Bois's discussion of "any peculiarities in the colored population of Greater New York" began with the sexual imbalance between black women and men, which was much larger than that found among African Americans in Boston or Philadelphia. Black women outnumbered black men five to four, largely because of what he described as a greater need for female domestics than male laborers. Second, most of the new migrants were young people in search of better jobs and fleeing southern white mob violence. Because of this unstable mix of young blacks, and with women outnumbering men, Du Bois warns that the North must now turn its attention to its race problem in a manner that is less "academic" and more in tune with that of the South. Otherwise, if southern race relations continued to decay and blacks became more disenchanted with their environment, then "into the large cities will pour in increasing numbers the competent and the incompetent, the industrious and the lazy, the law abiding and the criminal."[14]

From this point onward, Du Bois treads a precarious line, weaving from designating northern cities and white prejudice and discrimination as the culprits that pathologize rural blacks, to pointing to rural blacks themselves, pathologized by their own ignorance and incalcitrance, as sources of crime and maladjustment that defame the presence of law-abiding (*read*: northern-born) blacks, now unjustly defined by the actions of their migrating brethren. The environment of the Five Points, Tenderloin, and San Juan Hill areas were so inferior that any migrating blacks of good character could easily become tainted, and those already possessing inferior character would quickly become "professional criminals." Du Bois depicted the Nineteenth District, which housed five thousand blacks, half of whom were southern, as the spot where the pressures of city life were the hardest. Almost one-quarter of the mothers were widows and, in a veiled manner, he intimates that since most of the young men and women are unmarried and, being from the South, accustomed to early marriage and large families, there were probably larger than expected numbers of unwed mothers. This inference, and the struggles of widowed women as single heads of households, did not stem from Negro laziness; 99 percent of black men surveyed were employed. However, the chances of marrying and building families were severely curtailed by their patterns of low-paying, haphazard employment: three-quarters of African American men and women worked menial jobs. Some were rising, however; 10 percent worked in skilled occupations, and an entrepreneurial class was growing. Among what Du Bois would later term the "Talented Tenth" were ten lawyers, twenty physicians, ninety civil servants, one school principal, and almost forty teachers of African descent. Still, prejudice, discrimination, poverty, and crime defined daily existence for the overwhelming majority.[15]

Du Bois divides the black Manhattan workforce into quarters: out of 60,000 inhabitants, one-quarter "earn a good living" as domestics and laborers; half were just above the poverty line in similar jobs; and the final quarter, the "great, struggling, unsuccessful substratum" of African Americans and British West Indians, make up what Du Bois refers to as "God's poor, the devil's poor, and the poor devils." Out of this final number came those who, either by chance or their own flaws, made up the black criminal element. Here, Du Bois leaves room for analysis and speculation; these people may be at fault, or their environment may be at fault. He quickly changes direction, however, and states that 45,000 respectable Negroes, who were acculturated to their surroundings and living successful lives, should not be characterized by the 15,000 who were the criminals, the lazy, the immoral. These, he couches in his determinism, were the blacks who "have not yet succeeded and whom New Yorkers have helped to fail."[16]

Du Bois then returns to the environmental problems faced by Manhattan's blacks. The rents in the Tenderloin District, for example, were one to two dollars higher per month than whites paid for similar spaces. They were cramped, old, filthy, and lacked access to fresh air. To rent a better apartment meant moving to West 53rd Street, at the southern limits of San Juan Hill, where rents were even higher. Another problem was that of lodgers: Du Bois estimated that 40 percent of the black families in Manhattan rented to lodgers and, out of that percentage, only half were actually relatives. This meant that strangers were living in crowded situations with adults and children. His suggestion that the City and Suburban Homes Company should build the model apartment building as planned is poignant: this was the same company that, headed by Henry Phipps, finally completed the Tuskegee Apartments that Mary White Ovington would later occupy in 1908. Du Bois saw the construction of new homes not only as a necessity, considering the inferior housing in the area, but also a way to separate "the decent and vicious elements, which the lodging system and high rent bring in such fatal proximity."[17]

The rest of Du Bois's study focuses on the crime problem in the Tenderloin District and in San Juan Hill. Again, he walks the tightrope: considering how white discriminatory patterns of hiring, segregated housing, low wages, and inferior lodgings led to "general social oppression," while some blacks resorting to vice would be understandable since, under reasonable situations, Negroes were "law-abiding and good-natured." Yet, he cites the influx of southern blacks as the source of crime in black Manhattan.

> If we take a city like New York we find that continual migration and concentration of negro [sic] population here make it unfair to attribute to the city or to the permanent negro population the crime of the newcomers. Then, again, it has been less than a generation since, even in this city, negroes stood on a different footing before the courts from whites, and received severer treatment. In interpreting figures from the past, therefore, we must allow something at least for this.[18]

Du Bois then relays data collected since the seventeenth century to show that, before 1890, the proportion of black crime in New York City, even considering the unequal status of blacks historically before the law, had remained consistent with their proportion to the overall population. Why, then, had southern migration resulted in an increase in African American crime? One must "place [oneself] within the negro group and by studying that inner life look with him out upon the surrounding world," Du Bois advises. Consider the daily prejudice and degradation.

Consider that most blacks lived in a segregated, cloistered world, partly because of white prejudice, but partly of their own choosing. They had their churches and benevolent societies, various entertainments and schools. But their lives were claustrophobic and withdrawn; they "live[d] and move[d] in a community of their own kith and kin," far from the "rough edges" of prejudice and discrimination that cause them further pain. Within this cultural atmosphere, the migrant disorderly preyed upon the orderly. Du Bois feminizes black New York City to again warn that it would be unwise to identify all of her blacks as similar in character, to "suppose her a mass of ungraded ignorance and lewdness." There were definite divisions of class and status inside this African American and British West Indian community, with persons of substance and morals who "would pass muster in a New England village." Here, Du Bois harkens back to his own small-town Massachusetts childhood where he lived relatively free from the taunts and recriminations of racists and thoroughly absorbed the Yankee ethos. These southern migrants—these scoundrels, these lowlifes, this criminal element, the lazy, the immoral—these people represented neither Du Bois nor native black New Yorkers. "As we descend the social distinctions are less rigid," he explains, "and toward the bottom the great difficulty is to distinguish between the bad and the careless, the idle and the criminal, the unfortunate and the imposters."[19] One had to take the time and have the inclination to do so, however.

Mary White Ovington, Civil Rights Activist

Born in 1865 to a staunchly abolitionist, well-heeled Brooklyn, New York, family, Mary White Ovington stated that she had always felt that she "knew" African Americans without actually knowing any because, as a young woman, she had "known the possibilities of heroism in the race."[20] Her grandparents had been close friends of William Lloyd Garrison and Robert Bruce, and her father had left Henry Ward Beecher's Plymouth Church to become a Unitarian when he found that Beecher had become involved with a missionary society that, in turn, had had dealings with a slave owner.[21]

Ovington's knowledge of blacks had been largely imagined, but it was built upon her conviction of the unfairness of poverty and the paucity of worker's rights. Ovington did not valorize the poor—she found their living environments offensive. But from her revulsion she strove to do what she could and mobilized others around their plight.[22] Ovington's life had largely been one of ease, and she had taken the path of two years of formal education at Radcliffe after the requisite period of "coming out" into New York society. Her time at Radcliffe ended with a downturn in her family's financial status, however. Eschewing marriage or staying at home as a spinster taking care of her parents, Ovington became involved in the settlement house movement. Her initial social work began during her seven-year stint as the head of a settlement house in northern Brooklyn, where she worked among European immigrants. Her experiences at the Astral model tenements in the Greenville section of Brooklyn from 1895 through 1902 provided an eye-opening but frustrating education in the daily lives of the poor—eye-opening because she finally saw her socialistic and Unitarian perspectives in live action, frustrating because she could do little to change the stunted, unequal life chances of the tenement children. Her heart went out to the neighborhood boys that she attempted, with little success, to "culture." They were average, in her opinion; had they been born into more well-to-do Brooklyn families, they could have become businessmen whose earnings could have provided families with many of the same privileges that she herself had experienced as a child. She believed that the girls were doomed to follow in their mother's footsteps: working before marriage, then assigned the tasks of childbearing, child rearing, and homemaking on their husband's slim salaries as manual laborers.[23]

Ovington's fury over capitalism and inequalities of life in the United States led her to join the Social Reform Club (SRC) of Manhattan, a cross-class collection of intellectuals, workers, and businesspersons, where she met prominent socialists of the day: Josephine Shaw Lowell of the Charity Organization Society, William Dean Howells, and Leonora O'Reilly. It was through her association with the SRC that she underwent a change that motivated her leap from thinking about social injustices to activism. In 1901, the SRC sponsored a talk by Booker T. Washington, the "wizard" of Tuskegee who had become the best-known and most revered African American of his day thanks to his accommodationist stance toward southern whites and his silence on racism. Washington had been given the task of including the status of northern blacks in his speech. Ovington found herself appalled at the degradation that race and class had produced among blacks in her own city. "I had accepted the Negro as I accepted any other element in the population," she stated. "That he suffered more from poverty, from segregation, from prejudice than any other race in the city was a new idea to me."[24]

Instead of casting her support with Washington, however, Ovington became enamored with the forthright and radical writings of Dr. W. E. B. Du Bois, then an Atlanta University sociologist. She started corresponding with him in 1904 in an effort to learn everything she could about the southern and northern blacks and the racism they experienced. In Du Bois she found a kindred spirit in the cause of black uplift and was encouraged by his intellect, sociological methodologies, and idealism. Ovington told him it was her goal to open an interracial settlement house in Manhattan that would bring African Americans and other groups together for critical interaction and conversations over the nation's racial problems. He advised her that to do so, she would have to "meet with Negroes, and not shy away from them."[25] Her first foray into Manhattan settlement work began at the Greenwich House in Greenwich Village in 1905, where she voiced her concern that reformers had overlooked the needs of Manhattan's blacks and made it known that she would like the Charity Organization Society and other groups to support the creation of an interracial settlement. She also began a friendship with Jessie Sleet, an African American visiting nurse who later worked in Columbus Hill. Her association with Sleet and other black professionals became the base of what would become a unique perspective from which she could bring the black and white worlds together. With the backing of COS, she set out to find a financier to build the house and targeted Henry Phipps, who broke ground on the Tuskegee model tenement in San Juan Hill in 1906. He would not finish the building for almost another two years. Meanwhile, Ovington also began sociological studies of working conditions among blacks and published several groundbreaking articles.

Mary White Ovington's experiences in San Juan Hill are chronicled in her autobiographical *Black and White Sat Down Together: The Reminiscences of an NAACP Founder*. When she moved into the Tuskegee Apartments in 1908 (during her tenure, Phipps decided against turning Tuskegee into a settlement house), the building was the first and only modern edifice in San Juan Hill, boasting steam heat and sunlit, ventilated rooms, hot water, and fireproofing. Of greater importance are Ovington's portraits of life among the neighborhood's denizens. Warned by friends against her project, she even met resistance from her mother, whom she had to remind of the family's abolitionist past, and of Ovington's personal role as a "neo" abolitionist, fighting for the racial equality that still remained as absent in the early twentieth century as it had been in 1861.

Her memoir reveals that she never felt threatened or incurred any rejection from the area's blacks. What she saw was the need to expand the Tuskegee model to create needed proper residences, and to tear down the older, virtually inhabitable tenements built before the passage of the 1901 Tenement House Act. Slumlords charged unqualified high rents among the deteriorating dumbbell and double-decker tenements. San Juan Hill was, in her opinion, one step above the dangerous Hell's Kitchen to the south, which was then inhabited by "Irish gangster[s]." Besides obvious racial differences, what differentiated tenement housing in San Juan Hill from Greenwich House or the Astral settlements in Brooklyn was the cross-class situation that resulted from residential segregation, and the desperate conditions among the working class and the poor. "There were people who itched for a fight, and people who hated toughness. Lewd women leaned out of windows, and neat, hard-working mothers early each morning made their way to their mistresses' homes. Men lounged on street corners in as dandified dress as their women at the washtubs could get for them; while hardworking porters and longshoremen, night watchmen and government clerks, went regularly to their jobs. Race prejudice and economic necessity threw all sorts and conditions of colored people together."[26] Ovington's openness about the variety of characters she encountered in San Juan Hill mirrors the reports Du Bois had written eight years earlier, but with more precision and color. Instead of teetering between racialized apologetics and Boston Brahmanism, Ovington tacitly intersects racial prejudice with economics, showing that perhaps the lewd, the tough, and the dandies would have turned out differently had they had equal access to better employment and living conditions. Here, black rural culture is not the problem, even though Ovington acknowledges the presence of southern blacks.

Her primary concerns were for black women and their children. It was typical for black women to begin working as teenagers and continue to do so throughout their married lives, juggling menial jobs as domestics and laundresses with their roles as wives and mothers. This made for a hard life but, Ovington theorized, in the end, the black women of San Juan Hill emerged with better footing than their white counterparts because they were less dependent on males for financial support. While native-born white and European working-class women had men who may have brought home enough money from their roles as male heads of household, with their wives only working sporadically if they were out of work or injured, women in these situations lived precariously on the whims of men. If abandoned, they had to find work and were unaccustomed to balancing housework and child rearing with wage earning. As their children grew older, they might be able to rely on them to bring their wages home to help the family. However, after adult children left home, white women were even more dependent in middle and old age on their husbands and often faced destitution if men left or died. Black women's lives were harder, to be sure. Upon reaching working age, black girls were not expected to hand over their pay to their mothers and were left free to save or spend their money. After their children moved away, black mothers still worked, and could decide therefore at any time during their life cycle to stay in a marriage or go it alone, leaving them less prone to take abuse due to economic dependency. Still, the time spent working outside the home left their children on their own, and many who were brought before the courts for delinquency were depicted as victims of "improper guardianship." Yet Ovington was impressed by the cleanliness of black homes, however modest, and the good manners of black children.

Another concern for Ovington was how easily a black girl could fall into prostitution, first starting as a servant, then becoming a "sporting girl." Ovington once stated that the black women of San Juan Hill were like "round pegs in square holes" because their talents were squandered by a discriminatory labor system that valued their bodies, and never their brains. When Ovington wrote *Half a Man* in 1911, she estimated that more than 60 percent of African American women were employed in domestic service. For those who grew tired of cleaning white kitchens and bathrooms while "the mistress moves, flitting, in New York fashion,

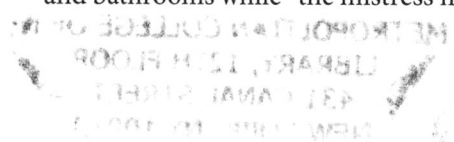

from one flat to another," the sex business was always open. In the evening, Ovington stated, after people came home from work and the sun went down, the carriages of the wealthy would cruise into the area looking for women. How many black women had fallen into prostitution, naively or knowingly? Ovington did not know. She simply bemoaned another example of talent going to waste.[27]

One could argue that Ovington's positive perspective on black culture in San Juan Hill was a result of empathy with African Americans and practical experience living with them. Her empathy and experience had matured over time through testing, from her upbringing as a Unitarian, her membership in the Socialist Party, her life in the settlement house movement, and her work as a writer and racial reformer. After leaving the Tuskegee Apartments when Phipps had changed his mind about making it a settlement house, she had been without a salary for eight months and had lived on savings. Undeterred, she helped create the black Lincoln House settlement in Brooklyn, and later became the only white member of Du Bois's Niagara Movement and a founding member of the NAACP. Ovington's descriptions come from experience: empathetic, but not overly sentimental. She acknowledges the promiscuity of black males, and how easy it was for young black women to fall into prostitution, considering their limited prospects and low-paying jobs. Nevertheless, her observations are salient: she not only observed black life in San Juan Hill—she willingly lived among the area's residents and respected them as human beings.

Frances Blascoer and Columbus Hill

In 1911, educators and private and public agencies in New York City questioned the Committee on the Hygiene of School Children about why so many children of African descent had been having problems in and outside of school. Their teachers strongly believed that these children's problems resulted from living conditions that were "unsanitary, immoral or wholly neglected conditions" and produced in some cases "a large percentage of immorality and weakened mentality."[28] Frances Blascoer, a social worker who also had been the secretary of the fledgling NAACP, was chosen to conduct a survey of the black schoolchildren in question and evaluate the public and private area agencies that were assisting them and their families. Blascoer had worked for five years among the Jewish and Italian populations on the Lower East Side and was thus accustomed to immigrant populations, and resistant to hyperbole or sentimentalism. This served her well. She conducted her research between December 1912 and December 1913. Her report revealed that the problems with truancy, stealing, and sexuality that were occurring among black students in the Tenderloin District, Columbus Hill, and Harlem were the same problems that she had encountered with other groups. She found that parents overwhelmingly supported her research. Blascoer also attempted to enlighten biased teachers, principals, and police officers who believed that black students needed special solutions for their problems because blacks themselves were racially problematic. Instead, most of their problems resulted from a poor home life, characterized by fathers who could not make a living wage so their wives could stay home and care for their children, and other psychological and emotional factors that were no less present than in other groups. In addition, Blascoer recommended that instead of judging individual children by an ascribed group identity and then attempting to help them with blanket programs, individual attention in the form of professionally staffed social recreation centers, visiting teachers, a school lunch program, efficient truant officers, and a training school for girls would better address existing problems.[29]

When contrasted with Harlem, a "normal community," Blascoer asserted that San Juan Hill was a place of extremes: either a "philanthropic or neglected slum, depending on the block." Accordingly, its inhabitants were "up-lifters and those to be in the process of being uplifted." Few blacks in the neighborhood owned or managed its stores, buildings, or institutions. Therefore, those who controlled the community were from outside San Juan Hill and had few relations with the area. The stores that existed lay along the "Avenue," and a few black-owned shops existed, but philanthropic model homes, settlement houses, and mission churches provided the foundation for the "up-lifter" or "uplifted" atmosphere of the neighborhood. Across from the model houses stood dilapidated Old Law tenements. Except for the Public Recreation Center between 10th and 11th Avenues and West 59th and 60th Streets, there were no entertainment facilities other than those operated by social agencies.[30]

Several social agencies and institutions worked in the area to serve black families, which helped mitigate the neglect by larger, private philanthropic associations. The Children's Aid Society operated the Henrietta Industrial School on West 63rd Street. Its evening trade school had opened in 1909 to train British West Indian immigrants.[31] At night, white female instructors carried on social work activities and conducted adult classes. Directly next door was St. Cyprian's Parish House and Chapel, a mission supported by the Episcopal Church. Black women attended sewing classes, where they made underwear and children's clothes that were sold in the neighborhood, with the proceeds going back to support the class. St. Cyprian's also housed a model apartment, which was open every day. On Thursdays, black domestics who had the day off would gather in the model flat to write letters, prepare dinner, and dance with each other whenever anyone played the piano. There was a milk station in the basement that supplied pasteurized milk for babies, and a laundry that employed neighborhood women for one to two dollars a day. St. Cyprian's employment bureau also worked to place West Indian domestics. The Lincoln Day Nursery cared for children from infancy through the age of two and fed them bread and milk twice daily. Although the nursery could house seventy-nine children, on most days only twenty-five to thirty-five attended. When social workers asked black women why they did not use the facility, they explained that they could not afford its ten cent daily fee (twice that charged at white nurseries), and that they had personal differences with nursery workers. Two other churches, Union Baptist, a black church, and a Moravian church, were also part of the community.[32]

Blascoer praised the work of these groups as vital, providing help on personal levels and creating a social buffer between the black community and large white philanthropic associations that either treated blacks benignly through smaller, segregated programs, or ignored them entirely. Blacks did not benefit from many of the services provided for other groups. When segregated opportunities were created for them, the programs went underfunded because portions of the monies given by the larger philanthropic groups did not always flow down to smaller, segregated agencies that dealt strictly with blacks. Blascoer cited the Big Brothers, Big Sisters, the AICP, the Children's Aid Society, and the Society for the Prevention of Cruelty to Children as examples.

From the paucity of programs and funding for black social problems came another problem: with so little attention paid to blacks, these larger agencies were loathe to hire and train social workers of African descent to work in black communities. Blascoer handles the problems of discrimination and prejudice deftly; while "differentiation," or segregation, might not be "objectionable" to all involved, philanthropic agencies could not possibly hold blacks to the same high professional standards that they expected from white social workers if white agencies themselves mediated who was hired or trained. And, she adds, if differentiation must exist, "the question arises whether it may not be both just and expedient for such agencies to create their own departments" to train black and white workers identically, but separately. This oversight had resulted in botched referrals and visitations, like the case of Mrs. R. that I described at the beginning of chapter 2. That Urban League visitor had been an untrained volunteer, and Blascoer believed her comments reflected a lack of preparation for what she had experienced.[33]

The National League on Urban Condition Among Negroes, the full formal title for the Urban League at the time, had been created by combining loosely affiliated agencies doing social work in 1911. It became a more united group in 1912 when the NAACP changed its purpose and left the care of social conditions to the League. The director's mission statement reflected the position that both black and whites members agreed that the "different problems engendered by the close contact of the two races in cities, must have, if they are to be solved, the careful study and sympathetic handling of intelligent and liberal-minded persons of both races."[34] The Urban League performed many outreach and clearinghouse functions, such as job referrals, housing investigations, a Big Brother / Big Sister group, and probation services for Negro male and female delinquents. The organization also believed that part of its work lay in being a clearinghouse for information, so that blacks could learn how to better use the services of private and public agencies. But the organization was underfunded and understaffed.

Moreover, Blascoer revealed that while some of its board members and most of the city's Negro leadership desired no programs that involved segregated services, the Urban League's official stance of intergroup cooperation did not match its patterns of segregated work.

Blascoer's report had lauded the efforts of the Community Organization Society, however, which included black social workers on its board. Social workers in the San Juan Hill neighborhood were known for their spirit of interracial collegiality. They had also organized to create the West End Workers Association. This group had done much to monitor and demand changes in police relations in the area. Overall, Blascoer believed the attitudes of these interracial social workers greatly alleviated the problems of African Americans and British West Indians because they did not rely on static definitions of black behavior. By comparison, workers at relief agencies tended to believe that most blacks could not be rehabilitated, and their efforts to help reflected this.

Black churches and other smaller groups tried to bridge existing gaps within black poverty by providing food, clothing, and assistance on a word-of-mouth need basis. But Helena Titus Emerson, a white social worker who coordinated the activities of the New York Free Kindergarten Association for Colored Children, upheld the idea that not only did blacks respond to rehabilitation efforts but that the changes were "almost automatic." Racial inferiority was not at the center of black urban problems. Instead, Emerson argued, poverty among black women created conditions that were deleterious to proper child supervision and nurturing homes. Emerson believed that black women needed better work opportunities, maintaining that "[t]he married women or widows with children to support, going out to work by the day as laundresses or house cleaners in white families, were out of work during the summer months when their employers were out of town, and much hardship resulted."[35]

The final "Needs and Recommendations" section of Blascoer's report also reflects this perspective that poverty was the primary issue. She saw the black child dealing with two problems: first, the need to master the difficulties of truancy, sexual promiscuity, and theft elucidated; second, the need to overcome the "certain restrictions apparently placed on him because he is colored," such as lack of access to better jobs and housing. The first part of the problem was not unique to African Americans or British West Indians. In all the immigrant neighborhoods where Blascoer had worked, she had seen good, solid homes usually producing "normal," solid children. This occurred more often when "efficient" mothers stayed at home and watched their children.[36] However, the ability of impoverished black mothers to stay home and watch their children rested upon fathers being able to earn a living wage—something that Blascoer addresses later when talking about racial prejudice. She does state that children with school and social problems could equally come from homes where poverty interrupted the normal processes of child rearing and child care (mothers who had to work outside the home to augment the salaries of fathers, or those who worked outside the home as single heads of households), as well as in situations with stay-at-home-mothers whose parenting skills were "inefficient." However, Blascoer cautioned that there were no unchallenged causal relationships between working mothers and delinquency or "inefficient" stay-at-home mothers and delinquent, troubled children. The problems of delinquent Negro children were not ones that could be overcome by blanket programs. Only individual attention from trained professionals like herself could adequately address black delinquency. For Blascoer, the process of using the unpaid, untrained volunteers of the past no longer worked.

The second problem of color, or racial discrimination, went far beyond institutional and agency boundaries but was, unfortunately, reflected in many institutional and agency attitudes and thus problematized the first problem of delinquency. American society had never addressed racial prejudice and discrimination, so it had never answered the question of whether persons of African descent should be completely integrated into its political, cultural, moral, and socioeconomic systems. Without attitudinal and systemic changes, Blascoer argued, "[t]he very social forces working in behalf of the handicapped of other races are in many instances not available for colored people." Considering that she had already stated that San Juan Hill's delinquency problems were no different from those seen in Lower East Side Jewish and Italian neighborhoods, it is also apparent that Blascoer saw and understood the complexities of racial, gendered, and classed inequalities as more than black versus white. From this stance, she was also able to add that in the true "polyglot" status of the United States, it would be unjust to declare where an individual's "disability" started and society's responsibilities began.[37]

Conclusion

The surviving social work writings of Mary White Ovington and Frances Blascoer, the New York sociological study by Dr. W. E. B. Du Bois, and Dr. S. Josephine Baker's memoir all provide crucial glimpses into how professionals, charged with providing services or critiquing provider services, viewed their work among New York City's poor and how they viewed the city's impoverished inhabitants. More specifically, their work and writings offer another critical insight into the private lives of women and children who lived in Columbus Hill and the Mulberry District. The "woman" question of the day—the lack of privacy accorded to the bodies of women and African Americans that Karla Holloway speaks of—intersected both the "Negro" question and *la questione meridionale*, the question of how to assimilate southern Italians, if it were at all possible. The women of Columbus Hill and the Mulberry District were, in the eyes of the most sympathetic reformers, racially gendered, impoverished women whose private reproductive and sexual lives came under public scrutiny, justifying intrusion and scrutiny because many saw them as embodying economic, social, or health threats poised to endanger the larger Anglo society. Moreover, in an era when adherents to the culture of maternalism judged women's cultural traditions for whether they met dominant cultural standards or fell short, the habits of these women and their children were squarely judged as problematic. Yet the health care and social work carried out among women and children in Columbus Hill and the Mulberry District were among the best in the world. How the work of maternalistic, professionalized health care played out in these neighborhoods, and how black and Italian women worked to shape the opinions of themselves, their motherhood, and the health care that they and their children received are discussed in the following chapters.

4

Culture in the City

In 1892—the same year that the sixty-seven-year-old orator, abolitionist, and activist Frances Ellen Watkins Harper published her first novel, *Iola Leroy*—Harper spoke before the Brooklyn Literary Society and delivered a speech titled "Enlightened Womanhood." Hazel Carby argues that Harper's prowess as a fiery public speaker had been honed over decades of speaking out against slavery, to the point that occasionally some whites in her audiences believed that she must have been a man dressed as a woman, or a white person darkened to look African American.[1] But the power of Harper's rhetoric came from the convergence of two deeply held opinions: she was a feminine-minded, race woman, and she was unafraid to speak on private subjects that she believed would help uplift the black race. She especially loved speaking to strictly black female audiences, which, from the tone of the Brooklyn speech, may have been the case on the evening of November 15.

Regardless of the nature of the audience, Harper lays out the foundations and reasons behind creating an "enlightened" spirit of motherhood among African American women. First, the gift of womanhood and motherhood emanates from God, and "into the hands of Christian women comes the opportunity of serving the ever blessed Christ, by ministering to His little ones and striving to make their homes the brightest spots on earth and the fairest types in heaven." Harper conflates the status of womanhood moving into motherhood as an eventuality. To Harper, this does not obviate black women working outside the home; she had begun publically supporting wage-earning women during Reconstruction.[2] Instead, Harper warned mothers to train their daughters *and sons* against the perils of sex outside of wedlock so that the home, through marriage, would become the "crown" of black female motherhood, "more precious than the diadem of a queen."[3]

Harper's emphasis on sexual purity within manhood as a counter to fornication or adultery is also a crucial aspect of African American womanhood and mothering; what mother, she asks, would not want "social purity" for both her daughters and sons because of equal love and concern for them? Her reference to social purity was probably coded language, as the term typically referred to the ongoing venereal disease epidemic of the late nineteenth and early twentieth centuries, and the social purity and later social hygiene movements created to combat the scourge of syphilis, which could sterilize women and endanger infected fetuses and newborns. That the social hygiene movement focused on female prostitution makes Harper's argument stronger. Even when considering the time period, her insistence that mothers protect their daughters by charging themselves and other women with preaching abstinence before marriage *to their sons* is powerful. Also, she deftly combats the prevalent stereotype that most black women were hypersexual carriers of venereal diseases. While she evokes sympathy from her audience by telling them that even that night, untold numbers of men lay dying "as physical wrecks, having burned the candle of life at both ends," and openly reveals how lust and untamed sex had "tainted their imaginations and sent their virus through their lives," she also acknowledges that some of the burden for venereal disease and out-of-wedlock births belonged to men and, by connection, to their mothers. This she makes clear when stating that God had blessed each mother with a tabula rasa, "an ignorant child" who had to be nurtured and trained to avoid the evils of the world.[4] This, then, is how Harper represented both Negro womanhood and motherhood to her audience: to be waged workers; to keep one's body pure and removed from wanton sexuality; to be selfless—to take up racially gendered roles that included the home and the public sphere, where young men and women would be taught to honor the race by honoring themselves and each other; and to conform one's expectations into doing whatever would be necessary to uplift the race through proper living and proper mothering. In Harper's rhetoric on black motherhood, no divisions existed between the private and public; to continue the advancement of the race, the "private" of black bodies must become public, and dealt with.

Much like Harper, public health reformers during the Gilded Age and Progressive Eras linked the preservation of social health to that of the bodies of women, starting within their families and extending outward into larger communities. The health and vitality of infants and children, and whether poor infant health or high rates of infant deaths boded ill for a U.S. social structure whose own vitality was predicated on healthy adult workers, led them to see a straight path from the uterus to the nation. The obverse were future unhealthy adults, infants or children whose lives were being jeopardized in utero, during infancy, or during childhood by mothers they deemed socially immoral, inept, or incapable of proper modes of childbearing and child rearing. This meant that women—their bodies and sexuality, roles, and expectations—occupied pivotal spaces in the Progressive Era discourses on public health and maternal roles. Individual female expectations and desires might mirror or run contrary to expectations of female roles in male/female relationships, families, social networks, and larger communities. But with education and supervision, some Progressive infant and maternal health reformers believed that the behaviors of racially gendered, impoverished women could change. With proper training and adherence, their minds could be uplifted. Within this process, their moral standards would grow to embrace the tenets espoused by reformers, and through learning proper childbearing and child-rearing techniques they would also better control their bodies and thus produce more viable infants. The privacy of the female body and of motherhood became virtually nonexistent.[5]

Racializing Motherhood in the Early Twentieth Century

In "Racialism and Infant Death," Richard Meckel argues that, to analyze the effects of racialized thought and practices on infant research and health campaigns between 1900 and 1920, one should approach them as "structured in two overlapping but essential discourses that, at least initially, were regionally distinct in evolution, foci and participants."[6] Meckel maintains that officials theorized "race" as a causation behind higher infant mortality rates among immigrants differently in the Northeast and in the Midwest. Most of these persons had migrated from European countries. The "racialized" attention that southern, central, and eastern (SCE) Europeans received from health officials stemmed from their numbers and the pressures they put on increasingly overloaded housing, sanitation, and water facilities—read in negative racial terms. But when municipalities and private organizations linked SCE racial identity to infant health and other health care programs, race was not viewed as a completely negative central determinant. Instead of being a justification to ignore high rates of infant deaths, officials poured money into research, milk and well-baby stations, and community health care centers. In its wake, this application of race for southern, central, and eastern Europeans left the largest number of health care programs created prior to the New Deal.[7]

The obverse occurred when health care officials applied race to blacks, however. As many of these same entities discussed black urban life and infant viability, they negatively applied racialisms in their concerns and questions regarding declining health among freed blacks and their descendants, and their migration into towns, especially in the South. Race became the negative explanation to many questions. Southern physicians and health officials surmised that post-Emancipation freedom and the absence of direct white supervision had resulted in the appearance of diseases and illnesses that were believed to have been absent under slavery; therefore, black ill health resulted from black racial inferiority, evinced in poor environments, behavior, and immorality. The health of black infants and children did not come to be seen as a separate case for study and health work than adult health until the late 1920s. This occurred even as environmentalists countered hereditarian racializations after 1900 by deducing that poverty, a lack of education, and malnourishment placed deleterious pressures on infant and maternal bodies, resulting in higher morbidity and mortality rates that could not be persuasively explained through theories of racial enervation. In particular, obstetricians sought explanations for high rates of fetal and neonatal mortalities in diseases, such as congenital syphilis, tuberculosis, and other diseases.[8]

While these empirical causations challenged long-standing beliefs in racialized health and provided the bases for some affirmative health care programs, they were cast onto a landscape already tainted with negative racial stereotypes, where race adherents still eagerly accepted the existence of congenital diseases in fetuses or infants, or the debilitated state of women's bodies, as outcomes of poverty, disease, or both, through a lens that further proved the existence of racial determination. In other words, health care changes that should have freed patients—particularly women—from preexisting racial group stigmatizations sometimes had the opposite effect in terms of representation—an example of unintended results. Congenital syphilis as a fetal or neonatal health hazard did little to separate women of African descent from some attempts to represent their bodies as degenerate, and the mothering of their own children as deficient, fueled by immoral lifestyles. Similarly, when southern Italians had already been depicted as tuberculosis carriers and syphilitic as well, it did not help, in a representational sense, to target the disease in their neighborhoods. Public health realities justified such moves, while popular cultural representations exploited what was already believed by many to be racially determined.

The Gilded Age and Progressive Era were times when the movement into urban areas coincided with and facilitated the expansion of scientific definitions and explanations for illnesses and diseases. In turn, representations of persons affected by diseases could also change. For example, by the end of the nineteenth century, the image of the consumptive patient had transmogrified from representations of coughing, translucent white male and female sufferers with a "wasting disease" that also marked their intellectual and artistic capacities to images of filthy, impoverished male and female immigrants who perniciously bred tuberculosis in tenements. Science had provided a new explanation for consumption, renamed when the tubercle bacillus was isolated and replicated in a laboratory, then revealed as a contracted disease, and surely not the "general systemic condition shaped by both the physical and moral attributes of individuals" or other causes as in the past. However, the scientific shift to a contagion also marked a shift in popular cultural representations of tuberculosis, from reluctant acceptance or even status in the older, more pervasive agrarian order to fear and stigmatization that coincided with an expanding urban order. As a contagious disease—albeit one where a single person in a household could be ill while others showed neither signs of illness nor traces in their blood—tuberculosis bore the frightening face of a selective killer that could attack anyone without explanation.[9]

In *Illness as Metaphor*, the late Susan Sontag maintains that when societies cannot explain or fully understand diseases, they have historically linked depictions or explanations of misunderstood and deadly diseases to subordinated, maligned groups via fear, ignorance, superstition, or simple blame. This partly explains the change in the popular mind with regard to who carried tuberculosis from who was susceptible to contracting consumption through some environmental cause or inherit the disease through one's lineage. Normally, control of popular representations rests in the powers of each society's dominant culture with regard to publication, dissemination, and retention. Thus, lacking control of mass-produced images, written or visual, individuals in stigmatized groups, and the larger groups themselves, may be depicted in popular culture as human representations or embodiments of particular diseases.[10]

But what happens when members of marginalized or stigmatized groups create and control their own representations of individuals in their same stigmatized groups? What would one encounter in the late nineteenth and early twentieth centuries if one read or listened to representations of African American women written by black women themselves? Would these images reflect or counter those constructed by the dominant culture? Could they do both? How would class or regional differences play out? What kind of mothers—actual, or potential— would one see?

In this chapter, I use cultural artifacts from literature, songs, plays, interviews, and folkways as popular cultural representations that show how some African American and British West Indian writers, singers, and everyday folk portrayed women and their private lives in their own groups during the Progressive Era.[11] In the previous chapter, the perspectives and representations of sociologists, social workers, and the head of a large urban public health agency helped shed light on how the ethos of maternalism, and its interconnections with science as a dominant cultural worldview in the United States, helped shape the health and medical programs that were created for impoverished black women in Columbus Hill. Taken at their most flagrant or benign, many in the professionalizing occupations of medicine, public health, nursing, and social work embraced these world views. It does not require a huge leap in thought to posit that they may have perceived the cultural traditions of their clientele as either merely stunted and in need of expansion, or borne of an ignorance that might have been teachable, hereditary, or even pathological. To counter and/or embellish these perspectives with feminine representations of womanhood and mothering from those in their "group" adds additional spice to what is already a complex, heady mix of voices, all useful in positing what African American and British West Indian mothers of Columbus Hill may have thought, and why they may have behaved as they did toward the programs created by white health officials and physicians.

Zora Neal Hurston's *Color Struck*

Novelist, playwright, essayist, and folklorist Zora Neale Hurston officially burst into the literary world during the Harlem Renaissance. She won several awards for her writing in 1925, which included a second place, best drama *Opportunity* magazine award for her four-scene play, *Color Struck*. Hurston's play carries an all–African American cast through the tale of a black male-female romance that occurs in Florida in 1900 and has a brief, aborted rekindling in 1920. Though no whites appear, panoptic whiteness is ever-present, but not consuming, because Hurston lets her characters choose the degree to which they let racism and whiteness influence their lives. Only Emma, the primary female figure in the play and the only mother, internalizes whiteness and racism through self-hatred because of her dark skin. She continuously accuses John, her boyfriend, of favoring lighter-skinned women, even though he loves her deeply and professes no interest in any other woman. It is Emma's fixation with her darkness, imagined slights, advantages accorded to mulatto women, and her deep desire to love the affable, committed John while fearing that he will leave her for a lighter-toned black woman, that leads to a tragic argument and their breakup. She views the argument as the final confirmation of her allegations.

> EMMA (*calmly bitter*). He went and left me. If we is spatting we done had our last one.
> (*She stands and clenches her fists*). Ah, mah God! He's in there with her—Oh, them half whites, they gets everything, they gets everything everybody else wants. The men, the jobs—everything! The whole world is got a sign on it. Wanted: Light colored. Us blacks was made for cobblestones. (*She muffles a cry and sinks limp upon the seat*).[12]

Twenty years pass. John leaves Florida for the North, gets married, becomes a widower, and returns to find Emma, his only true love. He rediscovers her as a single mother raising a sick little girl. Emma's self-hatred and self-centeredness are still shaped by the belief that her dark skin has corrupted her life chances—she believes that she has missed all the advantages and powers wielded by mulattas. In a sickening attempt to correct this injustice in the next generation, Hurston implies that Emma has a child apparently fathered by a white man, whom she never married. John enters Emma's home, little more than a darkened hovel with a few decaying pieces of furniture. As he explains what has happened in his life, she allows him to light a lantern. He asks her to marry him if she is unmarried. She answers yes, and John is interrupted by moaning sounds emanating from a filthy, disheveled bed.

> "Thass mah chile," Emma reveals. "She's sick. Reckon Ah bettah' see 'bout her." John takes it in stride that Emma has had a child, and immediately begins to call her "our girl." As he goes over and sees the child, he notices her fair complexion—she is a mulatto. "Talkin' 'bout *me* liking high-yallers," he retorts, "yo husband musta been pretty near *white*." Emma tells him that she never married, which John again dismisses as unimportant. "Our child looks pretty sick, but she's pretty," he says. "Think she oughter have a doctor."[13]

Hurston then spins the final strands of a web that is the life of a black woman, psychologically damaged, even more flawed as a mother than in the personal decisions that have shaped her life. John repeatedly begs her to leave to find a doctor, and even gives her money for cab fare as the girl's condition worsens. Emma is besotted with the idea of marrying John. In a trancelike state, she keeps asking John if he really loves her, and if they could marry the next day. She finally leaves, and as John ministers to her sickly daughter, she returns and flies into yet another jealous rage. "I knowed it," she screams, hitting him. "A half white skin," she yells, as she attacks him again. "Let me go so I can kill you. Come sneaking in here like a pole cat!" John stands silent momentarily, then realizes what has happened. Emma's self-hatred over her own dark skin and that of lighter women—even if the woman is her own child—has festered and only worsened over time. John flees, realizing that the woman he has loved for over twenty years is damaged beyond repair. The doctor pronounces the girl dead, and Hurston ends the play with Emma quietly crying and rocking in a chair as the stage fades to black.[14]

From the play's title, Hurston probably did not conceive and write *Color Struck* solely with a critique of black motherhood in mind. The title argues the existence of "color-struck" blacks, in this case a black woman, who constructs her identity, self-value, and relationships on gendered racialisms of white female beauty and black female ugliness. Moreover, she cannot accept the fact that a black man would prefer darker-skinned women to mulattas and light-brown-skinned women around him. Hurston uses being "color struck" to bring the problem out of the closet, and to warn blacks against conspiring in their own self-destruction.

Yet with Emma, more is at play than ruining her own life, or John's. In a symbolic attempt to achieve that of which the wrong parentage had robbed her, she creates what she desires and despises—a mulatto daughter—to share her loneliness. When the man whose love she had failed to reciprocate reappears to offer love, a middle-class life in Philadelphia, and marriage, she willfully sacrifices her daughter, even falsely accusing John of child molestation. What goes unspoken is the nameless child's life before that fateful night, and that relationship with Emma. How had Emma been raised—to accept her own beauty or lust after unachievable whiteness? Who had fathered Emma's child, and how? Had Emma allowed herself to be willingly impregnated by a white man, or had she been raped? Telling John that she had never married the father could have been admitting the truth, or shielding the shame of rape and fears of rejection. How had the child become ill? Is her illness and having a neglectful mother Hurston's attempt at the trope of the "tragic mulatto"? Emma was poor, but did poverty alone preclude access to any kind of health care until it was too late? And had Emma's transgressive interracial relationship—forced or otherwise—separated her from supportive familial or friendship networks that could have provided advice, financial assistance for medicine, and loving kindness? Or had Emma removed herself from contacts, preferring to wallow in the self-hatred that finally consumed her child?

Despite these and other unanswered questions, Hurston paints a woman whose choices ruin three lives and have a hand in the death of her daughter. The absence of other examples of motherhood in Hurston's award-winning play should not be interpreted to reflect choices in her own life—she never became a mother, but wrote about strong black mothers in other works. The character of Emma can be read as an aberration—a warning, a boogie-woman, of sorts, the creation of a racially gendered society. Yet Emma is potentially every black woman, and was probably many black women, to some degree, at the time. How internalized color partiality could cross and taint children, even to the point of causing illness and death, was itself a reminder that mothering often consisted of different problems for black women than for women of Anglo descent.

"Where's Mama?" African American Work Songs, the Blues, and Gendered and Classed Representations of Black Men and Women

"You won't find her here," would be Angela Davis's answer to the question above. As a musical genre, and even in its recording infancy when black female blues singers laid the foundation for the later male-dominated field, representations of motherhood, successful marriages, husbands, and children are largely absent from the blues. Unless the songs talk about failed marriages, cheating husbands or mates, dead mates, or soon-to-be-dead-if-you-don't-watch-out mates. Sexual themes ran through blues songs, whether sung by men or women, and as Davis explains, "Representations of love and sexuality in women's blues often blatantly contradicted mainstream ideological assumptions regarding women and being in love." If curious ears listened to blues songs for good mothers, or even potential mothers whose lives conformed to white or black mainstream ideals surrounding sexuality and women's bodies, gender roles, and individual women's or group expectations, they went unsatisfied. The situation was similar for the paucity of blues songs which lacked middle-class black male familial roles, even though one may hear men yearning for females who eagerly played "motherly" sexualized roles. In short, however, the blues songs of the Progressive

Era reflected the "social realities" in black gendered relationships among the poor and working class, realities that scorned accepted "uplift" mores, roles, and goals.[15]

But if black-constructed representations of parents, and particularly African American mothers or potential mothers, and their children are deliberately absent from blues songs, what else can the silence mean besides a disregard for bourgeois ideals that may not have fit black realities? The blues could also have meant an escape mechanism, a way for blacks who were desperately trying to conform to the ideals to blow off steam, to decompress, or to walk on the wild side. In short, the performance aspect of blues women such as Ma Rainey, Bessie Smith, and Memphis Minnie—along with the audiences—could have provided tantalizing spectacles for men or women who may not have fully "bought" the blues lines they were being sold, because the representations lay outside their realms of experience, or reminded them of from where they were trying to escape. People who may have heard the rhythmic beat and plainly spoken lyrics of black workmen's songs may have had no desire to join their manual labor but could have empathized with the words and how they used songs to work efficiently.

Thus, the absence of proper sexuality (veiled, heterosexual, and in the bonds of marriage), proper morals (circumscribed, and always under scrutiny), proper roles (responsible, pious, and selfless), and proper expectations (take nothing for granted, and look for all rewards in the next world) in blues lyrics, dancing, and drinking may have veiled the mainstream from the sight of critics. An old saying states that there was a thin line between gospel music and the blues. The blues and work songs gave African Americans who may have found middle-class values hypocritical or untenable a valued counter-narrative. There may have also been those who, while mimicking middle-class values, found resonance in bawdy, restless, or angry lyrics. They may have also at least momentarily reveled in the absence of the status quo and their tough struggle to achieve entrance. In essence, the blues were created by those on the edges of black society. African American poor and working-class men and women wrote and published few surviving works. Fortunately, the representations of black life contained in the blues and working-men's songs remains through early ethnomusicologist's efforts to record the lyrics and melodies.

African American Men's Work Songs

The songs of black workingmen carry on the traditions of class- and age-defined black male reputations. Work songs often reflected their acceptance of, and desire for, nurturing, motherly women who would protect and care for them, and be coworkers or even sole supporters. This came at a time when some black men viewed wives who worked outside the home as an attack against masculinity, even when their wives were educated and accomplished, and even if the family was experiencing strong financial need. Central themes in the songs of black male workers included their desire for black female fidelity, warmth, sensuality, and a willingness to serve their men, albeit financially, sexually, or emotionally. Some African American men represented themselves in work songs as sexualized, independent entities, embodying traits in opposition to those they expected in women. As I will later show in the works of black blueswomen, black male definitions focused on the importance of "reputation" in a white-ruled society rife with social, political, and economic inequalities.

> I ain't no miller,
> No miller's son,
> But do your grinding
> Till the miller comes;
> Tell me how long will I have to wait
> Or will I have to do a little hesitate.[16]

Other African American male work songs proffered the rhetoric of solitary, sexual pleasers—but admitted a weakness for womanly powers, particularly when contained in an aesthetically pleasing package. For example, the songs of Alabama workingmen spoke of what a "good" woman would do for a man: how she could make him straighten up and "act right." But good women are also capable of drawing men away from existing women.

> A good-looking woman make a rabbit
> Move his family to town.
> A good-looking woman

> Will make a bull dog join the church.
> A good-looking woman
> Make a bull-dog break his chain.[17]

The qualities of a "good" woman who could make a man "act right" (settle down, behave responsibly, and aspire to mature manhood status) are similar to those that would make the same woman a potentially good wife and mother—except the infidelity part. If the outward appearance of black women swayed black men's actions, then men generally sang of female differences predicated on outward, physical particularities. Brown-haired women were said to "drive a good man insane," but blonde-haired women (like the aforementioned "good-looking woman") would "make a bull dog break his chain."[18]

On the other hand, some African American male-centered folk songs took a woman's skin color to task, and reflected a preference for dark-skinned women: "It takes a dark-skinned baby / To make a preacher throw his Bible down." Again, black men often took pride in the dusky beauty of African American women, contrasting sharply with the white cultural preference for women of European heritage (a preference that, again, some men in the black community also valued):

> Some says yellow
> While others say brown,
> But for me I'll take the blackest in town.[19]

Similarly, the blues sung by African American men focused on their control over, or perceived ownership of, their women. Having a good woman was key to black male identity—a status booster that elevated even the poorest man over his peers. The blues recorded the pain felt when African American women left—abandonment, for another man, or in death.

> I had a good woman, I had a good woman,
> But the fool laid down and died;
> I had a good woman, but the fool laid down and died.
> If you got a good woman, you better pin her to your side.[20]

While work songs reflected the African American male desire for attractive, submissive, faithful, and nurturing female companions, representations of domestic violence against these same idealized women can also be seen in these and blues songs. Born into the ongoing prospect of discrimination, degradation, and physical violence at any time against African American men, some of their work songs reflected and advocated physical violence, masked as love, against black women. With sad irony, black women faced violence and degradation as much or more than their black male cohort, open to the possibility of abuse from the dominant culture, their own men, and other black women. These lyrics, overheard in 1915–1916 being sung by black workingmen in Auburn, Alabama, sum up a misogynistic worldview that equated manly love with total control over unruly women.

> If you're in love and your gal don't treat you nice
> Just pick up a big old stick and beat her all you might
> If my wife don't treat me right,
> I'll knock her teeth down her throat
> And walk the streets all night.
>
> If my wife comes home wid whiskey on her breath,
> I'll pick up a stick and beat dat heifer to death.[21]

Historian Darlene Clark Hine has long maintained that many African American women fled the South and migrated to other states because threats of rape and domestic violence were realities. Their movement signified a firm unwillingness to ignore and tolerate the violation of their bodies, regardless of whether the male perpetrators were white or black.[22] These work songs show that some black men may have used, tolerated, considered, or even found humorous the notion that misbehaving African American women should receive the physical abuse that their men thought they deserved. Tragically, what "misbehaving" meant was left in male minds to determine.

In short, the women represented in the working songs of black men were expected to conform to many of the dictates of middle-class feminine ideals: attractiveness, submissiveness, fidelity, warmth, and nurturance. Like diligent mothers, black workingmen expected the good African American woman to patiently accept or lovingly reform their wandering, lustful ways, raising them from adolescent wandering, laziness and philandering to full Negro manhood. It is less puzzling that ethnomusicologists often heard these songs from down-and-out menial laborers, or prison workers. Where they and the larger white society had failed them as black men, black women were to step in, as mothers of black communities, and guide them down the straight and narrow. The countercurrent of multiple sexual partners, male bravado, and violence against women reveals the complexities of black male and female interactions, something that many in the middle class would have rather left unspoken, or used as an example of how poor and working-class black women needed to be trained to be more womanly and pious to escape future beatings.

However, a few brave critics may have even called for black male-on-female violence to be exposed for what they believed it was: a tragic manifestation of love, mistrust, and control in a violent society. They may have even called for other men and women to protect vulnerable, beaten women. Black blueswomen took on the latter charge, singing about an alternative representation of womanhood and mothering that often met violence with violence, or initiated physicality on their own.

African American Blueswomen and Representations of Womanhood and Mothering

By depicting the experiences of women and men who lived lives usually separated from respectable moral standards, celebrated blues women like Gertrude "Ma" Rainey, Bessie Smith, and Memphis Minnie offered alternate representations of black womanhood. Their lyrics (and lifestyles) placed little importance on the mandates of black female respectability in black and white middle-class mores. Instead, they strode past the confines of respectability and transformed it by co-opting the male importance placed on "reputation." And, unlike their "uplifting and already uplifted sisters," they surveyed the racially gendered, classed, and sometimes sexualized landscape and uncovered its flaws.

First, as many middle-class black women had already discovered in their encounters with white women in social and religious movements, most of their white counterparts had rarely seen their claims of pedigree, money, or education, along with community work, as equal to or capable of reaching white levels of femininity.[23] Second, eschewing such examples of vanity, black blues women embraced the reality of many poor or working-class women's lives by claiming negative stereotypes of black female sexuality, anger, and gender relations, claiming their responses of strength or weakness as valid measuring points of female reputation that did not mean an internalization of racially gendered and classed inferiority. Third, they then simultaneously demanded and received respect from most who heard them—black women but, in particular, black men. African American blueswomen's lyrics show a knowing acceptance of ideology and reality. What represented femininity and womanhood from a middle-class perspective meant little or nothing within their arena of self-definition, female respectability and male reputation be damned.[24]

"Respectability" and "respect" were at the core of middle-class black women's literature, as well as their public and private lives. Only by keeping their inner lives and thoughts hidden could they protect themselves from repugnant stereotypes of hypersexuality and protect their bodies and those of their working-class sisters. Simultaneously, they believed their efforts at social work would uplift their benighted sisters to loftier levels of morality, thereby uplifting the race. Much was at stake for black women; much was outside their power. Yet if those with position and power failed to protect the bodies and offspring of poor and working-class women, what would be said about them and their movement? What would be said about the future of black race? Who would dare to fight back?[25]

Future salvation aside, few elite black female writers attempted to tackle the incendiary topic of black female sexuality, or the intimate relationships between black men and women.[26] African American blues women filled the void of the unmentionable. Also, most refined black women did not write about the lives of poor and working-class urban black women, newly arrived from the rural South or living in the South. Zora Neale Hurston stood out in this respect. Even if, behind closed doors, some of the same shenanigans occurred in the homes of wealthier African Americans as in the homes of their poorer brethren, the actions, or acknowledgments of infidelity and homosexuality, were

not openly discussed. Domestic violence, incest—these fell into similar states of silence. Black women protected their bodies, psyches, and honor from prevailing stereotypes by often hiding their thoughts and desires within a "culture of dissemblance."[27]

When cultural scholars Hazel Carby and Angela Davis mined the songs of African American blueswomen, they discovered that their lyrics revealed a proto-feminist consciousness and identity that existed among working-class black women during the first quarter of the twentieth century. This consciousness embraced and acknowledged their sexuality, independence, and empowerment—counter-representations of proper black womanhood. In particular, the lyrics that explored issues of black women's heterosexuality or homosexuality contrasted sharply with the images of bourgeois Negro womanhood as seen in the writings of middle- and upper-class African American women, as constructed through the age-old protective barrier of black female dissemblance and white female mimicry, and as manifest from the nineteenth century through the Harlem Renaissance.[28]

For example, Memphis Minnie, a popular but now largely forgotten black female blues singer, was noted for her rawness and salty language, for keeping it real, and providing vision into the African American working-class realpolitik for black women. These were urban or rural women, who sometimes, like black men, violated convention, hopped aboard trains bound for somewhere, and decided to take their lives into their own hands. These women may have been mothers, moving to another town to escape violence, to find better jobs, following a man, or creating a new life to later move their children into. Or they could have temporarily or permanently abandoned husbands, mates, children, and families. Minnie skirts no issues in "Nothing in Rambling"; she was born for the road and, until she finds the right man, vows to continue her traveling ways. She is a new prototypical black woman, a counter to the New Negro Womanhood of the Harlem Renaissance.

> I's born in Louisiana
> I was raised in Algiers
> And everywhere I been
> The peoples all say

Ain't nothing in rambling
Either running around
Well I believe I'll marry
Oooo, wooo, Lord, and settle down

I first left home
I stopped in Tennessee
The peoples all begging,
"Come and stay with me."

'Cause ain't nothing in rambling
Either running around
Well I believe I'll get me a good man
Oooo, wooo, Lord, and settle down.[29]

Minnie's coterie—dispossessed fellow ramblers—understood her. Women who felt confined, trapped, or resigned to marriages and motherhood may have felt a spark of what could be in these lyrics; they also may have shaken their heads in confusion or disgust. Minnie speaks of a paradox: a rootless, migrating woman who answers to no one but herself. Men (presumably) who are rooted desire her. Female listeners, tired or bored with everyday life, dream through her and perhaps find the audacity to uproot themselves for shades of the Promised Land. The notion of a black woman's rambling is nothing borne of shame, guilt, or judgment. It is evidentiary of unruliness and inspiring; Memphis Minnie needs no chaperone to justify her movement (as if two black women, however well-behaved or dressed, could completely dispel questions of their purity—as seen in the frustrated comments from the frequent train travel of educated, respectable black female writers of the Harlem Renaissance era as they traveled from literary salons in Washington, DC, to their work in Harlem). Nor would she probably care for such panoptic supervision. If she met one at all, a fellow traveling woman would have to be like her: rootless, wandering, and proud.

But Minnie acknowledges the dangers for black women on the road: "I walked through the alley / With my hand in my coat / The po-lice start to shoot me / Thought it was something I stole."[30] One initially accords hopelessness to black women who, away from the protection of family and friends, face the coldness of the white legal establishment on their own. Just below one's consciousness (and Minnie's; she never tells what happens or moans over her misfortunes with the law; more important are others on the highway: "Some is starving / Some is dying."), however, is the surety, however unpleasant, that were she home, dependent on the agency of family or friends, her complaint could easily have gotten someone else shot at or killed. So—minus the often illusory power of racial uplift to protect black female bodies and guarantee a better day, and minus gendered expectations of women's roles, especially as submissive, pious entities, Minnie and the others roll the dice and, outside the bonds of marriage—which seems a "whatever" on her scale of desires—stay on the road by choice. She exercises her freedom, however tenuous, in a threatening world as a black woman.[31]

More to the point are representations of African American women in the words of Gertrude "Ma" Rainey, the first blues queen (or king, for that matter). In "Don't Fish in My Sea," Rainey states her case and her womanhood: her man comes home drunk, and must be seeing another woman on the side.

> My daddy come home this mornin', drunk as he could be
> My daddy come home this mornin', drunk as he could be
> I know my daddy's done got bad on me
>
> He used to stay out late, now he don't come home at all
> He used to stay out late, now he don't come home at all
> I know there's another mule been kickin' in my stall

Instead of mourning a failed relationship, "kicking" the other mule who is apparently "kicking in her stall," or leaving for another man, she enlightens him as only Ma Rainey could: "If you don't like my ocean don't fish in my sea / Don't like my ocean don't fish in my sea / Stay out of my valley and let my mountain be." Very succinct and to the point: if he no longer desired her sexually, then leave her alone. There are no words expressing the desire to keep the marriage together for the children, or "What will the children and I do if you go?" Listeners do not know the status between these adults, or if children are involved. Apparently, these matters are unimportant. African American mothers in this compromising position had been expected to occasionally raise children as single parents for centuries if they, their husbands, or families were separated while enslaved. What Rainey will not tolerate in this song is being number two in her man's life.

She continues, lamenting this time that, on his part, their sex lives had been less than stellar, and nothing to shout about: "I ain't had no lovin' since God knows when." Rainey accepts no blame here. She claims to have been willing and able, and the fault lay at his door. Then, in a somewhat telling sentence that scholars have read as proof that some African American blueswomen were openly bisexual, she speaks her power: "That's the reason I'm through with these no-good triflin' men." Is she through with men all together, or merely those of questionable character? Either way, Ma Rainey has thrown down the gauntlet. And yet she balances her attack with the knowledge that both she and her former lover may come to rue his actions. "Never miss the sunshine 'til the rain begin to fall / Never miss the sunshine 'til the rain begin to fall / You never miss your ham 'til another mule's in your stall."[32] Short, and to the point: shape up, or be replaced.

It seems that the very outsider nature of the blues gave black women the vocabulary and opportunity to openly mourn the loss of their men without shame if they were singers doing tent shows, or women listening in the audience or singing to recordings in their own homes. In "You'll Never Miss Your Jelly," by Lil Johnson, a woman grieves over losing her man but schools him in the art of mutual loss once he finally misses that "jelly," or her sexualized body, that he had loved so much. The lyrics are graphic, for those who would understand the language, and leave little for interpretation.

> I woke up this morning with the blues all 'round my bed
> I woke up this morning with the blues all 'round my bed
> I felt just like somebody in my family was dead
>
> I began to moan and I began to cry
> I began to moan and I began to cry
> My sweet man went away / didn't know the reason why

> If you don't like my sweet potato what made you dig so deep
> If you don't like my sweet potato what made you dig so deep
> Dig my potato field three, four times a week . . .
>
> Just as sure as you hear me sing this song
> Just as sure as you hear me sing this song
> You sure won't miss your jelly till your jelly roller's gone [33]

That her man had liked her "sweet potato" so much that he had dug in her field deeply, "three, four times a week," does not establish what had been the nature of their relationship. Before someone could bemoan how such sordid lyrics of sex outside marriage (and sung by a woman) only served to bolster the stereotype that black women lacked sexual propriety and carried venereal diseases, the singer or a fan of the song could counter that the relationship could have been a legal marriage and the man had simply left for another woman. It could have also been sex outside of marriage. What really mattered was how black women were expressing their sexuality—how they enjoyed sex, how men enjoyed their bodies, how they missed sex with someone, and how that person would, in turn, miss their "jelly." This, probably more than guessing the hidden status of the relationship in question for its morality, upset blacks across class lines who supported uplift, along with Victorian stipulations that ladies, as they strove to be viewed, did not speak of such matters publicly. But the dialogue had already been opened and provided for those tired of keeping the difficulties of black womanhood under wraps.

If warning a man about the loving he would eventually miss did not work, African American blueswomen were not above threatening violence, in much the same manner as their male counterparts threatened them or other men. In Bessie Smith's "Black Mountain Blues," a woman laments losing her man—this time to a "city gal." As a result of losing the "sweetest man in town"—Black Mountain, a place where "a child will smack your face" and "babies [cry] for liquor and all the birds sing base," Smith tells her plans to all who will listen. She may be also giving a look into how some Southern black women deal with philandering men.

I'm bound for Black Mountain me and my razor and my gun
I'm bound for Black Mountain me and my razor and my gun
I'm gonna shoot him if he stands still and cut him if he run

Down in Black Mountain, they all shoots quick and straight
Down in Black Mountain, they all shoots quick and straight
The bullet'll get you if you starts a-dodging too late

Got the devil in my soul and I'm full of bad booze
Got the devil in my soul and I'm full of bad booze
I'm out here for trouble, I've got the Black Mountain blues [34]

"Black Mountain" is one of the few blues songs that mentions children, their behavior, and, by inference, the mothers who raise these unusual kids. Everything about Black Mountain is turned around: children attack adults, babies demand liquor, and birds sing in a very low key. This imagined rural area could later be transposed onto large cities where ghettoes were being developed: could such Black Mountain folks represent those that Du Bois and others saw each time they encountered a newly arrived southerner in the city, or heard of a stabbing, shooting, or beating? The mothers seem incapable of or even disinterested in raising their children to respect themselves or others. Will these later become the "black matriarchs" whose children become delinquents and malcontents? Smith lost her man to a city woman; could this man-stealing city gal be a match for any Black Mountain woman? In "Black Mountain Blues," women and men who listened to Smith got the message: two-timing men, an aggrieved, toughened woman, "bad liquor," a devil-filled soul, and a razor and gun did not make for a good time. Particularly for men who adhered to the black workingmen's blues that advocated violence against women, songs like Smith's "Black Mountain Blues" should have given them pause.

Thus, what can we say about African American, cross-class-created representations of womanhood and mothering during the Progressive Era? Although these examples are not exhaustive, one can see that Frances Ellen Watkins Harper's black women were still having a difficult time living up to their own ideals of womanhood and mothering. Through approbation, or even genuine care and concern, many black uplifters and reformers astutely pointed to the myriad problems the race faced in securing higher, protected status for black womanhood and educating black women in modern forms of mothering. Ignorance, carelessness, being given to drink, silliness, drugs, wantonness, laziness, impatience, and poor housekeeping were salient problems—but so were disappearing, violent, and uncaring men; good men laid low by poor wages, seasonal work, or no work at all; weakened or overworked female bodies that could not produce viable infants; diseased bodies that threatened fetuses; inferior housing; ongoing battles with racism, gender inequality, and class stigmatization.

In popular cultural representations of black womanhood and mothering, we see representations of Progressive Era African American women across class lines who found mothering problematic. One could argue that the voice of Frances Ellen Watkins Harper contains tones of resignation and calls for defiance. Resignation and defiance can also be heard in the songs of black blueswomen, even when they lost their men. Yet they seem to retain more of a hardened view of life that can still love, however flawed, and see the harshness of womanhood and mothering as real, a common status to be dealt with as best one may. Perhaps the obverse of the Bible is fitting when looking back at black female cultural representations: if much is expected of those blessed with much, then perhaps one may find more happiness in giving little when less is expected.

Cultural Representations of British West Indian Women

Finding similar representational artifacts of Jamaican and Barbadian women within their extant cultural histories is more complex, even when using surviving documents written by the educated elite. Moreover, no essentialized British West Indian culture or representations exist, or ever existed. Within the main migrating communities that made up Columbus Hill's West Indian populations were persons who were generally better educated than many blacks from the rural American South, often already acclimated to urban life, and prepared to "get ahead" in America's big cities, as well as rural, unskilled workers leaving their homes for the first time, or branching out from earlier labor migrations into the Panama Canal Zone and other places in the Caribbean.[35]

The differences between rural and urban life that influenced the pre- and post-migration representations and expectations of West Indian women were also reflected in the poetry of the time, but extant class differences emerged in their creation. Black West Indian poets espoused their love for an exoticized and idyllic rural Eden that contrasted with urbanity. Within these images of distant idealized island life were gendered metaphors that equated their lost paradise with beautiful, erotic women and fertile, nurturing mothers. In "O Little Green Island far over the Sea," Tom Redcam looks dreamily at the West Indies from afar, to where "My heart groweth tender, dear, far away land." He grounds his perspective of a longing immigrant presumably from England, the land he contrasts with Jamaica, his "little green island." As the "mother" of his soul, England is covered in glory and grandeur—"Truth, bare in its glory, with her deep self-control / With red in her flag, the white and the blue / For England is England, brave, patient and true." She is steadfast and nurturing; part of his identity will forever be rooted in her bosom. But the island of his remembered past brims with wildlife and gentle breezes, where the "West is aflame with the embers of Day," and where "lone peasant[s]" stride along highways of white.[36] This is the wildly romantic woman, the exoticized Jamaica. But can she be tamed into a responsible mother? Will she always be a Jezebel? Can she morph into a Mammy, or even switch identities at will?

The Jamaican poet Claude McKay also echoes this spirit of remembrance and longing. "So much have I forgotten in ten years, so much in ten brief years," McKay grieves at the start of his poem, "Flame-Heart." He mourns not so much for actually not living in the West Indies as for forgetting its delights—"I have forgot / What time the purple apples come to juice / And what month brings the shy forget-me-not . . . I have inflamed the days / Even the sacred moments when we played / All innocent of passion, uncorrupt." As with some of the lyrics of black blueswomen, McKay has purposefully left his love and now misses what he has left behind, and what other men now enjoy. But after a ten-year absence, would he encounter the same womanhood figure? Could she take him back? Would he ever return to never leave again? McKay paints a vivid portrait of loving times gone by, ones that might never have been as fulfilling as he actually experienced, but ones that the reader can taste, smell, and touch.[37] Here he lives in the past. He does not mention returning home to his lover and his mother until another poem, "I Shall Return," where he vows to go back to "ease my mind of long, long years of pain."[38]

The Jamaican immigrant's fondness for representations of all things colonial and British at the time cannot be taken too strictly, as seen in the excerpts from the above poems. Bilingualism and biculturalism became hallmarks of Jamaican identity that, however tenuously, often tied classes and genders together. Jamaican sayings used today come from oral traditions, passed down generationally from ancestors. They are meant to be instructional: to warn the listener about the pitfalls of life and provide wisdom to overcome them. They are also forms of social control, however: part of the arsenal of cultural capital used within the group to maintain standards of morality and proper behavior, and to be taken and used as the situation demands. Old sayings were also meant to place the onus of meaning on the listener; as with Biblical proverbs and parables, Jamaicans used sayings to put people in their place, to warn them of improper behavior or who not to become involved with, and how to extricate oneself from problematic circumstances. It is left to the listener, however, to glean whatever information was contained in the saying; to advance in the understanding of cryptic sayings displayed growth in wisdom and life skills.

Those who grew up during slavery or in British colonial Jamaica understood the sayings, which often reflected lived realities more than abstractions. At stake were social group norms and values; social control, as preached in these sayings, created a "subtle manner to prevent the violation of social rules and expectations, or to reestablish normative regulations where they might have been breached." No force was implied or needed in their use; psychological coercion came through the expectations of persons relinquishing individual desires in the face of group adherence to common values and norms.[39]

The use of Creole dialects to express old sayings stems from the plantation era: Afro-Caribbeans deftly created languages with linguistic foundations similar to those of their masters (English, Dutch, Spanish), and mixed in West African dialects to communicate with each other in "coded" terms, gibberish to white masters and overseers. Creole is still used extensively, but along class lines; lower-class Jamaicans and denizens of other Caribbean and West Indian islands still use and value Creole as their own: an evolutionized, syncretic mode of speech. Wealthier Jamaicans also use old sayings, sans Creole. In the Creole dialects, the pronoun *'im*, or "him," can mean male, but also can be genderless. In the same manner, "'im" can refer to nonhuman objects. Such is the elasticity of Jamaican Creole. Founded in Old English and West African languages, borrowing words from other lands, Creole lives as a testament to existence and survival during enslavement by the British and their later colonial rule. The following are examples of Jamaican proverbs, in Creole, which reflected late nineteenth and early twentieth century norms of social relations, especially relations between men and women, and aspects of womanhood and mothering.[40]

Reciprocation:
Rub ole wuman back, 'im mek yu tas'e 'im pepper pot. Do something good for a woman (rubbing an old woman's back) and she will respond in kind (food).[41]

Women and luck:
Wuman luck deh a dungle; foul cratch i' up. In Jamaican folklore, women are usually considered luckier than men, so much so that "it does not require much effort for the luck to surface." In this case, even though a woman's luck may lead to an unlikely place (a dung hill), she'll be lucky enough that a passing bird will scratch up whatever she needs—leaving her prize on the surface.[42]

Male responsibility for women:
Wuman a heavy load. Reflects female dependence on men; husbands' responsibilities to provide all their wives' needs.[43]

Derogatory or sexist sayings about women:
De three wuss thing a wuman tongue, wass-wass an' tambrin' tree. The sharpness of women's tongues is categorized to be as painful as the strong, springy, and thin branches of tamarind trees, which were used for flogging, and the dangers from wasp stings. Watson states, "To compare a woman's tongue with wasps or tamarind trees is therefore to imply not

only fury pouring forth, but also a devastating effect, ensuing from a woman's slander or malicious gossip."[44]

Wuman rain nebber done. "Woman-rain" denotes ongoing, unrelenting waterworks: the stereotypical response of nagging women who resort to unending tears to get their way.[45]

Wuman mout' an' fowl a wan. Another stereotype of women as ungrateful: "A fowl is said to show ingratitude after eating because it usually wipes its beak on the ground."[46]

W'en yu 'av' bad husband, no mek yu sweethaat caa' yu haafweh. This is almost simplistic in its honesty and humor; cheating women with bad husbands should watch their public behavior when with their sweethearts.[47]

Man bil 'ouse, but wuman mek de home.[48]

Man an' dawg; 'og an' pot-water; brown man an' rum. According to Watson, these groupings represent "affinities": men and dogs, hogs and pot-water, and brown men and rum.[49]

Ant follow fat, fat drown 'im connotes greed: you follow what you desire and it may lead to your end; in similar manner, *Ant follow fat, 'ooman follow man.* Ants and women both follow things they desire; will the same thing happen to women as ants?[50]

Children suck dem mudda when dem young, dem fada when dem ole. Gendered differences in offspring dependency, age, and timing.[51]

Drinking:
A drinkin' dame a special shame.[52]

The existence of a long, rich cultural heritage reflected in Jamaican folksongs stems from what culturalist Olive Lewin describes as the differences between climatization and the seasoning, or indoctrination, that enslaved West and Central African survivors of the Middle

Crossing endured within their eventual places of North American or Caribbean bondage. Climatization played a more important role in the perpetuation and resilience of African cultural memory in the Caribbean than in North America because the former climate and environment more closely mimicked that of West African lands left behind. Moreover, Lewin argues that, since white plantation owners in the Caribbean were largely absent, the "conditioning" or seasoning of African slaves would have been less traumatizing than that experienced by their brethren bound for North American slavery. Efforts to acculturate blacks for North American owners would have been more stringent because they would have had possibilities for closer, daily, intimate contacts with white owners and their families. Lewin writes, "In the Jamaican environment, African forebears would have found it possible to feel the presence of their gods and spirits, re-establish vital links with them and give succeeding generations the opportunity to experience a measure of cultural continuity. The colonial masters were primarily interested in amassing wealth and used the slaves to that end. No effort was made to expose the workers and their children to any form of education nor allow them time for any pursuits that were not in the interest of masters or related to their varied tasks." Thus, the memory of "gods and spirits" and other West and Central African cultural capital held dear survived longer in the generationalized memory of enslaved Caribbeans, remained more resistant to European cultures, and lived in a veneration of the past longer than in the collective memories of North American blacks, enslaved or free.[53]

Songs, then, became modes of entertainment and uplift, as well as information and resistance, for Jamaican slaves, and were often passed down to later generations. A song used by workers who built and hauled houses from place to place supposedly originated during slavery. In it, a victim of the sexuality of the slave system—Sally—was used to excoriate the privilege of light-skinned black women (female mulatto house slaves sired by white masters) while attacking their sexuality and perceived immorality, and its cadence aided in the pulling and pausing of house hauling.

> Sally was a whorin' mulatta
> Oh Sally.

> Sally was a whorin' mulatta,
> Oh Sally.
> Sally dweet (do it) a day,
> Sally dweet (do it) a night.
> Sally was a whorin' mulatta,
> Oh Sally.[54]

This male workers' song, handed down orally over the ages, had complex purposes and interpretations, depending on the singer and the listener. Obviously, the value of cadenced music as a metronome for work—especially backbreaking, unskilled labor—has been used since time immemorial, from powering slave galleys to the tramp-tramp-tramp of modern marching armies. It was also seen in the black male working songs from the Deep South. On the surface of "Sally" are black working-class male attitudes toward mulatto women and, perhaps in a more general sense, toward black women who embrace their sexuality with more than one man, or have sex with men for money. Further masked may be the anguish and fury held by black men toward white males, whose racially gendered power gave them access to any black woman, while the legal and cultural systems obfuscated their sexual roles in fathering children denied patriarchal protection and provision—the helter-skelter politicized process of sex for pleasure and chattel procreation. Even deeper may be a black male longing to behave in the same manner—with power to back it up. Regardless, these interpretations are one-sided, of course; missing are black female interpretations of this song. As with African Americans, representational perspectives are always important. Self-identification may always be shaped in some manner by group stereotypes and expectations of gendered roles that were created in the past, resistant to change, and much more complex than they seem on the surface.

Conclusion

Cultural artifacts provide a vital door into interrogating how women of subordinated groups have been represented in the past. Moreover, representations created by group members—especially, in this case, representations of women of African descent created by other black women—delve into intraracial, intragendered, cross-class, and cross-sexual meanings of womanhood and mothering that are often ignored, and which complicate existing dominant cultural ideals by showing alternative realities. The definitions of womanhood espoused by Frances Harper in 1892 overlapped existing Victorian ideals: some would argue that she merely adopted white middle-class dictates that even most whites believed blacks could never embody. But Harper took what was misconstrued as "for whites only" as a mirror into the private thoughts and lives of black women. She took the private and made it into a public clarion call for racial uplift by turning ideals on its head: the black race *will* survive because its women value their bodies, are capable of controlling their bodies and lives, and thus want to better equip their boys and girls for adulthood and beyond. Zora Neale Hurston's Emma results when the dictums of racialized beauty are internalized: a mother's privately held toxicity can destroy her child. The songs of black blueswomen stand on the periphery of black bourgeois tenets, but we also see that the Progressive Era black bourgeoisie may have had its own private secrets and troubles.

Yet, while giving public voice to what was considered private and unspeakable about women's lives in many black circles, the overall silence on issues of mothering reveals that, for most black women, problems existed that did not always need explication. Giving into the blues, even vicariously, could provide a needed respite from the personal and social expectations of living up to womanly and motherly ideals. Collisions of the private and public, in terms of motherhood and maternal and infant health, were daily manifestations of being black and female in America. We will see that in the next chapter on Columbus Hill.

5

Birthing in the City: Columbus Hill

On January 13, 1917, Bailey B. Burritt, the general director for the New York Association for Improving the Condition of the Poor (AICP), faced a dilemma. The results from the New York City 1915 mortality study, the first investigation of its kind, lay before him. While the overall infant death rate paled when compared to past statistics, the figures from one sanitary district elicited shock. Moreover, Burritt had already concurred, at the solicitation of Dr. Haven Emerson, New York City's health commissioner, that the AICP would coordinate public and private efforts to improve the district's situation.[1] Later, in a letter to Franklin B. Kirkbride, an AICP board member, Burritt revealed the human nightmare: in a black neighborhood on the west side of Manhattan, "more than three times as many colored babies are dying than in our average population."[2] About one year later, after instituting its health experiment in the Columbus Hill neighborhood, the AICP would name congenital syphilis as the culprit. New procedures would be adopted. Now, instead of black women being tested on an independent, inpatient basis at area hospitals, all pregnant black women would be forced to undergo syphilis tests as a condition of prenatal care.[3]

Only costly and extensive environmental work would change the infant health situation in the community, however. Burritt outlined the significant problems. First, although the neighborhood was blessed with two major hospitals, a health clinic, and city-run milk stations, it had no specifically colored health facilities.[4] Burritt wanted to create a health center similar to the Caroline Rest Home in Hartsdale, New York, where young mothers, weakened after the delivery of their babies, could rest in a pleasant rural setting while receiving proper training in infant care and modern hygiene.[5] But the cost of this would be exorbitant. More to the point was Burritt's request to fund a visiting nurse for the area. This would provide necessary supervision and education for black parturient

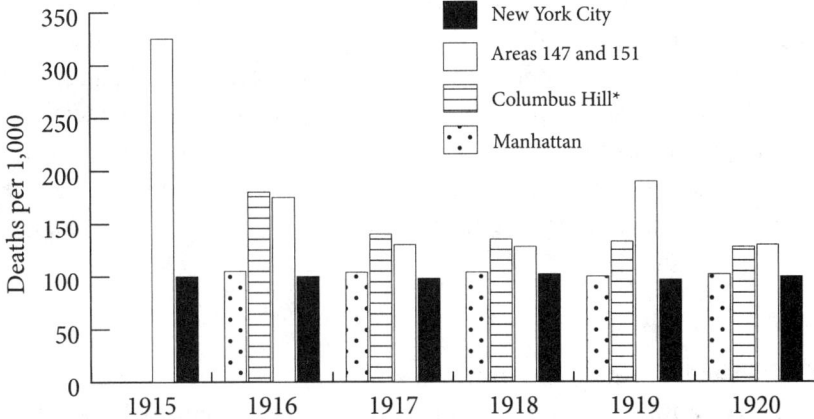

Figure 5.1. Infant mortality rates, 1915–1921. The data are taken from the Norman A. Holmes, "Sociological Survey of the Negro Population of Columbus Hill of New York City," photocopy (New York: Lincoln House Committee of the Henry Street Settlement, 1922), 8–9; William Guilfoy, M.D., and Shirley W. Wynne, M.D., *An Analysis of Mortality Returns of the Sanitary Areas of the Borough of Manhattan for the year 1915* (New York: New York City Department of Health, 1916), 15–18; and the annual reports of the New York City Department of Health, 1915–1920.

* The area consisted of native whites and Jewish, Irish, and Italian immigrants, as well as 1,800 blacks who lived outside "Columbus Hill proper." The 1915 data for "Areas 147 and 151" is for Area 147 only. Part of Sanitary Area 147 (created in 1920) corresponds to Areas 113 and 115 (created in 1915); part of Sanitary Area 151 (created in 1920) corresponds with Area 119 (created in 1915). The 1915 data for the borough of Manhattan are unavailable.

women and, later, for them and their babies in the first critical months of their lives. He also believed that Columbus Hill needed someone trained in "family social problems," since colored people were less likely to approach the AICP for aid than "the Irish or Italian, with whom we are dealing in such large numbers."[6]

Burritt got his wish. Kirkbride quickly spoke to the Westchester Association, a wealthy white philanthropic group, whose members agreed to fund the hiring of a nurse during the first year that the AICP coordinated its experiment with that of area hospitals and clinics in Columbus Hill.[7] The group increased its support to pay for an additional nurse in 1918. In that year, despite a pandemic of Spanish influenza,[8] Columbus Hill's black infant death rate plunged to 110 deaths per every 1,000 births, lower than the corresponding rate for native- and foreign-born whites living in the surrounding area.[9]

How were New York City and the AICP able to isolate data for a black section of a larger, racially mixed neighborhood? And why, with a focus on the race of the mothers and infants, were maternal and congenital syphilis chosen as the problems? This chapter explores the racialization of public health and health care in New York City and its effects on two separate but interlinked health demonstrations carried out after the city's first comprehensive health study in 1915.

The Racialization of Health Data in New York City

Challenges to how morbidity and mortality data should be collected had been a topic of interest among city managers before, during, and after the 1915 health survey. For example, Professor Robert Chaddock of Columbia University gave a paper before the "Vital Statistics Section" of the Association in Rochester, New York, on September 10, 1915. He outlined methods illustrating that, although one could never exert the same control over humans and their environments in real life as over subjects in laboratories, municipalities could make "[t]he City a Health Laboratory" by observing and investigating contributing health factors, their morbidities, and mortalities. Still, a crucial step was to "modify or control the factors which seem responsible for bad results and to observe the effects of these changes upon the mortality and sickness of the community." This methodology involved cities actively abandoning their old political ward boundaries, which they had previously used to glean morbidity and mortality data, for a shift toward smaller, homogenous sanitary districts, which would provide visible, empirical proofs of problem or healthy areas, undiluted and no longer hidden in large, amorphous voting blocs.[10]

This idea was not new. Dr. Frederick Hoffman, chief statistician for the Prudential Life Insurance Company, had vociferously advocated for this format three years earlier in a paper before the 15th International Congress on Hygiene and Demography in Washington, D.C. Hoffman had compared the data method used in the United States to that of European cities, and stated that, since the United States did not collect data by race, age, nature of death, and employment, it sadly lagged behind the more efficient European methods. While Hoffman, a well-known, respected physician and noted racialist, had predicted that African

Americans, like their Native American counterparts, were doomed to extinction because of their inherent inferiority and inability to supervise their lives, as reflected in their poor moral and health habits, Chaddock offered less hereditarian reasons for tracking illness, disease, and death by sanitary districts.[11]

First, Chaddock argued, such methodology would lead health care officials to a better understanding of factors that increased infant morbidity and mortality rates, such as environment (food, housing, sanitation, purer air, clean milk) and the "intelligence and income of families." Infant milk stations were first started by philanthropist and business mogul Nathan Strauss in New York City in the 1893.[12] They were already recognized as part of the public weal in the early 1900s. By providing area working mothers with pure, homogenized milk for their babies, the institutions' nurses also taught mothers "correct" feeding, clothing, and mothering techniques, recorded and monitored each baby's vital statistics (changes to height and weight, for example), and surveilled homes and housekeeping via visitations. This, Chaddock remarked, had resulted in decreased neonatal deaths resulting from bad sanitation and mothering mistakes. Moreover, by measuring districts over smaller areas, data were now spread more accurately, marking out troubled areas that would have remained masked in larger voting districts.[13]

Chaddock also maintained that it was important for municipal leaders to consider aspects of poverty, especially housing and other environmental factors, as causal links between human health, illness, and disease. The correlations between overcrowding and bad sanitation, malnourishment, impure air, and a lack of sewage removal were not new. With the last large cholera epidemic in New York City in 1866, sanitation became the bedrock of a new public health movement. Its roots extended back in time, however, emerging haltingly out of medieval European bouts with the Black Death; though ignorant of the modern scientific etiology of *yertsinia pestis*, the bacteria which causes the bubonic plague, cities had collected and burned the clothing of the dead, while those who could fled cities for the countryside. Other plague measures awaited: for those fleeing, military cordons attempted to block their egress or ingress; those entering cities by seaports encountered forty-day quarantines. These and other methods did not stop the plague, which raged intermittently over a four-hundred-year period.

The plague measures and the etiology of the disease itself did, however, challenge humoralism, or the accepted medical explanation for disease as having been brought about an imbalance of the body's four humors. By observing that human intervention and control over one's environment could lessen plague mortality, some began to see cracks in the ancient body of medical knowledge. Still, humoralism would survive into the nineteenth century, only to be truly tested by cholera and, from the 1870s onward, by the isolation of disease-causing germs, based upon the anti-humoral theories of the Paris School of medicine in the early nineteenth century.

The connection between environment and disease was brought to bear when John Snow, a nineteenth-century English scientist, studied a major cholera epidemic that wielded its savagery throughout England and continental Europe in the 1830s and 1840s. Imported from India by land and sea trade routes, cholera was no respecter of persons, but it especially seemed to have its way among the poor, living in impoverished, overcrowded conditions. Lacking the empirical proof that would come with later technological advances in microscopy, yet performing what was probably the first epidemiological survey ever conducted, Snow's meticulous backtracking and interviewing revealed who had brought the disease into which areas first; how it spread like wildfire among crowded dwellings; why it did not affect visiting doctors and nurses; and, most importantly, its oral-fecal etiology. Few believed Snow, because he could not present visual proof of the microscopic entity responsible for cholera. As a result, cities continued to institute tried but, unfortunately in the case of cholera, untrue plague measures that did nothing to thwart its spread.[14] The German School of medicine in the 1860s emphasized uniting chemistry with medicine inside laboratories, as the ability to refine microscopes that could truly show previously unseen matter increased. In France, Louis Pasteur isolated the bacterium responsible for rabies, and pneumococcus, staphylococcus, and streptococcus bacteria in the 1870s and 1880s.[15] Pasteur built the microbiological foundation that made possible Robert Koch's isolation of the tubercle bacillus, the final step in the creation of germ theory. This last discovery, in 1882, finally proved that tuberculosis was a communicable disease. Also in the last quarter of the nineteenth century, Max von Pettenkofer, a German scientist, began the sanitarian movement by combining Robert Koch's in vitro separation of *vibrio cholerae* with his belief that, like a flowering but hazardous plant, cholera grew underground in pools of contaminated water in alluvial soils, only to surface as miasmas, spreading the effluvia of cholera amongst unfortunate townspeople living in low-lying areas.[16]

In 1882, Italy—the site of many debilitating disease epidemics and the scientific center of malaria and, thus, the field of malariology and the advent of tropical medicine—was again attacked by cholera. The results were astounding: as in past events, cholera seemed to have a penchant for the poor, who lived in overcrowded, impoverished, unsanitary squalor close to the Bay of Naples, where their waste contaminated their drinking water. By contrast, the wealthy lived high above the plain and received their water from a fresher source. The lack of sewage removal meant that unsanitary water flowed into and contaminated groundwater. As a result of drinking cholera-contaminated water or cleaning fruit and washing clothes with it, residents ingested bacteria. This would not be problematic unless the person was malnourished and overworked, thus lacking the needed nutrients and, especially, stomach acids to kill *vibrio cholerae*. If the bacterium survived and traveled into the lower intestines, it died—and produced one of the most toxic substances known to mankind, which attacked the intestines, reversing the direction of cell absorption. Thus, instead of taking nutrients and water from the intestine and into capillaries, veins, and organs, the intestine cells sucked plasma from the blood, resulting in "rice water" diarrheal stools, which, being clear, were usually ignored by people living in dark, dank, cavelike dwellings. If someone touched rice-water contaminated bedding or clothing, then brought their hands to their mouths or to food, they could become contaminated. If the rice-water stool found its way into the drinking water supply, people could become contaminated. Those who worked with water—laundresses, in particular—became contaminated, as did fishermen and people who ate shellfish out of the bay. The resulting deaths were excruciating: blood, deprived of plasma and air, thickens to darkened, tarlike viscosity. Violent coughing and spasms began, to the point that muscles shredded under the force. Organs failed; the last one to go was the heart, deprived of oxygen. And this death could happen anywhere. Part of the terror behind cholera was its public nature: people died in the streets; someone who began a journey by train at the peak of health could die three hours later, already looking like an emaciated corpse. Plague measures did nothing to stop the spread of cholera. Authorities realized that, to quell civil unrest and restore the dignity of Italy (Naples was the monarchial seat at the time), something had to be done.

Paris had already been hit by cholera and, taking a lesson from von Pettenkofer's sanitarianism, had completely revamped its sewage system, torn down and replaced slum housing, and provided a cleaner water supply to its citizens. Cholera outbreaks had ended. Naples tried to copy Paris's success, marking out a fundamental urban revitalization plan that would do the same. However, the misappropriation of city funds, graft, and outright incompetence foiled the grand plans. Thus, when cholera hit Naples again in 1911–1912, although the death rate was lower, the city still suffered, especially the poor, who could not benefit from proposed changes that had not occurred. Still crammed into hovels, they died without impunity. And, to make matters worse, the Italian government and the newspapers purposefully hid the outbreak in order to hide graft and keep tourism alive. The U.S. government and the U.S. Public Health Service even participated in the charade. Agreeing with Chaddock's argument that better housing and environmental conditions were measurable factors that would decrease illnesses and deaths—along with rebuilding or building municipal sanitation and sewage systems, removing overcrowded tenements through legislation (as in New York City's 1901 tenement law), and providing clean water and better working conditions—larger cities adopted these methods after 1866 as a part of the U.S. sanitarian movement. Even so, as in Naples, much remained to be done to protect the populace from vector-borne or communicable diseases. The problem still remained: what conditions stemmed from heredity or environment? From where would the social will and the money come? How would one educate and control the seemingly uneducable and uncontrollable? And would the neo-Lamarckian tenet that positive knowledge, once imbued genetically, passes on to future generations, be enough to justify the time and expense?

Chaddock's third insistence—that sanitary district data would better track racial/nationalistic rates of health, illness, and disease—stemmed from his belief that one could not be totally certain which illnesses or diseases arose from heredity, which came from environment, and which resulted from an indiscernible mix of the two. In this sense, while straddling the swamp between racialism and environment, he did exhibit neo-Lamarckian predilections that mirrored many positions of social workers and so-called maternalists of the time. This genetic/environmental "wiggle room" left the door open for those Progressives who favored alleviating the adverse living and health conditions of the poor—the class-based perspective that he had already identified when calling for housing reforms:

> It is not enough to calculate the death-rate from tuberculosis for Negroes, Italians or Jews in the entire city. They may be susceptible to the disease or comparatively immune from it because of conditions from which they have come or because of racial characteristics . . . they may be affected by the new surroundings—where and how they live, what occupation they follow, their ignorance, and their changed habits and manner of life . . . [s]ome of the differences in health attributed to race may be accounted for by the environment—a factor more capable of modification in the campaign to improve health.[17]

By interrogating race and environment via class and poverty as critical and salient factors in municipal public health, Chaddock presented a more textured approach that, while not negating the common belief in racialized disease resistances and susceptibilities, did allow for the discussion of environmental factors and private and public works that could help alleviate some of the problems of the poor, as much as the public/private will could allow. Under the supervision of Dr. John S. Billings, who controlled the eleventh census of 1880 and advocated a change in methodology for collecting health and mortality data, and by redrawing city political wards into sanitary districts in 1893,[18] the move was on to refine neighborhood health data further by race, income, housing, and occupational patterns by the time of the 1915 citywide census.[19]

Therefore, Burritt's and Kirkbride's ability to focus the AICP's efforts on racially distinct neighborhoods stemmed from the statistical data collection method instituted by the New York City Department of Health in 1914. The idea to divide New York City's five boroughs into sanitary districts had, in fact, arisen before the boroughs outside Manhattan became New York City in 1898. In 1893, when the Department of Health had discarded its older ward divisions and separated the Manhattan and Bronx boroughs into 105 sanitary districts, Dr. Roger S. Tracy, the department's deputy registrar, stated that the reason for the switch from political wards to sanitary districts was to include "as far as possible, in each district the persons who were living under similar conditions as to race, nationality, social condition, housing, drainage and the vicinity of nuisances."[20] This would be reflected later in the changes, as well as in Chaddock's speech.

With subsequent divisions done in 1914, the city redrew earlier boundaries as populations shifted, further dividing neighborhoods as they were "voluntarily segregated," so that statistical data collection reflected the racial health in each district. According to William Guilfoy and Shirley Wynne, Health Department officials who analyzed the data from the 1915 infant mortality survey, the correlation of disease with environment and heredity provided public health officials, reformers, and philanthropists with statistical data that correctly reflected the health and socioeconomic needs of different racial groups.[21]

Despite the good intentions posed by advocates for redrawing wards into more manageable sanitary districts, a further perusal of Guilfoy and Wynne's health data analysis reveals that environmental concerns could mask hereditarian racialisms, or variations in the belief that humans, socially defined by such arbitrary designators as nativity, religion, skin color, culture, or phenotype, possessed inherited and distinctive health problems. For example, the black infant mortality rate that had initially stunned Burritt came primarily from Sanitary Districts 113 and 115, where people of African descent made up one-half of the population and lived in squalid, overcrowded conditions on the blocks of West 61st and West 62nd streets. A Lincoln House survey estimated that, of the 9,000 persons of African descent who lived in Columbus Hill, 1,641 lived on West 61st Street alone, with a resulting density of 656 persons per acre. Sixty-three percent of the apartments were categorized as "absolutely undesirable as habituous [sic] for human beings," whereas 21 percent were deemed "passable."[22] West 62nd Street formed the southern boundary of Sanitary District 119, another segment of the predominantly black area where Burritt wanted to expand the AICP's

Columbus Hill project. There, over half the black infants had died within their first year of life.²³

Both Guilfoy and Wynne agreed with Burritt's assessment of Sanitary District 115; they stated that, with its high black infant death rate and correspondingly elevated rates of infectious diseases and tuberculosis, "there is need of most intensive work in this district." The area's environment was remarkable for its "old type of tenement houses without any sanitary improvements," which housed the poorest of New York's poor. Their comments on Sanitary District 119 revealed their hereditarian bias, however. The prevalence of infectious and respiratory diseases resulted from the "well-known aversion of the negro to cold." Black infants died from diarrheal diseases because their impoverished mothers could not stay home but instead "go out to domestic services by the day." Unable to breastfeed, these women were "compelled to either place their infants in day nurseries or entrust the older children or to some old 'Mammy' in the neighborhood, any of which necessitates artificial feeding." To combat the health problems in Sanitary District 119, Guilfoy and Wynne advocated a breast feeding campaign, the creation of a combination day nursery / milk station, and "an effort to urge, if not compel" black women to place their babies in the day nursery while at work. They also suggested a tuberculosis campaign because, "[g]ranting that the Negro is highly susceptible to tuberculosis infection, there is no question but that the negro's [sic] manner of living is responsible to a very large extent for his susceptibility." If health officials could, "even in a small measure, overcome his carelessness and indifference," a decrease in the spread of the disease would result.²⁴

However, nine months into its health work in Columbus Hill, the AICP pulled an amazing switch, now targeting syphilis as the primary agent of black infant death instead of maintaining its initial focus on tuberculosis and other respiratory diseases.²⁵ Even when faced with statistical and epidemiological proof, they capitulated into racism; after all, most white physicians and scientists at the time perceived blacks as "a notoriously syphilis-soaked race."²⁶ Faced with the beginning of the Great Migration of African Americans out of the South, and the arrival of foreign persons of African descent upon U.S. shores, many northern, native-born white doctors eagerly relied on their southern counterparts for advice on a growing "Negro Problem."²⁷ The AICP followed the lead of other white organizations that funded and designed health demonstrations by retooling its work to conduct groundbreaking experimentation on syphilis and Negroes.[28]

The racialism and hereditarianism that may have undergirded this decision were but two modes of thought during the Progressive Era. Germ theory arose during an unstable period where sanitarian, eugenic, epidemiological, hereditarian, racialist, and environmental thought competed for supremacy among health care professionals, reformers, and the general public. Still, as revealed in letters, meeting minutes, reports, and statistical studies, the epidemiological and environmental concerns offered by public health officials, health care workers, and physicians often masked a hereditarian racialism, informed by gender and/ or class, that reflected the ability of Progressive Era white public health officials to temper their racialistic perspectives in a paternalistic ethos of professionalism, much as maternalists had done.[29] An analysis of the work done in Columbus Hill reveals that although New York City's health officials instituted an experimentation program that reduced infant morbidity and mortality, they often relied upon notions of black racial inferiority and the inherent hypersexuality of black women as the source of the impoverished neighborhood's health problems and the bane of publishing their health work results.

Social Inequalities, Germ Theory, and the Etiology of Disease

The nosology, or categorization, of diseases as separate and distinct in their identities and etiologies—their causes, transmissions, preventive measures, and possible cures—received a tremendous boost in 1882 with the discovery of the tubercle bacillus, the cause of tuberculosis, by German scientist Robert Koch.[30] Prior to Koch's work, periodic outbreaks of deadly contagious diseases bedeviled physicians and scientists alike. For example, cholera wreaked havoc in large U.S. cities in 1832, 1849, and 1866. As an important port of ingress and the nation's largest metropolis, New York City experienced the heaviest loss of life. Strategic yet temporal lessons were learned. Temporary public health boards, whose primary function centered on containing the spread of the disease through quarantines, were created in major U.S. cities. Their secondary focus lay in the removal from the streets of refuse, which resulted in miasmas, or foul air, that conveyed communicable diseases, or effluvia (microscopic, animal-like organisms). As trash, human, and animal refuse decayed, many sanitary reformers believed that miasmas carried effluvia, which could generate spontaneously. Sanitarians targeted those who dwelled in squalid tenements—poor native-born whites, blacks, and newly arrived European immigrants, especially the Irish—as the primary breeders of deadly communicable diseases.[31] The elitist scapegoating of subaltern groups as responsible for spreading diseases as a result of their presumed spiritual depravity and desire to live in filth and poverty became one crucial hallmark in the history of epidemics.[32]

The discovery of the tubercle bacillus disproved the spontaneous generative foundation of the miasma theory and formed the foundation of germ theory. Yet traditional modes of thought died hard. Although a small contingent of late nineteenth and early twentieth century scientists could prove that germs, or microscopic bacteria, possessed differing identities and generated from themselves and not from waste, most physicians, health officials, and laypersons remained wedded to sanitarianism. The new sciences of bacteriology and epidemiology faced formidable barriers, even within the scientific realm. It proved easier for physicians and health officials to believe that the illiterate, foreign, and unwashed masses streaming into American cities constituted a serious threat to the health of middle-class native white Americans than microscopic germs.[33]

The advent of epidemiology, and its fundamental ideological attack against sanitarianism, coincided with the scientific racialization of humans. Eugenicists deployed the burgeoning scientific methods of measurement and analysis to prove the empirical existence of racial hierarchies, and argued in favor of genetic breeding to protect the superior Anglo-Saxon race against enfeebled, degenerate, inferior races. Racial, gendered, and classed inequalities lay at the core of eugenic thought. Although definitions of "race" or "racism" must be historicized to reflect their dynamic social nature, as concepts of human differentiation based on familial or tribal lineage, phenotype, or nationality, racialism became accepted as fact in the nineteenth century. First socially and then legally justified by Christian monogenists as the will of God, and later, as science reached "religious" proportions, by Darwinian polygenists as empirical fact, scientists and physicians followed and shaped the prejudices of the masses and elites through craniometry, phrenology, and intelligence tests to chart levels of racial inferiority and superiority. People of African descent were consistently relegated to the bottom of the racial heap due to their inherent inferiority, and also "feminized" as a race.[34] But the European "white races" were also categorized and ranked by nationality as inherently separate and distinct, inferior to the Anglo-Saxon race. Hereditarianism grew in popularity during the dramatic influx of southern, central, and eastern European immigration that occurred from the 1880s through the Immigration Restriction Act of 1924. As presumed inferior European races poured into the United States and threatened the racial purity of native-born American whites, African Americans began their first concerted northern exodus from the Jim Crow South. Other nonnative blacks from the West Indies, Caribbean, and South and Central America soon joined them. It was during this era of racial migration and conflicting, yet complementary, ideologies of disease causation that health, and disease itself, took on a decidedly hereditarian, racialistic tone, often supported by health professionals themselves.[35]

This outcome was not inescapable, nor was it developed without a competing scientific perspective. As a counter to the harsh inevitabilities intoned by racialists, eugenicists, and hereditarians, environmentalists steeped in nineteenth-century sanitarianism argued that poverty helped determine poor health. In the case of Columbus Hill, they cited malnutrition, overcrowded, dank tenements, inadequate sanitation, and impure food, water, and milk as critical disease factors. These descriptive terms provide an accurate portrait of the neighborhood during the AICP study period from 1915 to 1924. The public and private will to transform an impoverished, poor and working-class environment in order to stave off the diseases that blighted the neighborhood and could easily pass to others remained another topic, however. Decency and philanthropy were tempered by the American ethos of individualism and self-sufficiency: give the poor too much help, and one replaces their dignity and independence with sloth and indifference.[36]

AICP Health Work in Columbus Hill

When the AICP decided to conduct its health demonstration work in Columbus Hill, it proposed to augment and strengthen the work already done by the Sloan Hospital and the New York Nursery and Child's Hospital, both of which provided pre- and postnatal care for blacks in the area. Delivery wards existed in each institution, but only the Nursery and Child's Hospital had outpatient services. Yet neither hospital provided a "field agency" that bridged the crucial link between hospital care and community health care education. In 1917, Dr. Haven Emerson, then commissioner of health for New York City, responded to Columbus Hill's black infant mortality problems by inviting the AICP to begin an educational nursing service for Columbus Hill's black inhabitants. The AICP opened its nursing service with two nurses and a doctor in the basement of the Vanderbilt Clinic. They coordinated their nursing efforts with those of the Lincoln House Branch of the Henry Street Settlement, which was located at 205 West 60th Street and housed seven trained nurses and a Mother's Club.[37] By educating mothers in their homes about proper nutrition, sanitation, and infant care, and by reminding syphilitic mothers of the importance of regular treatments and postnatal care, the AICP determined that a staff of mobile nurses could help decrease black infant deaths.

The AICP's Columbus Hill health experiment linked the resources and actions of many private and public agencies against syphilis as the primary source of infant and maternal deaths in the area. Several years after its experiment in the neighborhood had begun, at a 1924 meeting chaired by Burritt, the following independent groups that had been closely involved in the health work met to discuss what had been done, why, and what should occur in Columbus Hill's future: the New York City Department of Health; the New York City Nursery and Child's Hospital; the Vanderbilt Clinic; the Henry Street Settlement; and city-run milk stations. Still the AICP's general director, Burritt lauded the "unusual degree of cooperative effort" among the agencies that had made the experiment successful, adding that "I think there are now 95% of the expectant mothers in that district brought under supervision, and that, together with the other things that have been done, seem

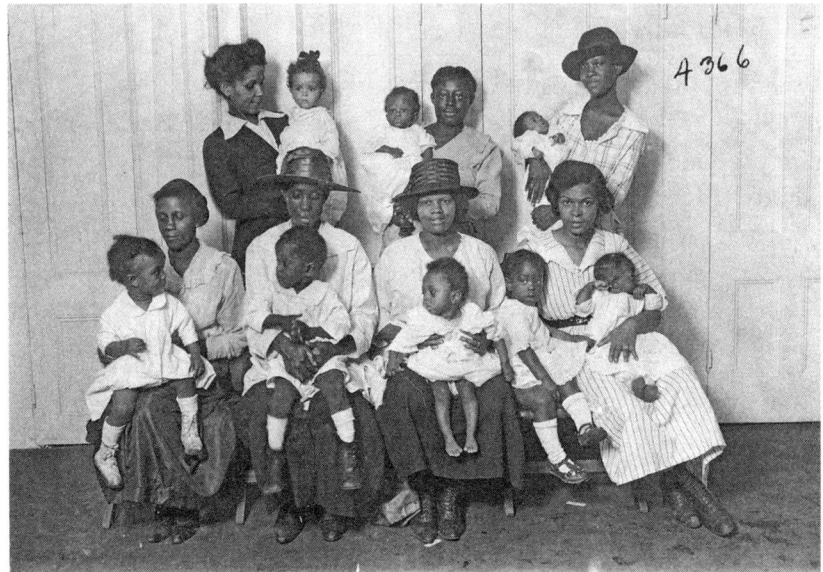

Figure 5.2. These Columbus Hill black women and their babies may have been some of the women who received pre- and postnatal health care from the AICP and its associated care providers. Creator unknown, "Columbus Hill Health Center Album, Developing Child Health via Community Organization," circa 1919, Rare Book and Manuscript Library, Columbia University, Community Service Society Collection, http://css.cul.columbia.edu/catalog/rbml_css_0547 (accessed March 2, 2014).

to me to indicate a good deal of work on the part of a large number of organizations."[38]

Miss Ethel Phillips, the AICP's nursing supervisor for the Columbus Hill project, then explained how the system worked. The AICP received its prospective prenatal cases from mainly the Nursery and Child's Hospital and the Sloan Hospital, for which the AICP supplied follow-up work. Presumably, since the AICP's experiment in Columbus Hill focused only on mothers and children of African descent, and since the AICP had already decided to limit its infant and maternal work to the effort to decrease mortality arising from syphilis-related infections, these referrals would have probably been black, either native-born or immigrant, and separated from the hospitals' other parturient clientele because of race. For these racialized cases, then, the AICP performed mandatory Wassermann tests to ascertain syphilis infections prior to providing prenatal care.³⁹ After receiving test results, the AICP referred any women with positive Wassermanns either to the Nursery and Child's Venereal Disease Clinic or to the Vanderbilt Clinic, which was run by the Columbia College of Physicians and Surgeons.⁴⁰ In addition, the AICP also received venereal disease referrals from area milk stations; these were sent to the Vanderbilt or Nursery and Child's clinics as well.⁴¹

Dr. J. L. Franklin, director of the Bureau of Child Hygiene of the New York City Department of Health, maintained that during the AICP's work, the black infant mortality rate for Columbus Hill had been almost twice that of the city in general, and the maternal mortality rate had been four to five times higher in the neighborhood than in New York City overall.⁴² Franklin O. Nichols and Ray H. Everett, both of the American Social Hygiene Association, agreed with Burritt that the anti-syphilis focus had been important, and that the Columbus Hill experiment had justified past and future health work. Everett went on to reveal that the Association had published most of John C. Gebhart's report on the AICP's results in decreasing the maternal transmissibility of syphilis and resulting infant miscarriages, stillbirths, and neonatal deaths from congenital syphilis the area.⁴³ Nichols agreed to its importance, adding, "I have been particularly interested in the handling of the so-called popular diseases among negroes [sic], like tuberculosis and venereal diseases. New York is getting an increased number of colored people from sections where they are not being adequately treated and I think you ought to be congratulated upon your experiment."⁴⁴

By 1924, the AICP still supplied only three nurses and one nursing supervisor to oversee Columbus Hill's parturient women; with such limited personnel, the AICP depended heavily on Henry Street Settlement nurses for assistance. Both groups worked in tandem to supervise black women who were expecting, encouraged prenatal visits and hospital deliveries, and provided postnatal care. For example, one month prior to delivery, both nursing units would handle prenatal care prior to birth. Afterward, Henry Street nurses carried the cases one month and AICP nurses looked after the patients for an additional month, until the mothers returned with their babies for their last examinations. All mothers and infants who had been under AICP care were forwarded to milk stations for additional training, and the "special feeding cases" were sent to the Nursery and Child's Clinic. Phillips stated that, as much as they could, the AICP attempted to provide postnatal care for their clients and the entire family, including a preschool clinic and a family welfare clinic from AICP or COS referrals.

She also revealed that several recent deportations of "some of the foreigners in the district where we find a great deal of illegitimacy [sic] and the unmarried mother problem exists" had improved the overall neighborhood. Phillips did not specify if the foreigners deported were of African, British West Indian, or European descent, but Gebhart's report stipulated that 58 percent of the mothers within the scope of the neighborhood's study were of foreign birth, with most speaking English and thus providing fewer "social barriers" than those from other immigrant groups.[45] Unswervingly, Phillips stayed on course, limiting the remainder of her comments to the task she had supervised for seven years: "Our problems are principally the venereal disease work. Of course, we haven't the facilities in the district for the cases. We should have free treatment for the men and evening clinics."[46]

To that end, the AICP conducted seven years of anti-syphilis work because its staff believed that infant deaths from syphilis occurred all too frequently in Columbus Hill's black community. When the AICP began its work in 1917, many physicians maintained that congenital syphilis, if left untreated in pregnant women and transmitted into the uterus during pregnancy, could cause sterility. Moreover, if pregnancies occurred, the sexually transmitted disease could also result in miscarriages, stillbirths, and early infant deaths.[47] Thus syphilis detection and treatment took on added importance with the area's health care providers.

This decision deserves explication, however; a brief overview of physicians' attitudes toward black health, and the debates surrounding the modes of syphilis diagnoses, treatments, and prognoses prior to the 1915 New York City health survey, may reveal why Health Department officials and the AICP viewed Columbus Hill's infant mortality problem through a syphilitic lens. Nineteenth-century physicians in the United States had racialized health by deeming black and white health patterns intrinsically different, based on perceptions of inherited white superiority and perceived black mental and physical inferiorities. The racialization of health reflected and supported a process that was occurring simultaneously in the field of science. As products of a racially stratified society, the work of both scientists and physicians often shaped social values, while scientists and physicians were shaped by existing societal prejudices and norms.[48]

White preoccupations with inherited, racialized health differences between blacks and whites began during the New World enslavement of Africans and their descendants.[49] By the antebellum era, white attitudes usually fell into two contradictory, yet mutually supportive, camps. When African Americans seemed impervious to diseases such as malaria or yellow fever, slave owners argued that black resistance to deadly diseases merely provided additional proof of their innate suitability for enslavement. When, on the other hand, blacks grew ill from certain diseases, whites alternately theorized that black illnesses stemmed from their "inherently weaker constitution" rather than from environmental causes. Either way, whites racialized health and health care and did not place black and white health issues on an equal footing. Starting in the latter part of the eighteenth century and lasting through antebellum period, white Americans increasingly viewed blacks as a separate species with acquired or innate abilities to resist the diseases that regularly decimated thousands of Europeans.[50]

For blacks, postbellum health care meant a shift from the slave owner as primary health care provider to the federal government, and later the state, as providers of health services. However, with the dawning of segregated "separate, but equal" facilities throughout the United States at the end of the nineteenth century, when blacks saw themselves denied equal access to adequate health care they actively took control of their own health care and medical training. Black women particularly stood out in the forefront as reformers, activists, nurses, doctors, and volunteers. Working with city, state, and federal agencies, they canvassed the rural South and urban tenements in an attempt to bring modern, scientific, and hygienic health care to the underfed and overworked.[51]

The gendered and classed aspects of racialized health, illness, and disease came into stark contrast in the early twentieth century. Despite scientific breakthroughs in germ theory, most in the white majority continued to regard black women and newly arriving southern and eastern European immigrants as threats to public health. In essence, while germ theory had explained the randomness of disease, older prejudices and beliefs in the immutable racially gendered and classed foundations of health and disease remained and frequently resurfaced, now justified by germs that, alarmingly, "have no color line."[52] Still, the social inequalities of the past slowly tempered, at least on the surface, thanks to Progressive reformers who cited the unhealthy environment in tenement districts as a primary reason for the spread of infectious diseases. Southern public health officials agreed with environmentalists but argued that blacks' ignorance of modern hygienic methods, and their inherent sexual immorality, laziness, and a general disregard for sanitation, revealed an apparent proclivity for poor health.[53] In the case of syphilis and other venereal diseases, whites genuinely believed that sexually transmitted diseases affected blacks more frequently and differently than they affected whites. Public health experts maintained that congenital syphilis would eradicate blacks, through either early infant deaths, maternal or paternal sterility, or both.[54] One physician who studied syphilis among southern blacks succinctly stated that within fifty years, an "unsyphilitic negro [will be] a freak, unless some such procedure as vaccination comes to the relief of the race, and that in the hands of a compelling law."[55]

Thus, environmentalism could easily transmogrify into racialism, or the two could comfortably exist as separate yet complementary modes of thought. Many northern physicians, when faced with an increased northward flow of blacks, relied on the experiences of their southern counterparts when diagnosing and treating black health problems, despite being generally more concerned with unhealthy environments than perceived racial differences as the causes of ill health and the spread of contagions.[56] Southern physicians who attended the National Conference of the American Public Health Association held in Jacksonville, Florida, in 1914 presented an array of statistics and anecdotes about the deplorable living conditions of southern blacks. They issued statements full of invectives aimed at negligent southern health officials who refused to educate blacks on matters of modern health methods and sanitation, the white public at large who remained in close contact with black servants whose illnesses endangered the white community, and the white politicians who had ignored poverty, poor housing, and bad food in black southern communities.

Despite the attendees having named critical environmental and educational flaws that exacerbated African American ill health, the debate swirled around whether black illnesses resulted from "genetic inferiority," social and economic problems, or both—with the latter being a manifestation of the former. Southern white health officials argued that the "negro health problem" had become "one of the 'white man's burdens.'"[57] Emancipation had "transplanted [blacks into] conditions of life which are entirely foreign to [their] nature," leaving them as "aliens" in a white society that, through "continuous and logical evolution," attempted to wrest its own race into modern health and sanitation practices. C. E. Terry, a physician in Jacksonville, Florida, blamed racial inferiority for blacks' ignorance and intransigence, and white health officials for the South's "negro health problem."[58]

Unmentioned and ignored in these "black" debates were skyrocketing rates of syphilis and other venereal diseases in the native-born white community, which loomed invisibly outside the furor over black health, diseases, and their effects on white society. Moreover, ever-increasing rates of venereal diseases among whites threatened to become an even larger hazard to the future existence of the white family. As always, racialisms hovered above the fray—people, and especially poor women, with any portion of African descent or, for eugenicists and anti-immigrationists, from any country they deemed racially inferior and thus did not meet their approval—were branded as probable syphilis carriers and dangerous to white males.[59] Racialism, however, *was* the fray. Whites recognized themselves as "raced" at the time, usually in terms of their Aryan/Nordic/Caucasian superiority over inferior races. White males were at the top of the biological pyramid of civilization and power; as their companions, white women occupied a lower status, but higher than other biologically inferior women thanks to their whiteness.[60]

Thus, at the turn of the twentieth century, politicians, reformers, theologians, physicians, and scientists argued that white "race suicide," as reflected in the reduced native-born white female fecundity rates, particularly among the "better classes," and perceived as the result of female selfishness, would only end if native-born, middle-class white women increased their birthrate and placed more emphasis on the family unit. As a disease that could lead to mental illness or death, postpone or destroy marriages, and result in parental sterilization or early infant deaths, syphilis infections in the native-born white community proved that the white race was in trouble.[61] To combat this evil, instead of concentrating on prostitutes and their clientele, social hygiene adherents and police and public health departments focused on prostitutes only, forcibly rounding them up for syphilis testing, treatment, and incarceration, while white males filtered into the darkness, looking for new sources of sexual pleasure and, in the process, taking venereal diseases home where "innocents"—white wives and their children—would become the latest victims.[62]

Enter the "Magic Bullet"

If human moral behavior proved intractable, threatening both home and society, then many physicians hoped that science could provide tests and cures for what humans would not resist. And science responded. In 1905, the German scientists Fritz Schaudinn and Eric Hoffman isolated the *spirochaeta pallida* (pale spirochete), the microbe responsible for syphilis. August Wassermann, with assistance from Albert Neisser and Carl Bruck, developed the means of detecting syphilis in blood serum in 1906 in a diagnostic test that still bears his name.[63] In 1909, Paul Ehrlich, another German scientist, ushered in the era of chemotherapy with the creation of salvarsan, an arsenic-based chemical compound that seemed on the surface to be the first effective treatment for syphilis.[64] Prior to Ehrlich's development of salvarsan, physicians had treated syphilis and other venereal diseases with mercury and other additives, given topically or in the form of a vapor treatment. Ehrlich boasted that the development of salvarsan issued in the era of the "magic bullet."[65]

The advent of salvarsan did not result in overnight agreement about its efficacy as a syphilis treatment, however; its high toxicity levels proved deadly in some cases.[66] Prior to 1915, the year of the first New York City Department of Health mortality study, few physicians agreed on how salvarsan should be administered, how large the doses, and with what frequency they should be delivered. Charges of salvarsan-related deaths began not long after physicians started using the drug. As early as

1913, Wilhelm Wechselmann, a German physician, argued that although he saw no direct connections between salvarsan and stories of arsenic-related deaths in general, physicians should be aware that the amount of salvarsan injected could result in untimely and, for physicians administering salvarsan, embarrassing, deaths. Wechselmann's study verified only twenty-one deaths from subcutaneous (below the skin) or intramuscular injections of salvarsan. Physicians who treated syphilitic infants administered salvarsan injections through scalp veins.[67] However, Wechselmann argued that undocumented and untraceable deaths may have resulted when physicians disregarded or underestimated their patient's physical conditions and injected too much salvarsan intravenously. Wechselmann stated that if an "unnoticed error" occurred before or during the salvarsan injection, these deaths were "rarely reported, and practically never [reported] by physicians who have given many injections."[68] As accusations mounted, Paul Ehrlich, the father of salvarsan, concurred that to avoid encephalitis haemorrhagica deaths, or deaths from brain hemorrhages, physicians must use small, initial doses of salvarsan, coupled with mercury treatments.

But other non-salvarsan-related problems coursed through the scientific community during the 1910s with regard to syphilis. In an influential 1914 article in the *New York Medical Journal*, Walter Baetz, a physician who had treated black males working on the Panama Canal, categorized syphilis as a "protean infection" that regularly went misdiagnosed and untreated because of its multiple manifestations. Often, he argued, syphilis misdiagnoses occurred as a result of the subjectivities of attending physicians.[69] Aside from the subjectivities of physical examinations in which doctors equated vaginal and penile skin rashes, lumps, and sores as proof of first-stage syphilis infections, positive reactions to Wassermann tests provided the only empirical, mistake-proof diagnosis of the disease.

Multiple Wassermann tests given to patients could result in both false positive and false negative results, often leading both physicians and patients to believe that the syphilis had disappeared or that the patient had been reinfected. As a result, laboratories themselves and the methods used to read Wassermann results also came under fire. By 1923, one year before the AICP published its study of its health work among black women and infants in Columbus Hill, Dr. H. H. Hazen, an influential syphilologist, issued a caveat to physicians treating syphilis cases. "Be quick to suspect syphilis; be slow to diagnose syphilis," he cautioned. He argued this because he believed that his colleagues placed too much trust in Wassermann results, and that "the diagnosis of this disease is often an extremely difficult one."[70]

Despite assertions of salvarsan-related deaths from overmedication and fears of subjective diagnoses, most physicians accepted salvarsan and neosalvarsan (the newer, less toxic, but also less effective formula developed by Ehrlich), when coupled with the older method of mercury treatments, as the only adequate means to treat syphilis.[71] Their proof came largely from personal experience and the medical reports of others. Physicians were also aided by Dr. J. Whitridge Williams's exhaustive study of more than ten thousand pregnant women and their infants. Williams administered Wassermann tests at the Johns Hopkins Hospital between the years 1916 to 1919. Overall, Williams attributed 26 percent of the fetal deaths that occurred during the period to syphilis infections.[72] He also maintained that black early infant deaths from syphilis occurred at a rate almost four times as high as the early death rate for white infants. His experimental procedures produced dramatic results. Certain that early syphilis testing and early treatment would result in a decrease in early infant deaths, Williams confirmed his theory: when pregnant syphilitic mothers received correct syphilis treatments, only 7 percent of their babies were stillborn or died within the first two weeks after birth. This result was a marked improvement from the 52 percent early infant mortality rate for syphilitic mothers who received no prenatal anti-syphilis treatment. Babies from a third group of infected women, who received "insufficient" treatment, posted an early infant mortality rate of 37 percent. From these results, Dr. Williams concluded that one-half of infant deaths that occurred due to syphilis could be eradicated with early detection and proper treatment. The Long Island Medical College in Brooklyn, New York, repeated and verified his results.[73] In 1916, Williams became the first U.S. obstetrician to mandate Wassermann testing for every pregnant woman who entered his clinic. Obstetric clinicians followed his lead. It would take another twenty years, however, before state and local administrations would require venereal testing for parturient women.[74]

Conclusion

The racialization of health and medicine, along with the overarching syphilis epidemic in the United States, the anti-syphilis campaign, and modern syphilis testing and treatments, created a complex backdrop for the importance of combatting syphilis in communities of African descent. These issues may have fueled the AICP's decision to forgo other disease-related and environmental causes linked to Columbus Hill's high black infant death rates for a solitary attack on maternal and congenital syphilis, even as the agency knew the existence of other environmental factors in the neighborhood that may well have caused higher infant and maternal morbidity rates. The results of the health work performed by the AICP and the alternate causal threat of tuberculosis will be discussed in the next chapter.

6

Health in Columbus Hill

Educated by their southern peers to equate syphilis with blackness, to view black health problems as environmental, racial, or both, and armed with Williams's results and anecdotal knowledge from personal cases, New York City's health officials, physicians, and nurses turned to the eradication of congenital syphilis in their effort to decrease Columbus Hill's black infant mortality rate. But this switch came over time.

Initially, when Bailey Burritt had hired Miss Price in early April 1917, he advised William Kirkbride that the Columbus Hill health demonstration would focus on alleviating infant diarrheal diseases, which were "considerably higher than that of the white population " and thus "the factor that we will expect to influence [the outcome] the most."[1] However, by February 1918, nine months into its work, the AICP revised its research focus to syphilis and revised its policy of requiring Wassermann tests only for pregnant black women admitted into area hospitals. Now, all expectant black women in Columbus Hill who approached them on an outpatient basis—"out-door" cases—were tested for syphilis. The increased testing revealed that "in nearly 50 per cent of the families we are finding positive Wassermanns." As a result, the AICP extended Wassermann tests and syphilis education to other family members besides pregnant women.[2] The AICP nurses either sought out pregnant black women during their patrols of Columbus Hill, women came in willingly, or cases were referred to them from the Vanderbilt Clinic or the Nursery and Child's Hospital. In any case, AICP nurses knew their mission: as stated in Burritt's meeting notes, "Our problems are principally the venereal disease work."[3]

The efficacy of the AICP's early syphilis work among Columbus Hill's black mothers appears questionable at best. In an AICP "Colored Prenatal" report extending from October 1, 1918, through September 30, 1919, out of a registered 350 parturient women, 212 delivered or "carried through confinement" during the period. They bore 198 infants under the supervision of two AICP nurses. By the end of one month, 190 babies had survived. Twelve recorded stillbirths occurred, with six deaths attributed to syphilis in the mothers. The report also lists three cases of abortions, two of which listed as the result of maternal syphilis. The AICP blamed syphilis as the culprit for four of the eight neonatal deaths. And two abortions, along with six stillbirths, may have resulted from congenital syphilis.[4]

These statistics can be viewed in conflicting ways. Overall, out of 208 potential live births, 198 survived birth: ten died via syphilis infections that resulted in six stillbirths. Another four neonatal deaths from syphilitic mothers and congenital syphilis also occurred; these four deaths, when added to four other non-syphilis-related neonatal deaths, results in the 190 neonatal survival statistic. Thus, ten of the eighteen deaths, or 55 percent, stemmed from maternal or congenital syphilis infections during the 1918–1919 period. One might argue, as had the AICP when it maintained that 50 percent of the black stillbirths in Columbus Hill had occurred due to syphilis infections, that the neighborhood's infant death problems had been correctly diagnosed. If syphilis had still resulted in six stillborn babies whose mothers had been diagnosed with syphilis and had undergone treatment, the disease might have easily claimed more lives had it been undiagnosed or untreated. However, since congenital syphilis supposedly claimed four out of eight neonates within their first month of life, one could also argue that maternal syphilis tests and their highly toxic treatments during and after birth may have cost infant lives. The salience of the AICP's argument that maternal and congenital syphilis represented half the stillborn and neonatal deaths could easily lead to a half-empty, half-full conclusion.[5] Even with claims of having administered Wassermann tests and syphilis treatments to *all* the pregnant black mothers under the AICP's care prior to October 1918, syphilitic black women still produced dead infants. And, considering the state of syphilis therapeutics at the time, anti-syphilis treatments may have killed viable black infants.

In a nutshell, the value of Wassermann tests and their validity often rested on laboratory readings, which could lead to false positive and false negative results; therefore, for many physicians treating syphilis, trust in or skepticism of Wassermann testing depended on one's faith in the laboratory that produced the results. Even then, experts suggested multiple tests during pregnancy and afterward (for the mother and child) to diagnose syphilis with certainty. By that time, however, multiple toxic treatments of arsenic compounds, mercury, and other additives may have profoundly affected cell tissue and organs in the mother, unborn child, and newly born infant. In other words, the AICP's forced Wassermann testing and syphilis treatments, even when done in good faith and accepted by black female clients as necessary and efficacious, may have done more harm than good.

To be fair, as previously stated, only a few persons in the Progressive Era health community doubted the effectiveness of salvarsan and neosalvarsan treatments and Wassermann results. In Burritt's 1924 meeting at which the principals discussed the progress of Columbus Hill's health work, Burritt asked Dr. Isadore Rosen, a noted syphilologist with the Vanderbilt Clinic, what the coalition should do next in order to foster "practical" control over syphilis in the area. As a leader in the primary institution that administered Wassermann tests and syphilis treatments to those in Columbus Hill, Rosen gave a rambling, somewhat coded response. Prior to Burritt's question, he had explained the work that he and Dr. John A. Fordyce had carried out by reading from a medical paper they had coauthored. "I might say here that the Wassermann is not always an indication of the presence or absence of syphilis, and we find that occasionally mothers come to us with active manifestations of the disease with the absence of a positive Wassermann. We find babies with active manifestations and negative findings, and if you are going to rely upon an absolute test during pregnancy you will sometimes be mistaken."[6] He continued reading, with the words "indicating great need for anti-syphilitic treatment during pregnancy as a protection with mother and child" handwritten by someone. Thus, while warning that Wassermanns could not absolutely indicate the presence or absence of syphilis, and chillingly adding that "if you are going to rely upon an absolute test during pregnancy you will sometimes be mistaken," those at the meeting apparently overlooked, ignored, or downplayed Rosen's comments, for Burritt's next query asked how they should proceed in treating syphilis. Confused, dejected, or merely musing aloud, those present—particularly Burritt—valued Rosen's input based upon his position and years of expertise.

When he finally answered Burritt's question, Rosen initially seemed to have forgotten his earlier comments and gave a more pragmatic, if disjointed, answer. He indirectly and candidly began answering Burritt by admitting that the AICP's follow-up work in Columbus Hill's black community had aided the work of the Vanderbilt Clinic (and thus the careers of syphilologists like himself at the Columbia College of Physicians and Surgeons), to the point that "[w]e have now a two-story building given over to us and we have now separate waiting rooms for men, women, and for our pregnant mothers and children." Still, he noted that even with all the changes, the clinic's "Social Service Dept. is almost wholly supported by private funds," and that "insufficient funds" had made work difficult. Then, returning to Burritt's original question and his own original doubts, Rosen again warned all present that "one test is not an indication of whether a patient has or has not syphilis, and it must be impressed upon the people that all babies should be brought back for reexamination." Nevertheless, he admitted, "I don't know of any better methods of prevention than is carried on at the present time."[7]

Hamstrung with testing, treatments, and therapeutics that fulfilled much less than had been touted by their creators, still, a focus on syphilis treatment and study had been very good for the researchers and tending physicians at the Vanderbilt Clinic, providing ample test subjects and, if moved by the spirit, ample avenues for caring work. Still, if Rosen deeply questioned the methods of syphilis testing and diagnosis at his disposal, other impediments may have added to the AICP's and Vanderbilt Clinic's overall lackluster progress in decreasing syphilis as a cause of infant and maternal mortality in Columbus Hill. First, and fortunately for unsuspecting clients, more false negative Wassermann reactions occurred than false positives. This unplanned blessing may have saved more lives from needless, highly toxic syphilis treatments than the treatments themselves may have prolonged. Second, as mentioned before, it behooved physicians to choose good serologists; as stated by one specialist, "it is probable that more attention should be paid to the laboratory worker than to the method employed."[8] Third, the treatment process itself became just as important as multiple tests; both could last for years. And, even by the mid-1920s, few physicians believed that anyone could be completely cured of syphilis, using current treatment methods.⁹ Getting patients to return for injections and subsequent tests proved difficult, if not impossible. Columbus Hill's nursing staff and Vanderbilt physicians bemoaned the fact that treatments and tests could not be forced upon syphilitic patients, their infants, or their family members.¹⁰ Black males afflicted with the disease were extremely problematic. In 1922, out of the 199 continuously treated and reported cases of syphilis, 137 of the infected were women, 47 were children, but only 15 were men. "Difficulty of obtaining man [sic] cooperation" was the explanation given by a social worker. The validity of the researcher's conclusion remains a mystery, but his statement pointed to a need for Columbus Hill's black women to form an equal partnership with their neighborhood health care providers.¹¹

Others also questioned how salvarsan and neo-salvarsan should be administered, and even laid blame on the media for unquestionably building up public expectations that an epidemic disease, left unnamed in polite circles, could be cured. In "The Impossibility of Curing Syphilis by Salvarsan Alone and the Dangers Arising From Insufficient Treatment," Dr. Charles M. Whitney of Boston fervently argued that, until the popular press had heralded the advent of Paul Ehrlich's "bullet" and its potential to obliterate syphilis from the human body and thus the world, the disease had had little public resonance. Reflecting general reluctance to discuss sexually transmitted diseases borne by human vectors, few people except infected carriers and their physicians discussed either syphilis or gonorrhea, or the threat they posed to public health during the late nineteenth and early twentieth centuries. With the creation of salvarsan, the "social hygiene" dilemma received new attention (which focused squarely on female prostitutes as syphilis delivery systems that infected unsuspecting male patrons, who then carried the disease home to "innocents"—wives and unborn children). Also, with the creation of salvarsan, Whitney argued that "the public was thus receiving its kindergarten education regarding the disease and its remedy" via popular culture and growing whispers. Physicians only added to the excitement as "[medical] journals were filled with enthusiastic articles describing [salvarsan's] marvelous results," embroidered with vivid photos of syphilitic lesions in their before-and-after states.¹²

Despite Ehrlich's claims, however, Whitney believed that, via salvarsan injections alone, and even with the subsequent disappearance of cutaneous lesions after patients received salvarsan injections, syphilis could never be cured. The media had wrongly inflamed patient expectations that salvarsan was a definitive cure for syphilis. Moreover, armed with salvarsan, its promises, and their own hopes, doctors often further misled patients to believe that a series of shots and the disappearance of first-stage lesions equaled a cure. Inadvertently, Whitney states, while the powerful drug performed excellently in removing lesions, when overused by repeated injections or, alternately, underused, if patients refused to return for follow-ups or physicians wrongly assumed that a few shots were all that were needed, syphilis could spread undetected over time into its second or deadlier third stage.

This problem was not new. Prior to salvarsan, patients with first-stage lesions would seek therapeutics from physicians who would have them return later to check for the appearance of second-stage rashes. If these rashes occurred, only then would a doctor be certain that the initial skin lesions had, in fact, been the result of a syphilis infection, and the patient would have been instructed that, with a long-term regimen of treatments, a cure would result. Of course, Whitney states, after a year of treatment and as "the secondary eruption soon faded, the induration about the primary lesion softened and gradually disappeared, and the secondary headaches, mucous patches and sore throat were rapidly relieved," the patient believed herself or himself cured and would not return. Usually, the disease would lie dormant and, upon its return in the third stage, would wreak horrible consequences. This led Whitney to assert that "our insane asylums are filled with its victims and our almshouses with blind and paralysed [sic] wrecks" because patients wrongly believed themselves cured too soon.[13]

In sum, Whitney stressed that "we know to-day that salvarsan alone does not cure syphilis but must be aided by the older and surer remedies," and he advocated against the use of multiple injections, which lured patients into a sense of false security, unless accompanied by older, proven agents, such as mercury with potassium iodide. Moreover, he maintained that too many salvarsan injections were injurious and dangerous. "It is not unreasonable," Whitney argued, "to expect that so large an amount of arsenic can be used without detrimental effects upon the kidneys and other organs, if repeated too often." On the other hand, he also warned that the underuse of salvarsan could have equally detrimental results. The problem of repetitive injections of salvarsan alone created false security in the patient and the physician. As syphilis spread unchecked into its secondary and tertiary stages, tests often resulted in more false Wassermanns, which led to more shots, which led to more syphilitic reoccurrences, more shots, and more Wassermanns. Eventually, any treatment would be too late. Yet, Whitney believed, accompanied by metals treatments and when "used with care and good judgment," the dangerous toxicity of salvarsan could be rendered "relatively harmless."[14]

Whether the partnership between Columbus Hill's African American and British West Indian women and local nurses, physicians, and social workers proved to be beneficial for all involved, especially for the physicians, depends upon perspective. As early as the 1870s, U.S. obstetricians realized that the prestige of their profession depended upon placing it on par with that of their European counterparts. In general, European physicians trained and taught at teaching hospitals, where poor patients, unable to afford adequate medical, became "guinea pigs." On one hand, their maladies and their very bodies served as training tools for medical students and new interns. On the other, they received better health care than the herbal remedies and nostrums to which they were accustomed. Armed with a ready supply of sick, indigent patients, medical schools that successfully persuaded hospitals that it was in their interest to align with them rose to the forefront of their field.[15] Again, perspective is a powerful thing.

After the turn of the century, New York City led the nation in the establishment of university-controlled teaching hospitals and, as importantly, university-controlled teaching hospitals that strategically aligned themselves with preexisting hospitals. Columbia University's College of Physicians and Surgeons, located in Columbus Hill, vainly sought a hospital alignment as early as 1908. Persuading hospitals to join with a medical teaching college often proved difficult; hospital trustees feared losing control over wards and patients. Funding was needed to sweeten the pot, and wealthy philanthropists gave the needed money.[16] In 1911, Presbyterian Hospital, which had already aligned with the Sloane Hospital, joined with Columbia College of Physicians and Surgeons. Vanderbilt Clinic already belonged to Columbia University through an 1888 gift from the Vanderbilt family. It officially aligned with Presbyterian

Hospital in 1928.[17] The New York Nursery and Child's Hospital, created in 1910 by absorbing the New York Infant Asylum, became part of the New York Hospital-Cornell Medical Center in 1934.[18] Thus, with the exception of the Nursery and Child's Hospital, medical teaching institutions controlled the remaining hospital and clinic used by the AICP for referrals by the time of the AICP's experimental health work.

The black women and infants seen by the AICP came under the control of the dean of the Columbia College of Physicians and Surgeons from the outset of the 1915 New York City Department of Health's mortality study. This meant that the syphilis work carried on at the Sloane Hospital and the Vanderbilt Clinic took on added meaning.[19] Syphilis research itself came under intense scrutiny after the United States entered World War I.[20] Reports on the levels of syphilis infections among soldiers—especially African American men—marked the first time that aggregate data were collected on the disease. For black soldiers, the racist predisposition of white army physicians led to faulty diagnoses and inequitable treatment. Fifty-eight percent of the black males in the army tested positive for sexually transmitted diseases. White males with venereal diseases were rejected from the service, a fact that the army conveniently overlooked when it asserted that all blacks were probably infected with sexually transmitted diseases and yet accepted them in service. Even the numbers of actual black venereal disease cases have been called into question by historians of science, since the high rates reflected not only the army's racial prejudice but also the poor preventive health care accorded blacks prior to the war.[21] After World War I ended, hospitals and clinics were left to carry on the venereal disease work. But many physicians balked at relaying the numbers and names of their syphilis patients to public health departments, fearing an intrusion of the public sector into the private lives of their patients.[22] Medical teaching facilities, aligned with private or public hospitals, gave venereal disease treatments an air of respectability through the banner of scientific research. True to Progressive Era thought, since the discovery of the syphilis bacillus, physicians believed that a true cure for all venereal diseases might be one research project away.

The proliferation of syphilis studies produced by members of the departments of Dermatology and Syphilology at Columbia College of Physicians and Surgeons underscored this hope. Diagnoses, treatments, and out-patient services at the Vanderbilt Clinic quickly increased after 1916. As these activities rose, Vanderbilt's space became overcrowded. In particular, the 1916 Dean's report of the College of Physicians and Surgeons stated that the "infirmary" at the Vanderbilt Clinic "has more than proved its usefulness . . . [and] therapeutics and [the] diagnosis of syphilis in the Departments of Neurology and Dermatology" also expanded.[23] By 1921, the influx of syphilis patients at the Vanderbilt Clinic necessitated expanding the floor space. In particular, the increase in new patients was marked by "the valuable work [done] among syphilitic pregnant cases and among babies with congenital syphilis." Moreover, the increased number of syphilis patients warranted enlarging the numbers of junior faculty in the department.[24] As Dr. Rosen would remark in 1924, Columbus Hill's syphilis work had done the Vanderbilt Clinic proud, showing a need for expanded services, space, and workers.

The pride spread when, in a 1923 report, the College of Physicians and Surgeons finally shared with fellow peers and alumni the medical procedures it had used to combat syphilis at the Vanderbilt Clinic. Patients with congenital or acquired syphilis had received arsphenamine (a type of salvarsan) intravenously or intraspinally, along with intramuscular injections of mercury. Children had received intramuscular injections of arsphenamine and mercury. Listed under the title "Miscellaneous" were various blood tests and vaccinations, including "tuberculin injections and tests." By 1923, the number of syphilis patients far exceeded the black inhabitants of Columbus Hill: patient visits totaled 32,067. Over 1,400 out of 5,241 new patients were treated for syphilis. Eighty of these new syphilitic patients were infants. More than 4,200 salvarsan injections and 6,600 mercury treatments were dispensed. Each week the clinic devoted one afternoon solely for the treatment of infants and children with congenital syphilis.[25] The following year, members of the Department of Dermatology and Syphilology, including Rosen, the AICP-related physician who had voiced concerns over the efficacy of Wassermann tests and syphilis treatments, published more than forty articles on syphilis and related dermatological disorders.[26]

Overall Results

In practical terms and when approached over time, it appears that the black female inhabitants of Columbus Hill experienced a slight benefit from this explosion in scientific knowledge in syphilis testing and treatment. During the AICP's 1917–1924 study in Columbus Hill, more than one in five (20.8 percent) black stillbirths and miscarriages stemmed from a syphilitic mother. Prior to the AICP's intervention in Columbus Hill in 1917, 24.5 percent of infants had been born to untreated, unsupervised infected black women. These pregnancies had resulted in stillbirths, miscarriages, or congenital syphilis. On its face, the 4.1 percent difference between the pre-1917 and 1917–1924 study data seems insignificant and calls into question the efficacy of the AICP's work and the truthfulness of its assertions. On the other hand, assuming the data are accurate, the decrease reflects a 17 percent decline from the pre-1917 rate. A decrease of almost one-fifth becomes something significant. One, then, must ask: If the numbers are valid, was the AICP correct in assuming total responsibility for the change?

A large share of the credit must go to Columbus Hill's African American and British West Indian women themselves, who took advantage of prenatal care that came with the mandatory syphilis testing, treatment, and nursing follow-up. Their diligence in acquiescing to invasive Wassermann tests and dangerous anti-syphilis treatments insured their delivery of a higher percentage of babies who survived their first, critical month of life. Much of this agency also came from sacrificing their time off from work, since visiting nurses commented on finding few women at home during the day. Thus, the key to reducing both the black infant and maternal death rates in Columbus Hill came more from prenatal care and education and less from mandatory syphilis testing and treatment. Comparatively, Harlem's black babies died at twice the rate of those in Columbus Hill for all cases, treated or untreated (67.5 percent versus 33.6 percent, respectively). Those who received no prenatal care in Harlem died at a rate three times higher than those whose mothers had received three or more months of prenatal care in Columbus Hill (67.5 percent in Harlem versus a rate of 20.6 percent in Columbus Hill's black community). Thus, Columbus Hill's black women benefited from prenatal care, a somewhat inadvertent benefit they received through mandatory syphilis testing and treatments, which may or may not have resulted in little positive good.²⁷

Moreover, the prenatal care they received not only reduced puerperal (childbirth fever) maternal deaths but also led to a decreased number of neonatal deaths. In a 1922 address to the American Child Hygiene Association's annual meeting, Dr. Louis I. Dublin, statistician for the Metropolitan Life Insurance Company, cited neonatal death as the most intransigent barrier that scientists, physicians, and health care providers faced in their battle to eradicate infant mortality. Early infant deaths generally resulted from five factors: malnutrition, premature birth, congenital defects, syphilis, and injuries that resulted at birth. Nationwide, early infant death varied considerably, influenced by poverty, poor sanitation, if the infant's mother worked outside the home, if she had access to prenatal care, and her knowledge of proper infant care. The level of neonatal deaths also increased in proportion to the level of infant mortality: areas with high neonatal death rates normally held higher rates of early infant deaths when compared to areas with low infant mortality rates.²⁸

Dublin cited the work of the Maternal Center Association of New York City, a group that worked in conjunction with the Henry Street Settlement, as proof that early infant deaths could be decreased through proper nursing and medical procedures. The early infant death problem had seemed statistically impervious to the tremendous health care dollars and work that had decreased infant deaths over the remaining last eleven-months of a baby's first year (deaths during this time were usually attributed to environmental causes that could be regulated through educating the mother about proper infant care and feeding). Comparing statistics for New York City in 1920 to those compiled by the Maternity Center Association in the years 1919–1921, early infant deaths from diarrhea and enteritis, and congenital malformations and debilities, were much lower for women whose babies were serviced by the Association than for New York City residents as a whole.

The lifesaving stopped there, however; early infant deaths from congenital debilities, syphilis, and injuries at birth still remained the same, or even higher, than the New York City total. Dublin believed that modes of home deliveries were of vital importance. To him, women whose babies had been delivered by midwives risked greater chances of early infant deaths. Inadequately trained hospital staffs posed an impediment to adequate prenatal care, as did institutions with inferior equipment and facilities. Therefore, according to Dublin's research, the work of the medical staff at each institution directly affected the life possibilities of infants in their first month.[29]

Tuberculosis and Blacks in the United States

The medical staffs that served Columbus Hill's African American and British West Indian community reacted less enthusiastically to tuberculosis as a threat to black health than to syphilis as a culprit. Blacks also seemed to have approached tuberculosis diagnoses and treatment with less than overwhelming zeal. Both the New York City Department of Health and the AICP began the early stages of health work in Columbus Hill armed with similar information: blacks seemed to possess inherent susceptibilities to syphilis and tuberculosis, which may have also reflected environmental influences. Racialists explained the former in terms that ran the gamut from moralistic to environmental, but the latter was thought to be caused first by heredity and later by environment, or a convergence of the two. During the nineteenth century, white physicians believed that blacks had possessed some quirky, hereditary internal mechanism that made them impervious to tuberculosis.

Southern white physicians founded their assertions on the plantation myth. Before Emancipation, they argued, few sources recorded outbreaks of consumption in the slave quarters; in fact, their absence sparked speculation that black blood was somehow impervious to the scourge that killed Europeans and their descendants handily. Moreover, at the mid-nineteenth century, consumption was considered by most to be a disease of creativity, beauty, and status—not something that enslaved African Americans would contract. During the antebellum period, top southern physicians, politically savvy as they surveyed the increasing economic, religious, and ideological gulf between the slave South and former slave North, and also cognizant of their powerful positions as experts of slave health and, thus, reasons why African Americans should stay enslaved, marshaled their medical knowledge into proslavery rhetoric. The rhetoric grew more intense as talk of secession grew. Key to their argument was the assertion that those of African descent were biologically inferior to Caucasians or whites; black/white health differentials were empirical facts of the black need for enslavement. The South's main medical slavery proponents, physicians Josiah Nott and Samuel Cartwright, had maintained that, since blacks were resistant or susceptible to some diseases that had opposite affects on whites, slavery was a just, humane system, providing essential supervision, work habits, and health care for a race that was physically and intellectually inferior to whites.[30]

Of course, what would later be classified as "tropical diseases" (yellow fever and types of malaria, for example) were used by proslavery southern whites—physicians and laypersons—as additional proof that blacks carried inherent resistance against humid, hot climate diseases that devastated whites. Ergo, the logic went, blacks were inherently created for laboring in tropical or subtropical geographical areas because they easily endured harsh climates and diseases that would kill whites; on the other hand, whites could deal better with cold and urbanized pulmonary diseases because their pulmonary systems were farther advanced than those of blacks, who needed to stay in the rural South, enslaved. Peoples of African descent did appear to be resistant to *plasmodium vivax* and *plasmodium falciparum*, the weakest and most virulent *plasmodium* (parasitic) strains of malaria, respectively; of the other two forms, *malarie* was rare in North America, and no record of *ovale* exists).

However, the reasons behind a perceived black inherited resistance to types of malaria both support and undercut the notion of separate, distinct African health. First, any humans lacking the Duffy antigen in their red blood cells possess a resistance to malaria; it just happens that almost all (90% percent West Africans and most (70 percent) African Americans lack this antigen. In fact, it is impossible for someone to become infected by a *vivax*-bearing mosquito vector unless his or her red blood cells carry the Duffy antigen. Apparently, many Europeans carry this antigen. Second, in addition to lacking the Duffy antigen, many African Americans may have also carried the sickle-cell trait or sickle-cell anemia itself. If so, the presence of the trait or the gene made them more resistant to, or even immune to, the deadlier *falciparum* form of malaria. So, in either scenario—red blood cells that lack the Duffy antigen and convey immunity to the *vivax* parasite, or an inherited sickle-cell trait or gene that conferred immunity to the *plasmodium falciparum*—African Americans appeared to endure much lower morbidity and mortality rates from malaria than local whites.

Yet most Europeans and their descendants who lived through the first few years of contact with disease-bearing vectors—the period of "seasoning," reported as early as the 1600s by English settlers in the Chesapeake Bay area—would also develop an immunity to *plasmodium vivax*. As whites replaced themselves with African slaves, and as non-immune Europeans came into the colonies and, later, into the young republic, this aspect of white seasoning became more class-bound and less visible, replaced by a fascination with an assumed total black resistance to malaria as another justification for enslavement as a valid distinction due to climate, disease, and African racial inferiority. Therefore, had they been really paying attention, whites may have seen blacks transferred from the upper South Piedmont *vivax* region (Virginia, for instance) in fact becoming infected by different malarial mosquitoes if moved to the Deep South *falciparum* areas—the South Carolina coastal Low Country or the lower Mississippi Valley. Depending on their hematological makeup, blacks could either become moderately to severely ill and recover, or die (resistance to *vivax* parasite in no way dictated resistance to the more virulent *falciparum*). As Todd Savitt has pointed out, even if immune to malaria-carrying mosquitoes in their region of Western Africa, once enslaved and brought into the Americas, Africans—like Europeans—actually underwent a time of seasoning if they dealt with vectors carrying types of malaria which their bodies had not encountered in the past.[31]

If, then, blacks may have inherited resistance to some types of malaria but, like whites, had to undergo seasoning for other previously non-encountered varieties, what about the white assertion that blacks had weaker pulmonary systems based upon a racialized flaw? As with resistance to malaria, African American susceptibility to lung diseases and infections of the respiratory system seemed apparent to most southern white observers of black health. Blacks were judged not only adaptable or amenable to humid heat but also desirous of such tropical and subtropical climates. Physiological differences (shallower breathing, large pores, and copious sweating to remove contaminants from the body, even nappy hair, which protected the head from the dangerous effects of sunlight and heat) were explained as either God-ordained or as human adaptation, passed on through heredity. However—as with the black and white seasoning periods for malaria—whites also manifested similar means of adaptation to extreme heat and humidity. Again, which group got stuck with laboring in what conditions became a matter or power, law, social custom and, thus, perspective.[32]

In the case of black respiratory susceptibility to cold, damp weather, on the surface the case seems less murky. There are specific circumstances that point to persons of African descent and their inability, when compared to whites, to ward off respiratory illnesses that stemmed from cold and damp, as well as other physical conditions, such as frostbite. In fact, the jury is still out on whether people of African descent possess an innate susceptibility to pulmonary and respiratory illnesses, or if environment plays a larger role in black adaptation to cold weather. Still, antebellum southern whites found their enslaved blacks curiously less susceptible to consumption than whites, even though blacks were viewed as more susceptible to lung problems. Part of the idea that blacks were different from whites when it came to consumption morbidities and mortalities originated from the popular notion that the pale, translucent skin, the emaciated, weakened body, the delirium and flights of creativity, and the ongoing, unremitting cough of consumptives were signs of inherited status, intelligence, and good upbringing among northern and southern whites. These racialized examples of consumption remained dominant until the 1880s, when massive immigration, the isolation of the tubercle bacillus, and the realization that consumption (now tuberculosis) was a contagion, challenged people to change their mode of thinking. Tuberculosis lost its glamorous hue, and instead became a sign of racialized and classed stigmatization, a scourge of those perceived as ignorant, illiterate, depraved, and poor—urban blacks and southern Italians.

Prior to the 1880s, however, when whites noticed what they construed as consumption in the slave quarters, they racialized it and separated it from what "whites" suffered. For example, the Negro Consumption or "Negro Poisoning," which consisted of extremely difficult breathing and sharp pains around the navel, was probably miliary tuberculosis— the most fatal form of the disease, in which tubercles erupt simultaneously throughout all the organs. This was also known as "galloping consumption," which seemed to spread rapidly among enslaved blacks and resulted in a high death rate. Moreover, scrofula, a disease that afflicted both enslaved blacks and poor whites as a "tubercular swelling" at the lymph glands and gradually ended in emaciating death, was not counted, along with miliary consumption, as a sign or aspect of consumption among antebellum slaves. When mortality figures from these illnesses are included, blacks died as often, or in even larger numbers, from consumption as whites. These facts are borne out by the 1850 mortality census, which indicates that blacks died from scrofula at twice the rate of whites, and by 1817–1836 figures from British soldiers in the West Indies, where West Indian black and white morbidity rates from scrofula were about even, though blacks died at almost three times the rate of whites.[33] Thus, while blacks may have exhibited both a "natural" and an adapted resistance to humidity and heat—an environmental resistance that whites could also achieve over time—and therefore exhibited more health and medical commonality with whites who also endured living in hot climates, there may be something passed on through the genes of peoples of African descent that helps them become more susceptible to respiratory diseases.

This supposed susceptibility must be contextualized, however. Considering environmental situations adds to whether an individual's body, regardless of color, phenotype, and ancestral origin, can successfully adapt to and fight off respiratory and pulmonary diseases and illnesses. Several theories are to be considered. First, like the native peoples of the Americas who had never encountered smallpox until the arrival of Europeans, the tubercle bacillus and pneumonia virus may have encountered "virgin soil" conditions in bodies of transplanted West African slaves who lacked European immunities. Second, enslaved blacks had to perform hard, manual labor under inhospitable conditions, wearing few clothes, eating a diet that ranged from limited to inadequate, and living in close quarters. These situations made their bodies ripe for respiratory diseases, even if they had had certain immunities to others. Third, working in damp, cold weather further compounded their vulnerability to congestive illnesses. If they did possess any inherent susceptibilities to illnesses exacerbated by colder weather, then malnourishment, overwork, crammed living quarters, and working in the damp made their chances of health and surviving consumption worse.[34]

Thus, Southern whites had been wrong when they deified the "plantation legend" and faulted blacks' inability to live without white enslavement as the root cause of their poor health after Emancipation.[35] After the 1890s, in particular, and the discovery of the tubercle bacillus, when the ever-increasing numbers of impoverished immigrants arrived on U.S. shores and bred tuberculosis in tenements, consumption transmogrified into tuberculosis, a social and scientific stigma, a contagion. Its earlier attractiveness as a mark of status and breeding soon disappeared. In the period that marked the upward trajectory of white racial hatred and intolerance in the South against blacks—particularly the strivers who dared compete and overtake whites financially and socially, as blacks moved from rural to urban areas within or outside the South— whites began noticing an increase in the numbers of black tuberculosis deaths. The period of the 1890s through the 1910s saw a deluge of medical journal articles, primarily written by southern white physicians, about this new "black scourge." As further evidence that blacks should remain inextricably tied to the rural South, and not on the roads as migrants to southern cities or (heaven forbid) northern ones, southern physicians—self-proclaimed experts on the distinctiveness of "negro" health—pointed to tuberculosis and, again, to the inherent black inability to handle colder climates or unsupervised urban living, as undeniable, logical proofs.[36]

Thus, no true consensus on the nature of consumption existed at the time, and many historians of science who have studied consumption as it existed prior to 1882 have found themselves equally bedeviled.[37] Physicians argued over its source, the method of transmission, or the most effective means of treatment. Post-Koch medical opinions swirled around the existence of a single causative agent responsible for tuberculosis, the fact that the tubercle bacillus could only be viewed through a laboratory microscope, and how human society should be reeducated and reconditioned to further its existence in a world of germs.[38]

In many Progressive Era minds, germ theory held the promise— though largely unrealized for decades—that if science could now reduce diseases to individual pathogens, cures would soon result. When none were created, germ theory adherents wedded epidemiology to older versions of thought. Sanitarianism, environmentalism, racialism, and epidemiology became not-so-strange bedfellows. Disease prevention became central to the overall debate. If no cure for communicable diseases such as tuberculosis could be found, those most responsible for disease outbreaks—urban, poverty stricken European immigrants and blacks—would be targeted for isolation, treatment, and forcible reform.

When white reformers and the public at large pathologized nonwhite tubercular victims, poor native-born white and nonwhite women, viewed as caretakers of the home and agents of home health care, became objects of blame and educational reform. In many white minds, "blackness" became the source of tuberculosis in blacks: native-born whites contracted tuberculosis from the rigors or "life intensity" of being at the apex of the civilization heap. Thus blacks only contracted the disease when they tried too hard to emulate whites.[39] Of all the European immigrant groups that entered the United States between the 1880s and mid-1920s, Italians probably endured more attacks than other migrating European populations from racist native white reformers and public health officials. Castigated as ignorant, dirty, and potentially threatening to the white public because of their high rates of congestive diseases such as tuberculosis and pneumonia, Italian immigrants suffered the brunt of white nativism. Again, the racialization of disease reared its ugly head—but this time, it was gender that became racialized and classed. Sanitarians, visiting nurses, and health reformers saw impoverished women of both groups as the key to preserving public health through educational reform. White illnesses emanated from many factors; black or Italian illnesses came from blackness, cultural ignorance, or filth. Women, as keepers of the hearth and cultural transmitters of knowledge in the home, stood at the center of the nation's urban tuberculosis problem.[40]

Tuberculosis posed a true threat to public health in post-1900 urban cities. In geographical areas where public health officials gathered statistical mortality data, they discovered that while urban blacks usually succumbed to tuberculosis at higher rates than their white counterparts, both groups seemed more susceptible to tuberculosis when confined to urban areas.[41] Racialism still existed in the minds of public health officials during the 1910s; still, racial heredity alone could not explain how descendants of both Africa and Europe increased in susceptibility to tuberculosis in large cities. Reformers, physicians, and health officials began shifting from racialism to consider the salience of environmental factors, such as poverty, overcrowding, overwork, and malnutrition as possible causal factors in the development and spread of tuberculosis. But if a provable causal link between poverty and tuberculosis could be established, why, some southern physicians asked, did rural whites and blacks suffer lower tuberculosis rates, with few blacks contracting the disease?

Antebellum white physicians had reported few cases of consumption in the slave quarters. Yet, in a study of consumption in seven southern states from 1849 to 1850, although blacks constituted 44 percent of the population, they suffered 37 percent of the consumption-related deaths. White southern physicians failed to view these figures as proof that rural antebellum blacks, often malnourished and overworked, contracted consumptive diseases at a higher rate than rural whites. Later, when both groups moved to urban areas, white consumption/tuberculosis deaths increased. For blacks, segregated in the worst occupations and housing, and facing malnutrition, the contributing environmental tubercular factors of poverty and malnutrition resulted in record high rates of black tuberculosis deaths.[42]

Tuberculosis among Blacks in Columbus Hill: An Alternate Causation

It is almost needless to say that Columbus Hill, an urban area ignominiously known for its high rates of poverty during the AICP's period of health work, also posted higher-than-normal black mortality rates from tuberculosis infections. The first attempts to provide Columbus Hill's black population with public health care began in 1906 when a black nurse established a settlement house in the neighborhood. Prior to that time, area blacks turned to women trained in roots and herbs and other sources of traditional healing. Their choice of traditional healers might have been personal, but few area hospitals admitted blacks, and white nurses refused to enter their homes.[43]

In 1900, New York City's Charity Organization Society (COS) broke the color barrier in previously segregated public nursing by hiring Jessie Sleet, a Canadian-born and Chicago-trained black nurse, as the nation's first paid black public nurse. Columbus Hill's black community became Sleet's personal territory from 1900 to 1909.[44]

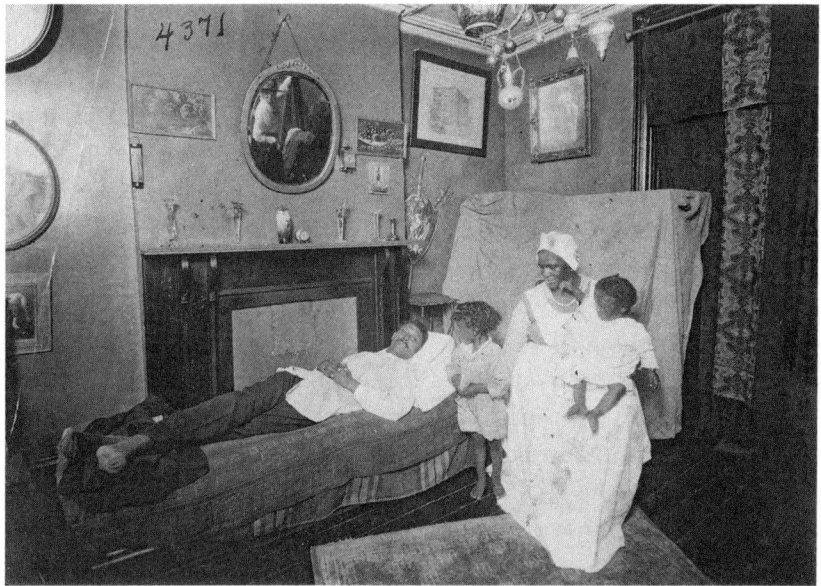

Figure 6.1. Jessie Tarbox Beals, "Columbus Hill Health Center Album, Man on Sofa with Family," between 1879 and 1950, Rare Book and Manuscript Library, Columbia University, Community Service Society Collection, http://css.cul.columbia.edu/catalog/rbml_css_0552 (accessed March 2, 2014).

In a 1901 article written about Sleet and published in the *American Journal of Nursing*, the writer revealed that during a two month period during the fall of 1900, Sleet "visited forty-one sick families and made one hundred and fifty-six calls . . . caring for nine cases of consumption, four cases of peritonitis, two cases of chicken pox, two cases of cancer, one case of diphtheria, two cases of heart disease," and other assorted maladies. She urged five of her black patients into area hospitals. The people Sleet served received long-overdue care. The writer relays the story of one consumptive twenty-seven-year-old woman called B.S. who struggled to support her three-year-old daughter and sick mother. They lived in a one-room apartment and all shared the same bed. After numerous visits, Sleet finally convinced the tubercular mother that, by sleeping in the same bed with her young daughter, she was endangering the child's health. The mother began greater efforts to protect the girl, opening the windows for fresh air as frequently as possible and covering her sputum cup with a rag. Although B.S. never asked for charity assistance, Sleet found her a domestic position. B.S.'s new employer felt pity for the family and found a medical specialist for her. B.S. soon saved enough money to repay back rent but died soon afterward.[45]

Sleet quit her COS "experimental" work in 1909. Prior to leaving, however, she published part of her research work a 1905 article titled "Tuberculosis among Negroes: A Report to the Committee on the Prevention of Tuberculosis." Sleet acknowledged the high rates of tuberculosis in Columbus Hill's black community but said that few public agencies realized the scope of the problem because many deaths went "unrecorded and unknown." More importantly, Sleet revealed the cultural dimensions of tuberculosis in the black neighborhood. "At the mere mention of the word 'consumption' suspicion is aroused, and the person questioned frequently becomes non-communicative," Sleet stated. She continued, "Many are of the opinion that there is a plan afoot to forcibly remove consumptives from their homes, and to place them in hospitals where the unfortunate need expect neither justice nor mercy." Sleet explained how, even for a black nurse, cultivating a high level of trust in order to serve the health needs of the black community remained difficult when tuberculosis was involved. She recalled the case of a "Mrs. W.," a domestic worker, whom she had visited; she stated her mission and asked if any in Mrs. W.'s family needed information or medical care for "lung diseases." Sleet's queries received negative responses. But, "after talking at considerable length . . . I decided to ask some direct questions. 'Have you any sickness in your family, or do you know of any sickness in the house?'" Mrs. W. cheerfully responded, "'I am thankful to say that this is a healthy house—everybody's well and hearty.'" With this admission, she asked Sleet to enter her home. They talked for nearly an hour before Mrs. W. placed herself next to Sleet and said, "'I'm going to tell you something and I don't want a word said about it, but my husband has it.'" Sleet states that she "pretended to doubt this." Further gaining the woman's confidence, as Sleet left, Mrs. W. confided that a young boy living upstairs also had "lung trouble." Sleet reveals that the cases of Mrs. W.'s husband and the neighbor boy both resulted in positive examples of tuberculosis.[46]

During her six-week study of tuberculosis in Columbus Hill's black community, Sleet discovered twenty-two cases of pulmonary tuberculosis (the patients were either under a private physician's care or receiving services through a health clinic) and ten presumably untreated cases with "alarming symptoms." Sleet revealed several lessons learned from her experiment. First, blacks viewed tuberculosis as stigmatizing because health officials categorized blacks as a group prone to tuberculosis infections, in addition to syphilis. Visiting nurses found it increasingly difficult to penetrate the black community's barrier of silence on the subject. Thus, data on tuberculosis infections in the black community may have been too low. Second, Sleet argued that public health nurses' door-to-door canvassing for tuberculosis cases would not work in Columbus Hill. Blacks would rarely volunteer the information that nurses and health officials needed, and Sleet admitted that "it would be quite impracticable for an official inspector to work as slowly as I did." Sleet solved her problem by visiting black ministers, who invited her back to speak before their congregations. This speeded up the process of dissemination and lessened the confrontational aspect of public door-to-door canvassing. Sleet also faulted undertakers who blatantly reported tubercular deaths as pneumonia so that survivors would receive death benefits from insurance companies that withheld funds from tuberculosis deaths. This practice had an upside: surviving families received badly needed money that lessened levels of destitution, particularly when insured male heads of household succumbed to tuberculosis. The downside occurred when families did not receive the fumigation offered by the city after tuberculosis deaths. Finally, Sleet revealed that many tubercular blacks who became too ill to work simply returned to the South to be supported by their families and friends, further exacerbating the spread of the disease. Sleet also blamed poverty as a cause for increased tuberculosis deaths in Columbus Hill. Poor housing, malnutrition, and the overworked condition of mothers—all contributing factors to high rates of infant mortality—also led to an increased black susceptibility to tuberculosis.[47]

Interestingly enough, the racialized renderings of blacks and tuberculosis trumped those accorded to blacks and syphilis when it came to the response of Columbus Hill's black community. When Columbus Hill's African American and British West Indian women, steeped in the trust and use of midwives in the U.S. South and in the Caribbean, abandoned their traditional use of midwives for modern delivery practices, and when the AICP, influenced by a tempered racism as much as by humanitarian, environmental or epidemiological concerns, mandated Wassermann tests for all pregnant black women, the black infant mortality rate and the rate of infant deaths *from congenital syphilis* decreased. However, syphilis-related infant deaths never accounted for more than one-quarter to one-fifth of deaths among Columbus Hill's black infants. It is hard to imagine that black women may have reacted more favorably to prenatal care contingent upon invasive and dangerous syphilis testing and treatments than tuberculosis testing; the racial stigma attached to tuberculosis must have paled in comparison to racially sexualized moralisms, masked beneath a protective blanket of scientific objectivity. In addition, women forced to endure venereal testing to receive prenatal care endured temporary stigmatization and embarrassment.

Yet syphilis is a sexually transmitted disease that can be hidden from the public, unlike tuberculosis; those stigmatized by public health authorities and society as tubercular could lose badly needed employment, housing, independence, and friends.[48] And tuberculosis was rife in Sanitary Districts 113, 115, and 119, where the common boundaries of West 61st Street and West 62nd Street housed most of Columbus Hill's black population. Physicians William Guilfoy and Shirley Wynne, the authors of the 1915 New York City mortality study, had already described Sanitary District 113 as an area where rates of pulmonary tuberculosis among blacks were triple that for whites in the area; district 115, where blacks made up 50 percent of the neighborhood, as an area with high infectious and tuberculosis rates in "need of the most intensive health work in this district; and district 119, where the death rate from tuberculosis, diarrheal diseases, and respiratory infections was twice that of the entire borough for children under the age of two. Both Guilfoy and Wynne had also issued a warning to the City with regard to Negroes and tuberculosis:

> The fact that the Negro is particularly susceptible to tuberculosis should not deter the Department from making an active campaign against this disease in the negro [sic] districts. Granting that the Negro is highly susceptible to tuberculosis infection, there is no question but that the negro's manner of living is responsible to a very large extent for his susceptibility, and if we can, even in a small measure, overcome his carelessness and

indifference, we should be able to secure a very appreciable decrease in the mortality of tuberculosis, and, indeed, of the other diseases to which he succumbs more frequently than his white neighbors.[49]

It would be unsupportable and dangerously pandering to negative racialized stereotypes to say that African Americans and British West Indians actually internalized the stigmatization of tuberculosis. But Mrs. W. had voiced real fears over public stigmatization nonetheless. New York City health officials approached tuberculosis reform zealously, playing on public fears of deadly airborne diseases through educational campaigns against spitting, sharing drinking cups, and fly swatting. They were also not above forcibly detaining those presumed infected, removing children from infected apartments, or sending the sick to tuberculosis sanitoria. Forced tuberculosis confinement occurred along strict racial and class lines in New York City. Simply stated, the Progressive Era was a time when health reformers believed that their construction of the public good far outweighed personal freedoms.[50]

One must also consider that the desire to avoid the infant deaths they saw around them provided black women with an urgency that allowed them to overcome whatever qualms they may have had about syphilis tests and treatment. Moreover, many may have desired syphilis testing and medication as a way to mitigate the pain and suffering caused by syphilitic infections. Just how committed they and their partners remained to the process is unknown. Dr. Thompson, a Vanderbilt physician who worked with the AICP, deplored how hard it was for them to get families to return for treatment. "I don't believe we have more than half a dozen records to study for a period of five years," he added. "If you can carry on and go through with children for the next ten years you could make a contribution that would be of tremendous assistance."[51]

Conclusion

The physicians who treated syphilis cases at the Nursery and Child's Hospital and the Vanderbilt Clinic may have been motivated by altruistic hearts as they faced a public health nightmare. Still, there was more than altruism at stake: a controlled scientific study of black congenital and acquired syphilis would have been quite a coup. As far as tuberculosis was concerned, medical experts had noticed a general decline in the disease decades before Jessie Sleet published her 1904–1905 study. But for urban blacks, rates of tuberculosis infection, the numbers of cases, and tuberculosis deaths would continue to outpace those for whites for several more decades. For whatever reasons (public health officials liked to think that their educational and medical programs led to its overall decrease), occurrences of tuberculosis had undergone a steady decline since the 1840s. By the 1920s, few physicians were concerned about anything more than creating a consensus around the diagnosis, description, and treatment of the disease.[52]

Yet few of the causal factors that led to higher rates of tuberculosis in Columbus Hill's black community had changed by the end of the AICP's health study. During the period from 1915 to 1920, reported black deaths from tuberculosis averaged 582 per 100,000, exceeded by only the tuberculosis mortality numbers in two other sanitary districts. Apparently, the stigmatization that blacks equated with tuberculosis remained, because health workers at the Vanderbilt Clinic complained that "few incipient cases [of tuberculosis] among the Negroes of the district were being reached by the Clinic."[53] As late as 1927, the AICP treated twice as many black families in Columbus Hill for tuberculosis than for syphilis: 21 percent versus 10 percent. A corresponding figure of 13 percent for malnutrition cases reveals that, along with the poor housing in Columbus Hill, another factor that figured in its high infant and tuberculosis mortality rates remained. The collaborative efforts of the AICP, the Sloane, Nursery and Child's hospitals, the Vanderbilt Clinic, and the African American and British West Indian mothers in Columbus Hill had worked to decrease its rate of infant mortality, believed to result from congenital syphilis. Yet environmental problems, the inadequate cultural methods of client contact used by public health officials and workers, and black perceptions of personal and social stigmatization remained.

Deaths from tuberculosis still haunted Columbus Hill's black community. Nevertheless, ironically, after only one year in the neighborhood, the AICP expanded its experiment into another district where tuberculosis, pneumonia, and other congestive diseases had created high numbers of infant and adult deaths. Thus, despite the problems encountered, created, or ignored, the health work performed by the AICP in Columbus Hill's black community became a model for the cutting-edge, lifesaving health demonstration in the heavily southern Italian Mulberry District in 1918 that will be discussed in the next chapter.[54]

7

Birthing in the City: The Mulberry District

Dr. William Guilfoy and Dr. Shirley Wynne worked for the New York City Division of Statistical Research; they compiled and published the 1915 New York City mortality study that had highlighted Columbus Hill's black infant and maternal mortality problems. In their analysis of the study's results, they suggested how the research could best be used in terms of health work and prevention. The city now used sanitary districts to define and delimit health, illness, and disease by racialized groupings instead of the old political ward districts. Data reflected and aided the racialization of science in the arena of urban public health, as well as how environments were shaped by and reflected landlord segregation and group comfort and loyalties, which combined to further racial stereotypes and class cohesiveness. As in the Columbus Hill case, residential segregation and group affinity may have made racialized data collection easier, but restructuring the city from voting wards to racialized sanitary districts also resulted in collected data that seemed a confirmation of racialized health, justifying racialized health work among a racialized population. The Department of Health and various organizations responded to the patterns of housing segregation and group affinity by coordinating health work to meet the specific needs of "sore spots," or racialized, impoverished, unhealthy neighborhoods that required immediate attention.[1]

Guilfoy and Wynne recommended that before the city tackled problem areas, "illness census[es]" should be taken to "serve the two-fold purpose of determining the amount of illness in these districts and of furnishing us [with] more correct detailed population figures," absent in the 1910 census. Furthermore, they advocated that the Department of Health should study areas with low mortality rates to determine why their inhabitants enjoyed good health and longer lives. Socioeconomic factors and housing, the number and quality of health care providers in an area, nutrition, and personal habits such as drunkenness were to be considered, measured, evaluated, and compared with those of sicker neighborhoods. With these processes and measurable factors documented, Guilfoy and Wynne believed that overall mortality rates calculated by sanitary district would help focus health care efforts on problem areas. Likewise, the tabulation of infant deaths, stillbirths, contagious diseases, and diseases/illnesses among school-age children by sanitary district would link preventive and educational expertise with the populations in most need.[2]

In May 1918, one year into the Columbus Hill infant and maternal health experiment, the AICP chose to expand its health work into Lower Manhattan's southern Italian Mulberry District.[3] At the time, many other New York City neighborhoods had equal or worse health concerns than those in Mulberry. Why, then, did a consortium of public and private entities, directed and supervised by an agency still buoyed by its first year of successful black infant death rate reduction in Columbus Hill in 1918, quickly target the Mulberry District as the next critical neighborhood needing immediate attention?

At first glance, Guilfoy's and Wynne's recommendations from the 1915 survey had probably seemed counterintuitive and had raised few, if any, eyebrows of those in the public health community, such as Bailey B. Burritt, general director of the AICP. For example, the health work that had begun in 1917 among Columbus Hill's black population had actually fallen outside the "illness census" prerogative because, in the results of the health survey, Guilfoy and Wynne had already identified it as a "sore spot," an area with inordinately high morbidity and mortality rates that more than justified immediate and coordinated health work.[4] Today, a growing number of sociologists are questioning the veracity of race-based statistical data and their use in studies in which researchers approach race as a biological certainty or treat race as a social construct that remains monolithic and static over time.[5] Even if the actual black morbidity and mortality rates had been halved, however, they would have justified attention to Columbus Hill's infant and maternal health problems.

Nevertheless, decades later, why the New City Department of Health and the New York AICP chose to initiate health work in the Mulberry District seems less self-evident than it may have at the time, and demands closer scrutiny. What may have been obvious during and soon after the survey era may seem illogical today, even when using the AICP's data and criteria. One obvious way to interrogate the differences between then and now is to question why people did what they did, and then backtrack and analyze their steps: to play "backseat driver," of sorts. For instance, unlike Columbus Hill, the Mulberry District was not included in the numerous "sore spots" that Guilfoy and Wynne had enumerated in their health report. More to the point, the Mulberry District could have easily evaded the Department of Health and AICP radar because of its comparatively better health. Instead, it became a larger laboratory for the AICP's work.

Simply put, the New York City Department of Health and the AICP targeted the Mulberry District for its next coordinated health work because of its racial and gendered distinctiveness. Public health officials viewed the overwhelmingly poor and working-class southern Italian immigrant community as a "racial grouping, typical of that found in New York and other large cities."[6] Moreover, to the AICP, since Mulberry's population was 95 percent Italian by birth and/or parentage, it represented a racially consistent area that was largely from southern Italy.[7] Second, they chose to focus on infant and maternal health, as in Columbus Hill. In short, the AICP considered the area virtually racially distinct, and its mothers and children thus ripe for measurement and study.

This is not to say that the neighborhood's inhabitants exhibited no chronic health problems. Infant deaths from pneumonia and enteritis, and maternal deaths from tuberculosis and pneumonia, became the AICP's initial foci in the area because they were serious issues. And, years later, the AICP and Mulberry Health Center and other facilities conducted health surveys and worked with public schools to fight childhood diseases, poor nutrition, and worker health, all areas of critical need.[8] Although the Mulberry District had numerous health problems, by the time of the printing of their report, Guilfoy and Wynne had inventoried and enumerated other neighborhoods with far worse health and environmental conditions.[9]

I believe that in answering the question "Why Mulberry?" the only justification remaining was the AICP's belief that Mulberry's racial and gendered distinctiveness made it the perfect next case to use what it had done in Columbus Hill's black population. At Mulberry's core was a population whose females preferred midwife to physician care, and the AICP used this preference to justify rupturing their traditional birthing methods. While there were residents in Mulberry with non–southern Italian backgrounds, health care officials viewed the neighborhood as an almost hundred-percent southern Italian community, and the prospects of conducting an epidemiological study among what they considered a pure racial group may have swayed public health officials' decisions. Their notions of health as racialized and hereditary reflected the white privileged-class world view of the day, one that was also largely accepted by the native-born white masses. This perspective, held by many men as well as women, coexisted as a contradictory yet complementary adjunct to modern technological discoveries, even as science increasingly gave credibility to the idea that most diseases and poor health also stemmed from complex convergences of environmental, physiological, and behavioral factors, which the ambiguous, catchall term "race" could not adequately explain. Moreover, these thoughts carried over into the womb—how women behaved before birth and afterward.

Race, Health, and the "Southern Problem" in the Mulberry District

Southern, central, and eastern European groups who migrated to the United States often found themselves—and the germs they allegedly brought—defined in a preordained, hierarchical system of identification and stigmatization. This definition was predicated upon centuries of evolving notions of identity, social control, reproduction, inheritances, and patriarchy in both the United States and Europe.[10] At the bottom of the European heap, one precarious step above peoples of African descent, stood the *contadini*—Italian peasants and townsfolk.[11] Historian Alan Kraut would argue decades later that, by the beginning of the twentieth century, public health officials, politicians, and social workers in large industrial cities—men and women with motives and perspectives ranging from benign and sympathetic to menacing and unreceptive—focused much of their attentions and efforts on the ever-expanding numbers of immigrants, especially those from southern Italy.[12]

Anti-Italian sentiments often mirrored those previously reserved for blacks. For example, Richmond Mayo-Smith, a professor of political economy at Columbia University, wrote in 1890 that Italians "[h]uddled together in miserable apartments in filth and rags, without the slightest regard for decency or health [and] present a picture of squalid existence degrading to any civilization and a menace to the health of the whole community." Years later, E. A. Ross, a sociologist and fervent nativist, raised the ante after a generally degrading and stereotypical description of their outer appearance, by concluding that "such people lack the power to take rational care of themselves; hence their death rate in New York is twice the general death rate and thrice that of Germans."[13] Even the New York AICP had its own negative attitudes regarding southern Italians, though its workers' opinions seemed less incendiary than those of their peers: this predominantly native-born southern Italian population created "greater difficulties than with other Italian groups" because of "national characteristics" that displayed "their clannishness, their known adherence to their native traditions and their natural suspicion" of authority figures. The AICP justified these perceptions by adding that southern Italians were more loathe to "participate in the American scene" than other groups, and also disdained U.S. citizenship.[14]

Notwithstanding these derisive opinions and the policies and actions resulting from them as anti-immigration sentiments spread, Italians—from any region, even the South—held the trump card of marginal whiteness, an identity not available to other immigrants of color or migrating African Americans and British West Indians. While deemed racially inferior to U.S. native-born whites, largely of northern European and British descent, they were white enough for assimilation attempts and could become naturalized citizens. Later, as the umbrella of whiteness spread to include "white ethnics" and as the definition of "race" constricted, eliminating nationalism and cultural traditions in exchange for nonwhite phenotypical differences, second- and third-generation Italian Americans and other non-Nordic European ethnics moved up the hierarchy to enjoy benefits of whiteness that their parents and grandparents could have only imagined.[15] Of course, the social change came as a double-edged sword: the older immigrants had shunned assimilationist efforts because they judged white American values, actions, and attitudes as antithetical to their own and found them severely lacking.

Younger generations may have suffered also, downplaying or ignoring their cultural heritage as the cost of becoming white.

Considering the strength and proliferation of nativist, eugenicist, and anti-immigrationist rhetoric of the period, who would speak for the other side and attack the quickly hardening strata of racial, gendered, and class inequalities, all justified and reified by scientific, public health, and social work expertise? Two physicians, writing twenty years apart. Attempting to temper the anti-Italian sentiments of the time that branded them, like blacks, as feared carriers of tuberculosis and syphilis, a prominent Italian-born physician named Antonio Stella, in a 1904 *Charities* article, strove to educate and reorient the thinking of the native-both Anglo American public health and social work communities. Later, in a further attempt to curtail the strict racialism of eugenicists and nativists in the 1920s, Dr. Louis I. Dublin, the chief statistician for the Metropolitan Insurance Company, measured immigrant mortality rates and discovered that Italians living in New York State and Pennsylvania were some of the hardiest of the newly arrived European races.[16]

U.S. health experts had considered Italians prime carriers of tuberculosis and syphilis. Stella countered their claims by arguing that Italians left Italy in states of relative health, only to reach germ-breeding grounds like New York City, where they contracted debilitating and life-threatening diseases.[17] Stella said Italians feared tuberculosis and other respiratory illnesses particularly because of their rarity in Italy: "Peasants so feared [tuberculosis] and its stigma as an almost certain death sentence that those infected would refuse to use a receptacle for sputum, preferring to spit on the dirt floor of the house as did healthy people."[18] The importance of a necessary ban on public spitting had begun in the 1890s; by 1900, the New York City Department of Health posted verbal and pictorial warnings to discourage spitting because the dreaded tubercle bacillus traveled in fresh sputum and, when dried particles floated in the air, kicked up among pedestrians and carriages, the germ entered lungs and began to spread. To thwart this public health threat, public spitting became an arrestable offence during New York's citywide anti-tuberculosis campaign. Visiting nurses who discovered the sick in their inspections on the street, and later visited their homes, demanded immediate lifestyle changes—mothers could not chew food and feed it to babies; any expectoration should be kept in a sputum cup; tuberculosis suffers should sleep by themselves in a bed near an open window. Serious offences against these and other rules could result in forced containment in tuberculosis sanatoria.

From the southern Italian perspective, the injunction to not spit hit particularly hard because customs supported the use of sputum to curse or bless. For example, applying sputum to the eyes of new born babies was a folkloric way of blessing and protecting against *malocchio*, the dreaded "evil eye." Italian mothers also employed spit for therapeutic uses and to protect against spells. Thus, as U.S. and Italian cultures collided, something as simple as spitting, dwarfed by the etiology of tuberculosis and its stigmatization, created an immediate and strident battleground between public health officials, visiting nurses, men in the street of any race or nationality, and the sanctity of Italian women as rulers of the *domus*.[19]

Along with denying that Italians were a tubercular race, Stella's insistence that Italians were not a syphilitic race was first tested at Ellis Island, New York City's port of entry for immigrants from Europe, Africa, Southeast Asia, China, the Caribbean, and Central and South America. Here, U.S. Public Health Service physicians deemed two positive Wassermann tests as proof positive of the syphilis spirochete, and the accused carrier would be denied entrance into the country.[20] In 1915, Ellis Island immigrants were used as experimental subjects for scientific research in syphilis and gonorrhea.[21] Later, in the Mulberry District, in 1922 and 1923, the Committee of Dispensary Development studied the neighborhood's health problems. Although they targeted the four major types of illnesses found (gynecological, "constitutional," nutritional, and respiratory and infectious), the researchers admitted that reported cases of "functional nervous conditions" may have resulted from venereal diseases or alcoholism. However, "the entire omission of alcoholic report and the scant mention of venereal disease suggests that this count [of 37 cases] is too small for functional nervous cases; all but one of these 37 cases enumerated are found in the age period [of] over fifteen years."[22] Without further concrete, believable data, the accusation that Italians, like blacks, were a "syphilitic race" seems to have been merely the judgmental dream of racists, nativists, eugenicists, and those who accepted modern science without question. With regard to tuberculosis among Italians, however, Stella believed the proof did not lie in epidemiological morbidity and mortality data tabulated by city boards of health. These data, he maintained, were "very fallacious," purposely kept low to allow the unfettered movement of impoverished Italian workers, yet kept high enough to fuel racist stereotypes.[23]

In the end, industrialists' needs for inexpensive labor trumped the views of anti-immigrationists and eugenicists who feared "race suicide" and the views of public health officials who feared the impact of germs on the native white population. But the advent of sociological and epidemiological studies provided city health officials with significant ammunition that fed both pro- and anti-immigrationists' desires and fears. For example, in the early 1900s, while the New York City Department of Health ranked Italian tuberculosis mortality rates as the tenth worst in the city (far behind the rates for persons of African or Irish descent, who ranked first and second, respectively), Stella believed that the true impact of tuberculosis lay among the infected, not the deceased.[24] New cases often went unreported due to fears of stigmatization. Correspondingly, when comparing the tuberculosis deaths of Italian youths under fifteen years of age with their cohorts from other races, Italians ranked second in tuberculosis-related deaths. With such high mortality figures among the young, Stella perceived that if New York City investigated and enumerated the prevalence of the disease by its rate of infection, Italian adults would reflect the same statistical condition as Italian youths.

Stella also believed there were other pertinent factors at work—movement within New York City and emigration, poverty and poor housing, and overwork. The challenge in adequately tracking the prevalence of new cases of tuberculosis, and thus the infectious spread of the disease, was that new cases went unreported, and infected persons moved to other tenements, other areas within New York City, or returned to Italy.[25] Lacking valid, unmanipulated health statistics, Stella pointed to everyday tenement life as the foundation of Italian health problems: poverty; overcrowded living conditions; close working spaces in dank, airless factories; hospitals and dispensaries that bred diseases; and departing steamships that carried Italian "birds of passage" back to

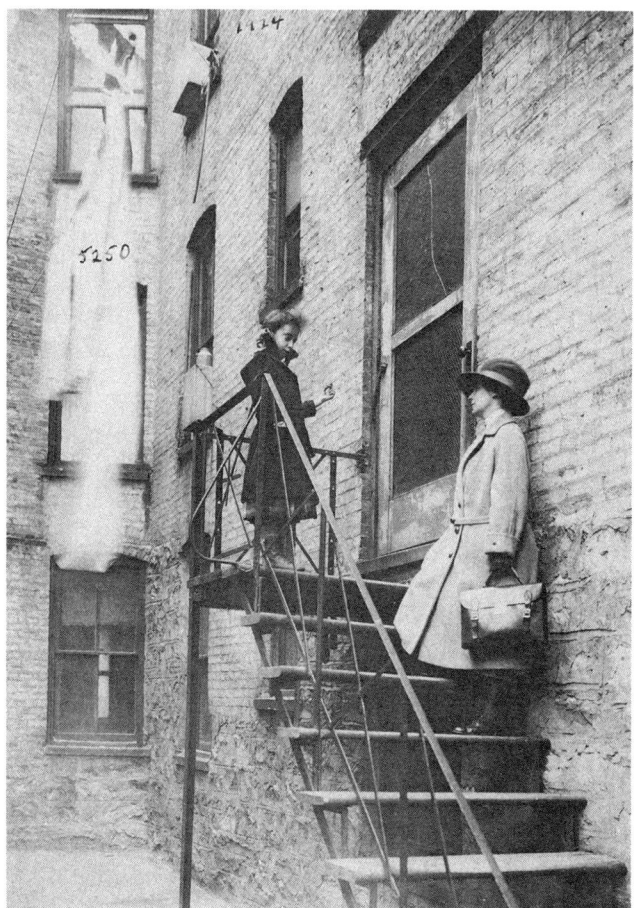

Figure 7.1. A white visiting nurse talks to a young Italian girl on the back steps of a tenement in the Mulberry District. Alfred Tennyson Beals, "Mulberry Health Center Album, Visiting Nurse on Tenement Back Stairs," circa 1923, Rare Book and Manuscript Library, Columbia University, Community Service Society Collection, http://css.cul.columbia.edu/catalog/rbml_css_0058 (accessed March 2, 2014).

their homeland, "with glistening eyes and racking coughs." Instead of returning to better health in sparsely populated rural Italian areas, they encountered "a quicker death."[26]

Stella blamed the urbanization of a primarily rural population and its experiences with overwhelming poverty and unsanitary housing and work conditions as causal factors in the prevalence of tuberculosis, particularly pulmonary tuberculosis among returning Italian immigrants, instead of infected steerage habitations.[27] This counterargument mirrored that taken by black public health nurse Jessie Sleet in 1905 in relation to the rampant tuberculosis among Columbus Hill's black population: the inhabitants were not merely more susceptible carriers because of their race, but carriers racialized by health workers and made susceptible to tuberculosis after migrating into a poor urban environment. In addition, the stigma of having tuberculosis kept many from revealing their ill state.[28] Like Sleet, Stella argued that Italians were not biologically or "racially" prone to tuberculosis; while many among the first-generation of immigrants succumbed to the disease, those who had stayed behind in Italy lived to an old age, absent the scourge of tuberculosis. Furthermore, first-generation Italian Americans seemed to have higher rates of immunity to tuberculosis, suggesting that those who survived their initial post-migration contact with the disease and successfully procreated passed on immunities to their young. In addition, he maintained that the tubercle bacillus found the emaciated, overworked bodies of southern Italians (particularly women) an ideal breeding ground.

Therefore, Stella consistently and forcefully believed that the prevalence of socioeconomic inequalities among the post-migration southern Italian poor and working classes explained the prevalence of tuberculosis among their "race." Occupations that required inhaling dust or air particles that contained dried, infected sputum resulted in tubercular infections—irritated mucous membranes and overworked lungs. And living and sleeping accommodations exacerbated the effects of dangerous work conditions: there was a paucity of pure, circulating, uncontaminated air because too many people lived and slept in tight, cramped spaces.[29]

Like Stella, during the 1920s, Louis Dublin echoed the importance of environment; unlike Stella, he also considered the effects of race in terms of individual and group health by measuring the mortality rates of European immigrants in Pennsylvania and New York State. Dublin directed his study at eugenicists whose fixation with the "relative vigor" of foreign races immigrating to the United States had been fueled by their concerns over "the character and potentialities of the various groups which are making the American of the future." Dublin attempted to explain why, in a wealthy, industrial nation with decreasing mortality rates across racial lines through age 45, the U.S. death rate for men and women over age 45 steadily increased, even as the age 45-and-over death rate declined in comparable nations in northern Europe and Britain. He hypothesized that overall national data, which pooled the mortality of native-born U.S. persons with that of less vigorous immigrant races with higher morbidity/mortality rates, had produced the escalating death figures.[30]

Dublin devised a four-step process to test his thesis. Initially, he constructed mortality tables on the death rates for each race living in New York and Pennsylvania, in 1910, per age group and gender. Since many recent immigrants landed and stayed in the Northeast, data reflecting the racial mix in New York and Pennsylvania would be highly valuable. From this foundation, he then tested the first premise of his theory: if foreign races came into the United States in a healthy state, this would be reflected in their mortality rate by age; since many entered as adults, if racial differences reflected *or* determined morbidity or mortality differentials, these should be eventually seen in national mortality rates.[31]

He found this premise to be partly true: for ages 10 through 44, there were virtually no differences in the mortality rates for the foreign-born and those born on U.S. soil with foreign parents. However, the same could not be said for those between 45 and 64 years of age: the mortality rates for foreign-born males and naturalized or U.S.-born males with foreign parentage was almost 50 percent higher than for their U.S.-born and parentage counterparts; the mortality rates for foreign-born females was 64 percent higher. The death rate differentials continued into old age, although they were smaller.

Thus, the life expectancy for a ten-year-old native-born white male would differ from that of a foreign-born boy of the same age. But the difference would be seen in post-45 mortality rates: the foreign-born boy would die sooner. To Dublin's thinking, since most immigrants entered the United States as adults, their disparately higher rates of death reflected a "lower vitality than the native stock" that manifested itself in the later years. This decreased racial vigor could be seen in the increasing mortality rates for older adults. Thus, adding immigrant mortality data to the overall U.S. numbers "can have only one effect, namely, to increase the death rate at the middle ages of life and at the older ages." [32]

Dublin next enumerated how the differing races ranked hierarchically by mortality and age. At the top were Russian- and European-born Jews who, Dublin theorized, exhibited longer lives and fewer health problems because they were already acclimated to city living and, particularly, to urban poverty and disease. He viewed the existence of Russian and other eastern European Jews as an asset to the American landscape when considering the deleterious effect of other immigrant groups and their bad health; "They increase the longevity of the total population rather than decrease it," he commented.

At the opposite end of the morbidity and mortality spectrum were Irish immigrants, whose shortened life expectancy (male or female) was less than that of Negroes within the same data registration areas. Irish males and females died at a rate of twice that of their native-born white counterparts. Moreover, their mortality differentials started in the prime of their adult lives: between the ages of 25 and 44, Irish men died at three times the rate of native-born white men; Irish women within the age range died at twice the rate of native-born white women. In addition, Irish women living in the United States could expect to live seven years longer than Irish men of the same age. Dublin targeted health and environmental causes for their inordinately high mortality rates: pneumonia, tuberculosis, and violence.[33]

Although Italians ranked lower than Russian / eastern European Jews and Germans, Dublin believed them to "have very favorable death rates in New York State and enjoy a good expectation" for longevity and health. Italian men seemed healthier than Italian women. While the men had lower mortality rates attributable to tuberculosis, cancer, Bright's disease, and heart disease than native-born white males, they had much higher death rates from pneumonia and violence. Italian women, on the other hand, succumbed more from tuberculosis and heart disease than their native-born white female counterparts; like Italian men, they also suffered higher morbidity and mortality rates from pneumonia. Despite the higher rates of illness and deaths when compared to native-born white men and women, and the fact that Italian women were more sickly than Italian men, Dublin had high hopes that they would further acclimate themselves to American urban living.

He already believed that although the climates of New York and Pennsylvania drastically differed from "the warm south" of southern Italy, migration had aided Italian health, and "the Italian-born live longer and suffer less from most serious diseases in their new abode than in their home country."

Unlike Stella, who denounced "race" used by those who stigmatized Italians for their poor living environment, Dublin's conceptions of the effects of "race" versus environment are interesting to note. Unlike dyed-in-the-wool, strident racialists, he accepted the powers of poverty, malnutrition, disease, and ignorance, and how they directly affected health and thus mortality. However, like sidestepping hereditarians, while acknowledging the power of environment he looked past it to glimpse some racialized essence that distinguished groups from each other and determined their "vigor," despite environmental change. His proof of both stances can be seen in his test case: Jews. Dublin's handling of Russian Jewish longevity and disease resistance tacitly accepted that some of his eugenicist audience may have embraced anti-Semitism, while others may have pointed to poor environment and the possibility of acculturation and assimilation in the distant future. He pointed out that, out of all the racial groups in his study, Russians constituted 560,000, or about 20 percent of the foreign-born New York State population, and a little over 6 percent of "the total white population." What came next—the fact that most of these Russians were Jewish—probably alarmed anti-immigrationists and anti-Semites who feared Jewish hordes, real or imagined, and in no way considered them "white," despite naturalization and immigration laws, the latter of which was soon to change with the passage of the restrictive Johnson-Reed Immigration Act of 1924.[34] Dublin explained that "both males and females of this race have an expectation as good as the native born of native parentage; in fact, the males are slightly better than the native stock." Old habits proved hard to shed completely: Dublin broke the mold with his admiration of Jewish resistance to disease and ill health; still, he gave the ultimate reason as group or racial "vigor."

Despite Stella's contentions that race could not determine health, even he would have agreed that, for whatever nature or nurture reasons, Italian women seemed to lack a necessary "vigor," especially during their childbearing years. Both Stella and Dublin perceived that impoverished Italian women were hit particularly hard by these factors. Public health officials, eugenicists, and nativists believed they bred unhealthy children too frequently, worked outside the home or expended their last energies in cottage work, performed too much housework for family and boarders, and suffered from poor nutrition.[35] Stark health differentials by gender and age existed among southern Italians living in the Mulberry District. Italian women between the ages of 15 and 45 (their prime childbearing years) were two to three times more likely to become ill than their male counterparts. However, by omitting the numbers of female deaths from puerperal disease from the calculations, the gender gap within this age group became almost equal. Clearly, childbearing in conditions of hardened poverty took its toll. Childbed fever usually occurred in clinic or hospital deliveries—a fact that may have hardened the Italian female resolve to resist abandoning midwife deliveries. Later, as they neared the end of their fertile years, between the ages of 35 and 55, Italian women were still more likely to become ill than men. Only in old age (over 55) did male morbidity and mortality rates overtake those of women.[36] As Louis Dublin agreed two decades later when regarding the failures of prenatal care among the poor, Stella's solution to decreasing tuberculosis deaths among southern Italians entailed raising their socioeconomic status, and it probably would have worked. In the minds of Stella and Dublin, an infusion of money into better housing, better working conditions and wages, and better nutrition would lower Italian susceptibilities to pulmonary tuberculosis and limit the disease's spread.[37] However, this public shift from individualism to taking care of the poor, only years away from becoming reality during the Great Depression, would receive only slight attention in the 1920s—poverty and poor health would still increase. Furthermore, a governmental shift from limited care for the poor (in widow's pensions until the Depression) to care for families with or without a male heads of households that extended past a bare minimum, seemed highly unlikely. Instead, prior to the 1930s, monies collected by private entities such as the AICP, the COS (its sister organization), and the many groups and clubs that donated money to both would have to suffice in terms of prevention, supervision, and education about illnesses and disease.

The Roots of Midwifery in the Mulberry District

That the AICP would use infant and maternal health issues as an "entering wedge" to gain admission into a culturally closed Italian community seems, in retrospect, calculated and pernicious at worst, and perhaps pragmatic at best. But these extremes and the wide range between have deep historical roots. Beginning in the mid-eighteenth century, colonial and U.S. physicians and broader medical and scientific communities looking to establish themselves and their professions benefited greatly by using the work of birthing to shift what women had considered a natural occurrence—supervised by midwives, or assisted by female relations or neighbors—to a "pathological," life-threatening event that required the strict intervention of trained men schooled in the medical arts.

This ascendance of science and patriarchy eventually challenged many Americans' overarching confidence and reliance on God as the wellspring of health and protector against illness and accidents. In addition, the colonial, and later American, world view did not conflate witchcraft with midwifery, unlike England, where "women's lore" or "white witchcraft" formed the basis of English perceptions of midwifery and childbirth. For example, during the fifteenth and sixteenth centuries, European midwives came under the attack and control of the Roman Catholic Church during the Inquisition; if a baby died, the clergy and believers accused the midwife of witchcraft. Instead, in the American colonies, Protestant leaders forbade midwives to use witchcraft. This led to the absence of the European link between midwifery and witchcraft. With this absence, little remained that made female midwives different from male practitioners. Over time, as Americans placed less faith in Providence as the sole determinant of infant or maternal survival, and with no gendered link between witchcraft and the practice of midwifery, science and its male practitioners gained importance and power over the act of childbirth.[38]

Mid-eighteenth-century changes in parturient technology also threatened the work of midwives. In particular, the French method of pelvic measurement during birth and the English creation of forceps aided in the shift toward male-controlled birthing. The French and English methods differed, however; while French practitioners took a theoretical stance and received their training from female midwives, their British counterparts adopted a more practical "trial and error" method of experimentation and were trained by men with limited natural childbirth experience. These male physicians had only experienced complicated births, as socially upheld norms of sexual indecency kept them from normal births. On the other hand, many midwives experienced hundreds of successful, uneventful births. This disparity led medical men to view pregnancy and childbirth for its pathological potential, and not as natural or even spiritual. Male intervention also justified charging higher fees for deliveries than those charged by female midwives.

Until the mid-nineteenth century, midwives delivered most of the babies born in the United States. The first "granny midwives" and "doctoresses" were enslaved Western and Central African women and their descendants, who passed on their cultural knowledge to each successive generation. Free and enslaved blacks and free and indentured whites revered black women schooled in the art of midwifery. In the slave South, for example, African American midwives delivered most babies, black and white, and these women also held high status in slave communities.[39] European midwives also brought their training with them. However, they did not create formal midwifery schools like the institutions where they had trained in their homelands. In a manner much like that of black midwives, European women passed on their knowledge through experience. In 1765, William Shippen, a physician trained in Britain, created the first formal midwife-training facility in Philadelphia. Shippen focused on delivering the babies of the rich and created a "lying-in" hospital for poor women, which was used to train obstetric doctors and midwives. During the nineteenth century, a few midwifery schools were created in the Northeast and Midwest; however, overall obstetrical training for midwives and physicians was poor—sketchy at best, and nonstandardized. As southern, central, and eastern European immigration increased during the late nineteenth century, the numbers of formally trained European midwives expanded in the United States.[40]

Thus, as the use of forceps and the fees of male physicians increased, childbirth became gendered, racialized, and classed. Midwives eschewed forceps as a male contrivance and continued using their smaller hands to position infants in the womb. They also charged less for services they considered natural and part of being a woman. As a result, they increasingly serviced only poorer women. Male doctors justified their use of forceps and charging more because they thought, as trained men, they were more capable than women of the rational thought needed for the medical arts, and had received the scientific training. Moreover, as men continued to use forceps, they further separated themselves and their patients from the poorer masses as physician deliveries became a sign of white middle- and upper-class status.[41]

Thus, obstetrics became the first field of medical specialization in the United States: male-controlled, interventionistic, and wedded to the "birth as pathology" perspective. By the early twentieth century, midwives increasingly bemoaned the consequences of physician excesses and the medical establishment's attack on trained and "granny" midwives increased their worries over their future as health care providers. Forceps deliveries often resulted in serious injuries to parturient women and their infants: vaginal tearing; the increased occurrence of puerperal (childbirth) fever, a serious, life-threatening infection; and cranial damage in newborns. Even with these serious physician-created problems, a cacophony of voices—primarily, yet not exclusively male—grew, railing against presumed midwife ignorance and incompetence. New York City stood at the forefront of the midwifery debates.[42]

Therefore, the midwife issue that the AICP encountered was not a new one, especially within the Italian community, where women retained their preference for midwives throughout the 1920s.[43] Prior to 1907, New York City health officials knew that immigrant women preferred midwife to physician deliveries, because of tradition, accessibility, and affordability, and had agreed that midwives could legally practice their trade as long as they provided the Department of Health with two physician letters of recommendation and "a certificate of good moral character." No further supervision or monitoring followed unless clients submitted complaints. Apparently, this system had worked until, in the minds of officials, the numbers of European midwives trained in midwifery schools dwindled when compared to untrained and sometimes illiterate practitioners, as the flow of southern, central, and eastern European immigrant populations into New York City increased.[44]

In response, New York City began its war against untrained midwives by requiring them to register with the Office of the Registrar of Records in 1907. Later that same year, the state legislature mandated that midwifery fall under the control of city boards of health. New York City responded by placing the licensing of midwives under the purview of the Bureau of Child Hygiene in 1909. Medical inspectors controlled the new registration system; they canvassed communities, identified midwives, and explained the new changes under the law.

At first, women who had received formal training at European midwifery schools, such as those in Italy, Germany, Austria, and Denmark, chafed at the notion of supervision and the need to be licensed by the Department of Health, even if the law had been created to eliminate their untrained competitors. The process of "scoping out" midwives, demanding their presence at the Department of Health to register legally, and the registration process itself, probably offended many qualified women who saw themselves as professionals, new laws be damned. In particular, the new registration form may have fueled their resistance by requesting the level of education attained by midwives, place of training, whether the midwives had ever been arrested (and if so, why), and other personal information besides their names, addresses, and marital status. Furthermore, the Department of Health demanded that applicants had to include signatures of two physicians who knew them and had supervised their work. Finally, as with the old registration, a "layman" (preferably a cleric) had to vouch for each midwife's character. When (or if) approved, the registration enabled a midwife to work legally for one calendar year (unless clients lodged complaints or the midwife was arrested or "accused of criminal practice," usually performing abortions), had to agree to monthly inspections of her home and adhere to hygienic methods, proper (or improper, to some midwives) equipment, and character. And after one year, the process began again.[45]

In 1913, the New York City Department of Health increased its vigilance over midwives by creating a special Division of Midwifery and, in the same year, Bellevue Hospital instituted its School for Midwives.[46] Dr. S. Josephine Baker, head of the New York City Bureau of Child Hygiene, had targeted all midwives for mandatory licensing and training, believing that most were ignorant, untrained, and presented health hazards to women and their newly born children. Implied was the notion that the heavily Italian immigrant population was filled with racially lower-class—and thus lower-quality—people. This posture, repugnant to most today, was commonly voiced: "As the character of immigration changed, the class of midwives also changed," stated Dr. Rosalie Bell in an article about how the Department of Health supervised its midwives.[47] Other health care officials took a milder tack, focusing on eliminating the incompetent while creating working alliances with European formally trained midwives and those who would be trained at Bellevue.[48] Public health care workers desperately needed links between their blossoming modern, official system and its more traditional clientele, and many welcomed any means of establishing truces with trained midwives and their client populations, a sentiment reflected in the 1924 AICP pamphlet on its Mulberry work.

At best, midwives who supported the work of the New York City Department of Health and various private organizations, like the AICP, provided crucial validation for these agencies, as they dealt with often hostile and dismissive immigrant populations. In much the same manner as enslaved women before them, many women in these foreign-born communities accorded midwives positions of cultural power and influence, which gave their opinions more weight than those expressed by native-born whites who wielded official power and influence. At worst, if midwives ignored or dismissed the overtures of the public health coterie, at least officials could rejoice that, with stricter licensing measures and the establishment of the Bellevue School of Midwifery, the help given to parturient women was safer and more hygienic than before. The reality lay somewhere between, as public health officials and workers, trained and untrained midwives and their clientele fought for power and control on a daily basis.

In fact, the Bellevue School had been created specifically to provide modern training for midwives and better health care for immigrant neighborhoods that preferred midwife deliveries. Also, officials perceived that the immigrant population had already outpaced the capacities of professionally trained midwives and obstetricians. Even prior to its opening, hospital officials realized that "the 'thoroughly prepared' midwife was to continue functioning in the community" where she would "[tailor] health care delivery to the desires of the family."[49] Still, as midwife licensing tightened, their numbers decreased; in 1913, for example, fewer than 1,400 women held midwifery licenses in New York City. Twenty-six percent listed Italy as their birthplace.[50]

Moreover, since the AICP had considered its maternal work the "entering wedge" of health care to the entire family, once trained, the midwife "could be an excellent liaison for community and health team goals."[51] Thus, in the same manner, Italian female clients could laud midwives in both traditional and modern senses: traditional female birth deliverers whose access to their bodies did not violate cultural norms and bring disrepute to women and their families; and acceptable authority figures trained in the modern methods of midwifery. These characteristics of trained midwives may have elevated them within the community without doing critical damage to untrained practitioners. Bottom line: Italian women preferred midwives, formally trained or not. The agency displayed in this private decision meant their adherence to midwife deliveries constituted resistance against native-born white attempts to acculturate and assimilate them by controlling their bodies.

By the early 1930s, when formal reports revealed that physician deliveries accounted for more infant and maternal injuries and deaths than those of midwives, midwives could finally reap what their care and professionalism had sown. However, with the Depression and an effective war against midwives, the validation came too late. By then, urban Italian women and many first-generation Italian Americans or Italian-born women who had already delivered at least one child by a midwife or had had a prior good experience with a physician delivery had switched to prenatal care and physician deliveries in hospitals.[52] Nevertheless, during the 1920s, most of Mulberry's female population had successfully ignored and dismissed physician deliveries as an approved alternative to midwives.

Yet there remained the equally pressing issue of prenatal care concomitant with the midwifery brouhaha. In 1914, the year prior to the first citywide mortality study, Drs. S. Josephine Baker and Philip Van Ingen (later president of the American Association for the Study and Prevention of Infant Mortality) warned infant health advocates that neonatal mortalities were inextricably tied to the health of the mother before delivery, and that any efforts to decrease neonatal mortality rates must address the health of prospective mothers. This stance, taken by influential leaders in the fields of public health and infant health, marked a critical change in how advocates should tackle the problem of infant deaths. Until that point, they had only concerned themselves with educating and supervising mothers' postnatal care of infants. But Baker's and Van Ingen's argument meant that infant health advocates must now expand their attention to include the bodies of parturient women.[53]

Medical authorities had speculated for centuries that a mother's health influenced the viability of an infant. Just how, though, had remained a mystery. Notions of Victorian propriety made women loathe to submit to vaginal or even stomach inspections. The mid-nineteenth-century rise in women physicians and training schools had addressed this particular problem. Yet, despite intuiting a link between pregnant women's health and that of their infants (however ambiguous and unexplored the connection), infant welfare activists decided early on to ignore prenatal preparation and instead focus on postpartum education and supervision, or training women to become better mothers by hygienically controlling their babies' environments. This, activists believed, would eliminate the two most frequent causes of infant mortality: the diarrhea and enteritis that stemmed from bad milk and improper or tainted food.[54] So, by the late nineteenth century, and with the mortality data that now came from expanding death registration areas, concerned physicians and reformers had already drawn the outline for changes in infant feeding, arguing that, particularly in poorer urban areas, infants who succumbed to gastrointestinal disorders had died from improper feeding methods.

The connection between infant deaths and bad milk or food did not come easily: until the late nineteenth century, scientists had no concept of bacteriology and its causal association with gastrointestinal illnesses, and even death. At first, climate was blamed, for, since the American colonial era, observers had known that something was different about the American climate and its effect on infants and the very young during long, hot summers. Gastrointestinal disorders were considered "infant cholera," and *cholera infantum* had killed many babies. The dying process was particularly difficult to watch: constant crying, vomiting, and diarrhea; extreme dehydration and malnutrition coupled with the inability to ingest and keep down needed liquids; eventual coma and death. Until the 1840s, physicians believed that infant cholera resulted from a humoral imbalance and bad food; after the 1840s, environmental causations leading to ill health came into scientific vogue; later, bad air replaced bad humors and their link to bad food. Historians believe that the ultimate cause of infant cholera was either bacterial or viral, but physicians and scientists lacked the knowledge and means to deduce the cause for several decades. And even later, old perceptions died hard. For example, concerns over bad air and its effect on urban infant health grew during the sanitarianism of the 1860s and 1870s, and remained even when the scientific community gained knowledge of germ theory, bacteriology, and epidemiology. But the potency of bad air paled when compared to concerns over bad food and milk. Even as mid-nineteenth-century "pediatric theorists" had admitted that breast milk was best for infants, they had begun work on artificial options that would move the task of feeding babies away from mothers and into science.[55]

One further step remained—proving the connections between science, infant feeding, and good infant health. This required the rise of pediatrics as its own medical field by the 1880s, no longer a lowly subspeciality of eighteenth-century obstetrics—a valid medical field, but with its own identity and validation problems. This shift occurred as the numbers of orphan asylums and children's hospitals expanded, providing pediatricians with hands-on clinical training. Victorian ideas about children and childhood changed as well, with adults now seeing childhood as a unique time in human development. Moreover, pediatricians approached the care of children holistically, as the move toward specialization grew in other medical fields. To validate itself, however, since the eighteenth century, the male pediatric community had had to prove to the larger public that most women lacked the necessary knowledge to feed and care for infants and children. In his famous essay on child care, William Cadogan had spoken for many male pediatricians when he admitted that childrearing "has been too long fatally left to the management of women, who cannot be supposed to have the proper knowledge to fit them for such a task."[56]

Pediatricians then linked poor feeding methods to all the ills that could afflict a child. To do this, they joined the ranks of experts considering the benefits of proper nutrition. U.S. infant theorists learned of the importance between nutrition and good health from their English and German counterparts, then quickly spread the word. Male physicians had already worked on creating artificial mother's milk that equaled or surpassed the real thing. To finally have the validation of the European scientific community that nutrition *did* influence health justified the movement toward scientifically controlled nutritious baby foods and pediatric supervision of child care, which were given as solutions to the problems of gastrointestinal disorders and high infant morbidity and mortality rates in urban areas. Pediatricians and infant health reformers focused their energies on polar opposites: wealthy women were too "overcivilized" and neurotic to mother properly without counseling and supervision; poor women were too uncivilized, impoverished, and overworked to mother properly without counseling and supervision.[57] Rich women received private care; reformers aided poor women (especially those who could not / would not breast feed because they worked) via publicly and privately funded milk stations, pure food and milk campaigns, and the postpartum supervision by visiting nurses. Prenatal care, built upon theories of women's general incompetence in child feeding and child care, their general lack of scientific or medical knowledge, and their general need for expert supervision, became the next logical step.

But in 1922, when Louis I. Dublin analyzed the progress made by U.S. infant mortality reduction activists, he found their efforts lacking. In a critical paper addressed to colleagues of the American Child Hygiene Association and in his role as the chief statistician for the Metropolitan Life Insurance Company, Dublin charged that while infant health experts nobly and pragmatically focused on teaching women how to correctly feed their babies, the poor languished, having received little concrete help to alleviate environmental conditions that could protect their children's lives. The passage by Congress of the Sheppard-Towner Act of 1921 had given funds to educate women about birthing and child care. However, the monies allocated were small, and some states refused them totally because Sheppard-Towner required matching funds before the release of federal monies. Physicians who had fought against its passage had finally seen its wisdom, adopted its educational techniques, and made Sheppard-Towner irrelevant and redundant. Before the decade of the 1920s had ended, the Sheppard-Towner Act had succumbed due to a lack of funding.[58]

Regardless of the efficacy of Sheppard-Towner's mission to train and educate new mothers, it did not provide funding to help families survive.

Neither states nor the federal government provided adequate financial remuneration that could have improved living environments and saved mothers' lives and those of their children—not in the form of stipends, better housing, higher wages, or food. Additionally, U.S. society failed to view mothering as a job, deeming "work" a largely male prerogative or, when a female activity, one performed prior to marriage and childbearing. Most people still perceived childbearing, child rearing, and housework as women's duties or "work," but not real, paid men's work. Dublin concluded that while the focus on child feeding, though admirable, had done much to decrease total infant deaths from the ages of one month through one year, neonatal, or early infant, deaths, and stillbirths were more resistant to change and had been virtually ignored by reformers and health care professionals. These deaths, Dublin argued, constituted "losses . . . so large as to justify the keenest interest not only on the part of members of this association but of all engaged in public health work." In sum, efforts at educating and training parturient and post-natal women in better feeding and childcare habits had resulted in virtually no reduction in neonatal deaths across the country.[59]

By 1922, neonatal deaths made up half of all infant deaths. These babies died from malformations, congenital diseases such as syphilis, birth injuries, or complications resulting from premature births. But Dublin focused on the stillborn, because officials had "all but forgotten to consider them as deaths," and few registration areas recorded their numbers or the particulars surrounding their deaths. In effect, hundreds of thousands of babies were stillborn without public recognition or concerns over why they had died. Moreover, Dublin argued that many of the contributory factors that resulted in neonatal deaths also affected fetal health and may have caused stillbirths. He revealed that although only 7.6 percent of infants (almost 200,000) had died in their first year of life, fully half of those had died in their first month. Still unrecognized were the stillborn, which Dublin estimated at 109,000 deaths—almost equal to the total number of neonatal deaths.[60]

Determined to reeducate physicians and public health officials to extend their attention to stillbirths, Dublin argued that if one added the numbers of stillbirths to that of neonatal deaths each year, the composite number would exceed the total number of neonatal deaths from tuberculosis and other infectious diseases.[61] Moreover, many of the factors that later led to neonatal deaths also contributed to stillbirths—inferior environmental and socioeconomic conditions, poverty, poor sanitation, parents who lacked hygienic skills, and poor obstetric services.[62] Yet most in the scientific and public health communities had turned their backs on both neonatal deaths and stillbirths, frustrated over their inability to reduce the numbers of deaths they understood little about. Dublin charged them with fatalism, as revealed in a 1917 quote from prominent British writers on the subject:

> Just as in every packet of seeds there are some that do not germinate, and in the young of every flock there are some that do not survive, so it may be suggested that these deaths represent Nature's failures, and man with his present knowledge cannot hope to prevent this loss. . . . We see here natural selection in operation, uncontrolled and uninfluenced by man's efforts, steadily eliminating the unfit, and we realize how shallow is the argument sometimes brought forward that by preventing infant deaths we are in the long run injuring the natural physique by interfering with natural processes.[63]

Dublin believed that, in effect, public health experts faulted nature for large numbers of early infant deaths because traditional thinking regarding causal factors for early infant deaths did not hold true—and this confounded and frustrated them. For example, the data collected from overall infant deaths painted urban life as a primary culprit in most infant mortalities—experts had known for years that, generally speaking, cities produced more dead babies. However, neonatal death rates remained consistent, whether the data came from urban or rural areas. This seemingly contradictory evidence had led many experts to discount environmental factors in early infant deaths, and instead blame neonatal deaths on fate, nature, or Darwinian evolution.[64]

Dublin countered, arguing that, contrary to existing expert opinion regarding the absence of any substantive etiologies for neonatal deaths, many of the same environmental factors that produced overall infant mortalities (those occurring between the first and end of the twelfth month of life) also had negative, disturbing influences on parturient women's bodies and the viability of fetuses and newborns. These variable factors resulted in many stillbirths and neonatal deaths. To prove his thesis, he constructed a series of pertinent questions. First, were stillbirth and neonatality rates consistent: Were they "fairly constant and not subject to considerable variation?" No. There were fewer variations in early infant deaths than in deaths that occurred during months one through twelve. This neonatal variability in deaths came as a shock for many infant experts. For Dublin, the variability suggested a wide range of socioeconomic factors that could have direct and serious influences on early infant life and pre-birth viability.

> There seems, from the facts available, to be good presumptive evidence that factors possibly associated with social and economic conditions, with sanitation, housing facilities, family income, industrial employment of the mother during pregnancy, the hygienic intelligence of fathers and mothers, and the character of obstetrical service, and so forth, are in some manner influential in giving rise to this variation from place to place and from group to group. All of these may be responsible for some part of early infant mortality. In any case, before a negative conclusion can be drawn, it will be necessary to eliminate each one of these items as a possible cause.[65]

Dublin's second question sought any possible correlations between areas with high or low neonatal mortality and overall infant mortality rates; in other words, do areas with high overall infant death rates also post high neonatal death rates? Yes. In particular, places that exhibited significantly high neonatal mortality rates also had high overall infant mortality rates, and vice versa. The answers to these two questions convinced Dublin that neonatal deaths and stillbirths could be prevented if health care officials and physicians placed as much emphasis on the bodies and environments of parturient women and newborns as in teaching postnatal women how to feed their babies. Prenatal care seemed to be the answer.

To test his thesis and premises, Dublin tracked the "practical work" done by the New York City Maternity Center Association (MCA) health demonstration, performed in collaboration with the Henry Street Settlement house from 1919 to 1921. The MCA, a voluntary public health association created in 1918 to supervise maternity centers throughout Manhattan, provided visiting nurses under the direction of physicians, and education and care for the city's poor.⁶⁶ Its goal was to see if prenatal care—then a decade-old, yet sporadically used system still under development in many areas of the nation—could decrease early infant deaths and stillbirths in poor immigrant neighborhoods. Over a twenty-seven month period, nurses and physicians diagnosed, tested, and treated over 8,700 pregnant women and their babies. The process began as women came to the MCA seeking information or assistance, or as visiting nurses combined home visitations with clinic trips. Central to the process was urine testing for albuminuria, preeclampsia and eclampsia, syphilis, and other maternal conditions or diseases that could potentially harm women or their babies.⁶⁷ The prenatal processes extended up until the period of confinement; since the MCA had no facilities or personnel for deliveries, women delivered wherever and however they chose. After delivery, the MCA took up where it had left off, now performing postpartum testing, treatment, and education.

That the MCA focused on urine testing to deduce potential maternal or infant health hazards marked a shift in targeting prenatal health problems and adducing their deleterious effects on women and their babies. As Dublin stated, the MCA and Henry Street Settlement were set on "controlling the albuminurias of pregnancy," or the diseases or conditions that could be deduced by urine testing. Even in 1922, physicians could infer from a positive urine test detecting albuminuria itself (or how damaged kidneys leak the protein albumin into the urine) that the expecting woman might have serious medical problems ahead, and that a stillbirth would likely occur. Today, we know that albuminuria signals the possibility for diabetic kidney disease. Also, traces of albumin in the urine can reveal a propensity for heart disease or hypertension in women—all critical diseases that could have harmful effects on maternal or infant health.⁶⁸ Preeclampsia and eclampsia were also feared, largely because, unlike albuminuria, the etiologies or causes of the conditions were (and still are) unknown. Preeclampsia, or toxemia, is an illness that occurs only during pregnancy; it starts with the tearing away or damaging of the placenta, or the sack that holds the fetus and provides its protection and nutrients. As a fairly common condition, preeclampsia affects fully one in ten pregnant women, with symptoms and results that are usually mild, but can quickly escalate into eclampsia, marked by seizures or fits and comas. Particularly at risk are women who are pregnant for the first time; pregnant by a new partner; over the age of thirty-five; suffer from diabetes, hypertension, or kidney disease; have a family history of the illness.[69] Preeclampsia and eclampsia obviously could wreak havoc on the bodies of pregnant women. The loss of oxygen and nutrients through damage to the placenta could also result in serious mental and physical problems for babies, or stillbirths.

The results from the MCA / Henry Street Settlement's two-year prenatal health demonstration seemed to indicate that high rates of neonatal deaths and stillbirths were not a naturally occurring inevitability, and that adequate prenatal care could save fetal and early infant lives. Dublin pointed out that the maternal mortality rate for eclampsia declined proportionately by 33 percent of what was normally reflected in general, with only three out of nine women dying as a result of the illness. Just as important, only 5 percent of women whose urine had tested positive for albumin had miscarried. Malformations resulting from congenital causes also declined. In addition, the women of the study delivered one-third fewer premature babies than the overall premature delivery rate for New York City.[70]

Yet, as Dublin lauded the work of the MCA, he warned that much more could have been done; there had been no decreases in neonatal deaths arising from congenital syphilis, dystocia, and other birth injuries, or congenital debilities.[71] He maintained that these illnesses and conditions still resulted in infant and maternal deaths because the MCA had no control over where the women in the study had been confined or had delivered. As a result of this lapse in supervision and control, half of the women had chosen home confinement with physician or midwife deliveries, while the other half had delivered in area hospitals. However, some of the cases who had undergone hospital deliveries had contracted septicemia from the improper use of non-sterile equipment or unwashed hands. As Dublin himself admitted, "The benefits resulting from good prenatal work were lost through the breakdown of the obstetrical service."[72]

The MCA / Henry Street prenatal work also fell short because too little attention or importance was placed on congenital syphilis. Unlike the women of African descent in Columbus Hill who had had to undergo mandatory Wassermann testing and syphilis treatment to receive prenatal care, the parturient women of the MCA's study were simply encouraged to receive Wassermann testing. Of those who came forward, the MCA actually tested few and administered even fewer follow-up syphilis treatments. While autopsies confirmed only seven deaths out of one thousand births as resulting from syphilis, fifty-five deaths were attributed to "congenital debility," a loosely amorphous catchall phrase where Dublin admitted that "a considerable proportion of these deaths may rightfully be charged to syphilis. This accounts largely for the unsatisfactory results in the rate from dystocia," he added, "as a factor in early infant mortality." So, despite the emphasis in Columbus Hill and the AICP's four-year work with congenital syphilis as a factor in stillbirths and congenital diseases among black women, or the earlier pathbreaking work done by Dr. J. Whitridge Williams at Johns Hopkins Hospital on maternal syphilis transmission to infants in which all parturient women, regardless of race or class, underwent mandatory syphilis testing and treatment, the MCA and the Henry Street Settlement chose to overlook the possibilities of congenital syphilis as a source of infant mortality among their population. As a result, Dublin believed that the oversight made moot any prenatal care given to mothers or infants suffering from this disease.[73]

Dublin articulated another problem area, charging physician negligence or errors that caused or resulted from dystocia, or "difficult labor." In general, painful or abnormal labors could come from physical abnormalities in a woman's birth canal, weak contractions that would not allow the cervix to open adequately for birth, or fetal misalignment in the birth canal.[74] In some physician cases, however, Dublin argued that doctors had actually damaged women and infants through intervening in the birth process with forceps. Midwives had also leveled this charge against male obstetricians. Here, Dublin stands out for warning what few in the medical community would openly say or admit at the time. He charged physicians with the overuse of invasive birthing tools and techniques, maintaining that

> there is the possibility of reducing early infant mortality through the discouragement of instrumental and other interference with the mechanism of labor. An inquiry among representative obstetricians in the United States and Canada early in 1921 suggested that there has been an increase in recent years in the used of artificial means to hasten labor, and that this

practice is often accompanied by disastrous results to mother and child. The death rate from injuries at birth could be appreciably influenced by a change in this phase of obstetrical practice. In fact, the whole problem of improving the mortality record of early infancy depends upon the betterment of obstetrical service the country over.[75]

Had obstetricians heeded his indictment by lessening their practice of forcep-aided deliveries and cesarean sections, they might have reduced the rates of infections that led to puerperal fever and septicemia, birthing malformations, and deaths.

Conclusion

After its success in Columbus Hill, the AICP moved its next health demonstration into the Mulberry District, perhaps without considering that what it had accomplished with one group of impoverished women might not work with the next. In a period when race was perceived as biological and self-evident, race was race and women were women. Even more broadly, as with their existence in the United States and, more narrowly, with the neighborhoods in which they lived, the reproductive organs of racialized, impoverished women were viewed more narrowly as problematic sites that needed control—white, male, professional control. The southern Italian women and midwives of the Mulberry District stood in their way. To control the former meant eradicating the latter. To control the Italian people meant controlling the birthing practices of its women.

This, compounded with racialized attitudes toward gendered and cultural traditions held by Italians and issues of disease susceptibility, was the status of midwifery vis-à-vis obstetrics before and after the AICP started its health demonstration among the Mulberry District's Southern Italian women. The AICP chose to move its health demonstration into the Mulberry District because of the racial makeup of its inhabitants. What we will see in the next chapter are the results of the AICP's health work, which gave some reason to celebrate and others reason to mourn.

8

Health in the Mulberry District

In its ongoing effort to assimilate southern Italians in New York City by controlling their birthing methods, the AICP made certain that the public health community would understand its mission when reading *Protecting the Mother and Child* by defining its prenatal health care in the Mulberry District as an "entering wedge" into the community.[1] As such, the AICP's entrance into southern Italian families and the community's health through the bodies of women and children constituted the rupture of meanings and traditions, and a subsequent influencing of familial and community power relations. Mulberry women and their children stood at the core of the Department of Health's and the AICP's racialized, gendered, and classed health perspectives, and the health officials' larger social need to control and contain contagions, ill health, and maternal assimilation—the cultural and social locus through which Italian families and communities assimilated or resisted the Anglo American world. The Department of Health and the AICP tried to extend their power and domination over immigrant neighborhoods through infant and maternal health. In exchange, the Mulberry District's inhabitants received exceptional health care—though it was often created and administered by officials and workers armed with the dual intentions of assistance and control. By coordinating with other neighborhood facilities, the New York City Department of Health and the AICP created the Mulberry Health Center, conducted an in-depth community sickness study—the first of its kind in New York City—and by 1923 had developed health care programs for preschool children. In the meantime, the AICP's presence challenged female and male familial and community traditions in ways previously unknown.

The Mulberry District and Public Health Care from the Southern Italian Female Perspective: Prenatal Care

When the AICP attempted to control southern Italian women, it quickly ran into a wall of resistance. The women of the Mulberry District preferred the use of midwives over physician deliveries throughout most of the 1920s. During the period of the late nineteenth and early twentieth centuries, the professionalization of medicine, provable scientific etiologies or the causes of diseases, the massive migrations of poorer populations within the United States, the movement from rural areas into cities, the ascendancy of women's rights campaigns—all these and other factors worked to challenge and ultimately change women's birthing, feeding, and parenting methods. The 1910s stand out as the decade during which New York City and other major cities around the nation began all-out campaigns to license midwives as a means to improve immigrant health, modernize the profession, and control midwives' actions. Simultaneously, medical schools, the American Medical Association, and powerful physicians such as J. Whitridge Williams and Thomas De Lee, campaigned for the eradication of midwifery as a practice. Obstetricians would replace them.[2]

Therefore, New York City's 1915 citywide health survey, the health campaigns that began in Columbus Hill and the Mulberry District, and the stances of accommodation and resistance taken by the African American, British West Indian, and southern Italian women within these neighborhoods occurred as public health care officials and physicians began championing the principles and benefits of prenatal care and physician birthing. Public health officials and infant health activists sold the change from midwives to obstetricians as a natural, necessary progression from well-baby clinics, milk stations, and the visiting nurse supervision of new mothers. From their perspective, when they looked at convincing Italian women to switch from midwives to white physicians, midwives stood in the way. Would the traditional embodiment of women's privacy and familial reproduction become part of this sea change, or would the powerful, modern medical establishment drive them from their craft?

The Department of Health and the AICP initial programs of prenatal care in the Mulberry District encountered stiff resistance from mothers and midwives that crested early and waned over time. It fell far short of its goals, but not from any laxities or hesitations from public health officials, physicians, or nurses. Their failures lay within the professional controversy surrounding debates over and changes to pregnancy care and birthing methods, and the fact that, regardless of the controversies, Southern Italian women wanted nothing to do with Anglo physicians and hospital births. First, the Mulberry Health Center and the AICP supervised only half the births in the area from 1918 to 1928 because many Italian women simply ignored their overtures, refusing prenatal care and retaining their traditional preference for midwives.[3] Their preference for midwives obscured their hatred and fear of hospitals; years later, even Italian Americans—the second generation—still dreaded the thought of delivering in hospitals. In her study of the birthing patterns of Jewish and Italian women whose children were born between 1920 and 1940, Angela D. Danzi found that strong anti-hospital beliefs had been passed on from their mothers and other older female kin. She discovered that "[t]hese attitudes ranged from an outright distrust and fear of hospitals for *any* treatment to a belief that childbirth in particular did not warrant a hospital stay."[4]

Second, when evaluating whether to continue its prenatal service in the Mulberry District in 1929, the AICP questioned the logic of such work "in an area where the racial stock seems to keep down the mortality rate in early infancy." Staff members lamented that, despite all their efforts to change Italian women's birthing habits, in 1927 68 percent of the neighborhood's women had used midwives, a rate five times greater than midwife use for all of New York City (13 percent).[5] The AICP had been accustomed to how readily Columbus Hill's black women had accepted prenatal care and physician deliveries—mandatory Wassermann testing and treatment. The difference in attitude must have been infuriating.

Yet southern Italian women accepted the tenets and intrusiveness of public health care workers to help their preschool and school-age children.[6] This ability to simultaneously reject and accept modern health practices tied directly into the new identities that southern Italian women forged in New York City—reevaluations of traditional notions of self, reflected in sexual, cultural, and civic terms. As the private and public health agencies had relied on negative stereotypes of black women, they also negatively stereotyped southern Italian women as ignorant and superstitious, having relinquished any power they possessed to violent, abusive men. They therefore expected Mulberry women to accept change and accommodate prenatal care and physician deliveries. The health agencies never really invested the time and patience needed to set their preconceptions aside and listen to the women. Yet public health officials, physicians, and nurses correctly gauged the high value that southern Italian mothers and fathers placed on older, healthy children and their ability to learn, work, assist their families, and have a brighter future.

Thus, at stake, for public health workers, reformers, and immigrant communities were differing expectations regarding acculturation and assimilation. The Department of Health and the AICP, in short, did and did not know, or care to learn about, the population they served. They failed in some areas and succeeded in others. Generally speaking, southern Italians harbored a great disdain for authority figures, stretching back to harsh dealings with *padrone* and bureaucrats in Italy. The *contadini* from southern Italy constituted diverse ethnic groups whose languages differed, yet their approaches to health care remained similar. Drawing on customs and folkways, southern Italian women perceived and treated illnesses and diseases differently than U.S. health care providers and reformers. They revered folk remedies and often disdained the advice of doctors and nurses.[7] Southern Italian women's responses of resistance and accommodation, taken together, reflected the new identities they crafted as modern, urbanized female citizens who kept some traditions while abandoning others.

The Mulberry District and Debates Surrounding the Boundaries and Directions of Infant and Maternal Health: *Protecting the Mother and Child*

Beginning in 1918 in cooperation with the New York City Department of Health and the Bureau of Child Hygiene, and culminating in 1924, the AICP's health experiment in the Mulberry District produced data that were published in several public health pamphlets, of which *Protecting the Mother and Child* most directly reveals how the agency thrust its experiment of scientific childbirth and mothering, or its "entering wedge" of public health, education, supervision, and control, into southern Italian families via mothers and infants and, subsequently, into the larger Italian community.[8]

The pamphlet's foreword, written by Bailey B. Burritt, characterized the AICP's infant and maternal work as a health demonstration, created to prove that "a well rounded health service for mothers and children" coordinated and supplemented "existing facilities where they are inadequate" and provided total care if facilities were nonexistent. The AICP defined its prenatal work as the "keystone" of the health work it had provided for more than five years within the Mulberry District. During this period, its work expanded to include preschool children, with the opening of a children's examination clinic and the start of full-service preschool health work in 1923.[9] This dual-edged health care strategy was both educational and preventive, focusing on stages from identifying women from their earliest stages of pregnancy to children before they entered public school. The AICP hoped that, as in its Columbus Hill experiment, an overwhelming majority of pregnant women would willingly visit the Mulberry Health Center (formerly the Mulberry Community House and renamed in 1922) for more than three months prior to delivery to receive what the AICP considered optimal prenatal observation, supervision, and health care. Afterward, the agency believed that these women would return with their two- through six-year-olds for nutrition, dental, and health examinations before the children were enrolled in school, where the Department of Health would assume health care responsibility.[10]

The Mulberry Health Center essentially began with the AICP's prenatal experimental work in the neighborhood in May 1918, conducted by its staff nurses. Nutrition courses and economic relief help began on September 20 of that year. One year later, the AICP's central office was working busily in the area, operating an observation center for children in a New York Diet Kitchen Station, as it continued the teaching of proper infant, child, and nutrition classes and offered prenatal services and "fresh air" assistance for those vulnerable to foul, close tenement air. The actual Mulberry Health Center came into existence in 1922 at 256 Mott Street. The Mulberry Community House—created in 1920 and later renamed as the area's Health Center—had already absorbed the AICP's relief work with the poor, the examinations of prenatal women and children, dental care (provided by the Columbia University School of Dental Hygiene), and nutrition courses. In 1921, the AICP devolved its school-age dental work from the Community Center to P.S. 21 and 106, schools previously covered by the AICP's dental work.

The years 1922–1924 saw the Mulberry Health Center's creation and the further decline in the AICP's services. Simultaneously, the Center added other departments, such as one for adults operated by the AICP and the Dispensary Development Committee. In addition, following the earlier advice of William Guilfoy and Shirley Wynne after the 1915 citywide study, two morbidity and social service surveys were conducted in 1922 and 1924. These occurred as the AICP rethought its centrality in the neighborhood, and as other health care institutions picked up more of its work. By the third neighborhood health survey in 1927, and at the end of its anti-rickets and school dental programs, the writing was on the wall. The Mulberry Health Center ended its prenatal and infant services and preschool clinic in 1928. In a review of its work at its ten-year anniversary, the AICP congratulated itself for the "distinctive character of the health service provided" to Mulberry. When it compared the neighborhood with other health centers that had majority-Italian clientele, the AICP believed that the Mulberry Center stood out for its examination system, the large amount of time physicians spent with each client, and the percentage of clients who returned annually. By the AICP's own criteria, the Mulberry Health Center had been a resounding success.[11]

Yet all had not gone smoothly in the Mulberry District. Chief of the obstacles encountered by the AICP was what it termed the "midwife problem," or the dogged persistence of its foreign-born clientele's preference for midwives. Both midwives and their patients continually challenged the modern medical practices and institutionalized power of the AICP and the Department of Health. The AICP acknowledged that the Italian women's choice of midwives over physicians stemmed from their retention of traditional cultural practices. They also admitted that, when it came to the fairly new practice of prenatal care, persuading "a perfectly healthy mother to go to the doctor long before the time for delivery seems to many a preposterous suggestion." Midwives proved no more trusting or understanding of this novel approach than their patients, since it was their practice to administer women's deliveries

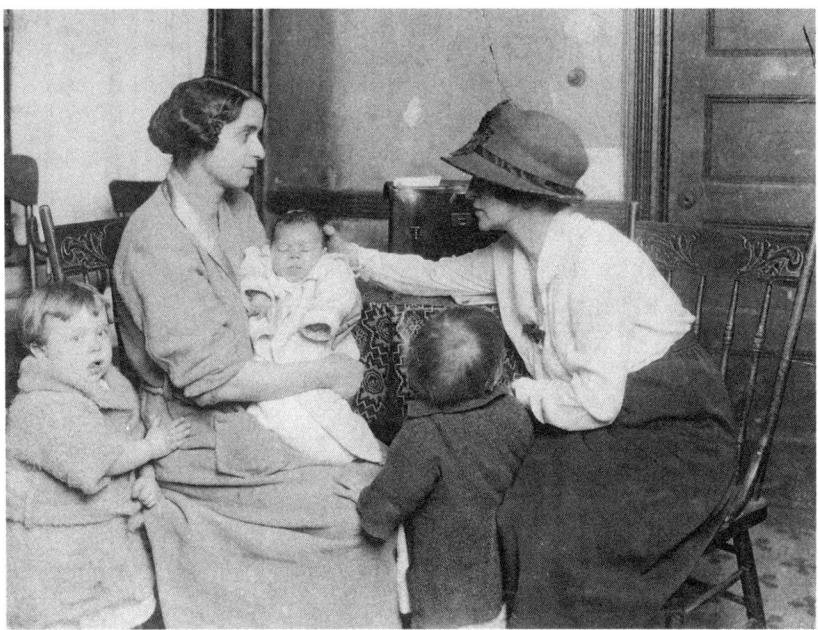

Figure 8.1. Alfred Tennyson Beals, "Mulberry Health Center Album, Visiting Nurse with Mother and Three Children," 1923, Rare Book and Manuscript Library, Columbia University, Community Service Society Collection, http://css.cul.columbia.edu/catalog/rbml_css_0600 (accessed March 2, 2014).

apart from the prying eyes and opinions of men—or women—from outside the Italian community. That these inquisitive, judgmental, and opinionated non-Italian and native-born white American strangers wanted to supervise Italian women and their midwives only made matters worse. To add them and prenatal care to the mix before a birth occurred made no sense whatsoever.[12]

Despite these roadblocks, the AICP said it overcame cultural midwifery traditions and claimed a critical victory over time, as reflected in its *Protecting the Mother and Child* pamphlet: "At first, the midwives were disposed to look with suspicion and apprehension upon the work of the prenatal nurse." It added that Italian midwives jealously guarded their status and positions within the community and "feared that the prenatal nurse, through her intimate relation with the mothers of the district, would interfere with their practice." The AICP had reason to be concerned over competition. As of the 1924 publication of the pamphlet,

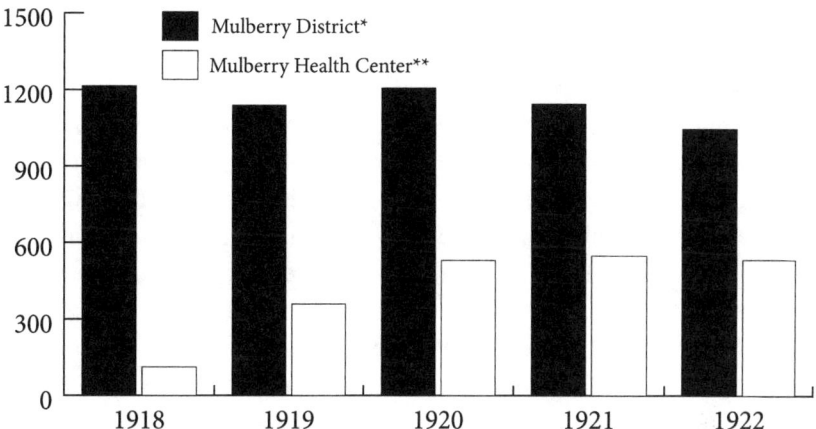

Figure 8.2. Birth rates for the Mulberry District, 1918–1924, comparing actual birth numbers for the area to those under AICP care.

 * Although the 1918–1922 Mulberry District birth data is contained in the AICP's own internal ten-year study of its work, the study states that the "number of births were taken from the records of the New York Department of Health," which should constitute raw data for the neighborhood. "Vital Statistics of Mulberry Health Center, 1915–1925; Part III—Comparison of Birth Rates for Mulberry and New York City, 1915–1925," 11; data taken from "Table VI: Birth Rates for Mulberry Health Center, 1915–1925."

 ** AICP care. This data comes from *Protecting the Mother and Child*, 6, "Table IV—Amount of Prenatal Care for Mothers Delivered during Each Year in the Mulberry District." The data period extends from May 1918 (the 113 AICP delivery number compared to the number for prenatal care reflects the fact that the AICP recorded only five months of births) through October 1, 1922. It is important to separate both sources of these data to graphically see the southern Italian preference for midwife deliveries in Mulberry during the first five years of the AICP's prenatal care and deliveries. Yet "Table III—Number of Deliveries of Mothers Under the Care of Mulberry Prenatal Service Compared with the Total Births Reported for the District" calls the AICP's numbers into question. Here, the district's total births for 1918 and 1919 (New York City Department of Health data) are the same as those which, according to the AICP's "Vital Statistics," originated from the Health Department. The 1920 data for the neighborhood's total births differs by 100 in both publications (1,107 versus 1,207—easily a typographical error), and in *Protecting the Mother and Child*, the 1921 and 1922 Department of Health numbers are estimated, which fits for the publication date (1924, while the "Vital Statistics" publication date is 1927). These differences are not problematic; the numbers of births given as "under our care" are, however, increased in the Table III graph from the data given in Table IV. Yet the AICP states that both reflect the number of mothers delivered by the AICP who had been "under their care," receiving prenatal care that varied from none to three months or more. Even when length of time (for example, in 1922 and for a period of only nine months, the AICP lists 453 mothers whom they delivered and who had received prenatal care, while, for the same year and in another table, 532 cases are listed as delivered, 47 of whom received no prenatal care, resulting in 485 who received prenatal care—the additional 32 babies may have been delivered over the missing three-month period), other data differences have no logical explanations. John C. Gebhart, *Protecting the Mother and Child* (New York: New York Association for Improving the Condition of the Poor, 1924), 5–6.

it reported that midwives had delivered 68 percent of the 1,761 cases in which the mothers had received at least one month of the AICP's prenatal care.[13]

During the same time period, fewer than 2 percent of Columbus Hill's black mothers underwent non-physician deliveries; to receive prenatal care, all had to undergo syphilis testing and, between 1917 and 1923, only five had received no prenatal care.[14] The reasons for the stark difference, of course, reflected their racially gendered and classed positionality within U.S. society, and their particular group identity and agency. Black women who had been denied equitable, modern health care with whites in the American South, or who had struggled to find good health care in the British colonial West Indies, quickly surveyed the landscape of the public health system in New York City and, perceiving themselves removed from some aspects of their usual Jim Crow and British colonial obstacles, demanded admittance and equal treatment.

At the other end of the spectrum were southern Italian women, carrying a distrust of officials and yet courted by the public health community because of their European "white, but not *really white* heritage" that left them in a state of what Robert Orsi has aptly termed "in-betweenness."[15] They also had to deal with racialized, gendered, and classed stereotyping. However, they exercised their identity by clinging to past practices and exercised their agency by ignoring the demands of white clinic nurses and physicians. Thus, even with data that at times has made me scratch my head, the AICP had to admit that midwives delivered more than half the Italian babies in the Mulberry District during the 1920s, and that Italian women and their midwives eschewed prenatal visits for traditional care.[16] Nevertheless, in its 1924 pamphlet, distributed to agencies across the country, the AICP steadfastly maintained that Italian midwives no longer feared visiting nurse intrusions as unwelcome advances into their territory. In fact, the AICP stated that "in many cases the midwife became a staunch ally of the nurse."[17] Considering that midwives held sway over the southern Italian women who preferred their care at least through the 1920s, they probably did not see AICP nurses or physicians as intrusive or threatening.

Therefore, the next obstacle faced by the AICP was getting Italian women to come for prenatal care. The AICP encountered stiff resistance initially. In 1918, the agency recorded 1,215 births within the District, of which only 16 percent of the mothers had received AICP prenatal care. By 1924, however, as the number of births in the Mulberry District declined to 1,100 (an estimated statistic), the percentage of women under AICP care had risen to 41 percent. Correspondingly, the length of prenatal care given to expectant Italian women increased over time, as more women reported for medical appointments prior to delivery. As a result, the AICP remarked that although the client response fell far short of its 100 percent goal, "[t]he influence of the service has therefore gradually spread through the neighborhood."[18] Over time, the AICP believed that its "entering wedge" would triumphantly rupture the closed southern Italian community through the bodies of its women and infants. But that never occurred during the first ten years of the Mulberry Health Center.[19]

The audience for the AICP's publications—other private philanthropic agencies and groups, social workers, public health care providers—may have tempted it to "tweak" or enhance data that, when compared with its internal studies, looks a bit different. Or, perhaps its methodologies of data collection and collation changed over time—though, to date, I have seen no record of this. Yet, even in a study of its own work between the years 1920 and 1925, the AICP knew that its Mulberry data (and thus the efficacy of its work) could be skewed by "nonresident" use of the area's facilities.[20] This became evident when, using 1920 census data to calculate 1920 infant birthrates, the number of births reported for both the Mulberry District and New York City were much higher than the U.S. census data for children under the age of one. This, the AICP admitted, begged the question: Which data should it use to represent and calculate its delivery and prenatal work—that representing the mean infant birth data per thousand of the population, or the birth data per thousand reported births?

The two methods of data collection differed radically. Resident births and deaths, as data collected by the New York City Department of Health, were credited to the mother's borough of residence. Public health authorities and sanitary districts, however, made no attempt to allocate nonresident births and deaths to the actual borough where the mother resided. This resulted in erroneous data; neighborhoods with good health facilities attracted women and children from other neighborhoods and boroughs. Thus nongovernmental statistics could reflect higher birthrates per population, yet lower death rates/1,000 live births, because these infant deaths were not usually recorded in the same neighborhood or borough where the births had occurred. In 1920 alone, the New York City Department of Health recorded 255 more infant births within the Mulberry District than the data collected by the Health Center. If the discrepancy occurred due to the fluidity of families moving out of Mulberry's three sanitary districts, this could result in a population and infant birth differential between the Health Center and the city (as argued internally by the AICP). And, along with this discrepancy, if the Mulberry Health Center and city differed on how they interpreted the boundaries of the sanitary districts, unequal statistics would also result. The truth of either theory remains unknown. Regardless, the AICP stuck with the public health officials' standard of measurement—infant deaths/1,000 live births—to measure its health work until statewide census data could provide the numbers of infant deaths per population for 1925.[21] This position, of course, would reflect high birthrates and lower mortality rates for the area.[22] Either would engender data that could simultaneously enhance or diminish the success or failure of their work.

Nevertheless, the AICP agreed upon one thing in its internal 1920–1925 study: while generally mirroring New York City's overall infant death rates and their causes, those that occurred within Mulberry had been "consistently higher, [and had] shown more violent fluctuations." Both statistical groupings, however, had recorded a steady decrease between 1923 and 1925, so that the infant mortality data of the final year was one-third lower than that of 1920.[23] Also, the AICP claimed that another difficulty in ascertaining the efficacy of its prenatal program was the fact that the Mulberry mortality rate for infants under the age of one week and under the age of one month was lower than that for the city and the U.S. Birth Registration Area.[24] It found this problematic because it contended that it should have been able to attribute this to its prenatal program, but admitted that the data might be incorrect (particularly if considering the resistance of Italian mothers and their midwives to prenatal care).[25]

On the surface, one bright ray of success seemed to be Mulberry's lower neonatal mortality rate when compared to that of greater New York City, as reflected within the U.S. Birth Registration Area. In

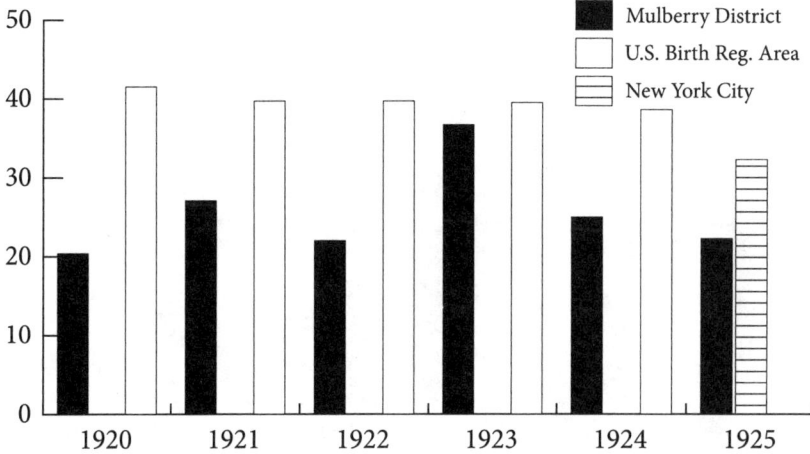

Figure 8.3. Mulberry Health Center infant mortality rates, 1920–1925 compared to New York City and U.S. Birth Registration Area neonatal death rates per 1,000 births.

Protecting the Mother and Child, Gebhart declared that one positive result of the AICP's work could be seen in the reduction of neonatal deaths during the period of 1918–1924.[26] Yet, in the unpublished study of the AICP's 1915–1925 work, when the corresponding 1925 Mulberry neonatal infant mortality rate for babies under the age of one week and under the age of one month was compared to the Mulberry rate for 1921, the decrease for both groups was only 2 deaths/1,000 live births. This led the AICP to question privately how well the prenatal program was running, since the purpose of its demonstration was to further prove the efficacy of prenatal care and the fact that it had tied prenatal efficiency to a decrease in neonatal deaths. In fact, the neonatal death rate did decrease within the Mulberry District, cresting in 1923, and falling by 1925. Still, the 1925 neonatal one-week-and-under mortality rate was 11/1,000 live births, compared to 13/1,000 in 1921, while the one-month-and-under death rate for 1925 was 22.3/1,000, scarcely more than the 22/1000 rate in 1922.

The graph in Figure 8.3 only shows the neonatal (age one month and under) mortality rate for New York City in 1925; the 1918 rate was 35.4/1,000. According to the AICP, the City was missing the corresponding neonatal death rates for 1920–1924. The U.S. Birth Registration Area neonatal death rate was unavailable for 1925 at the time of the study's

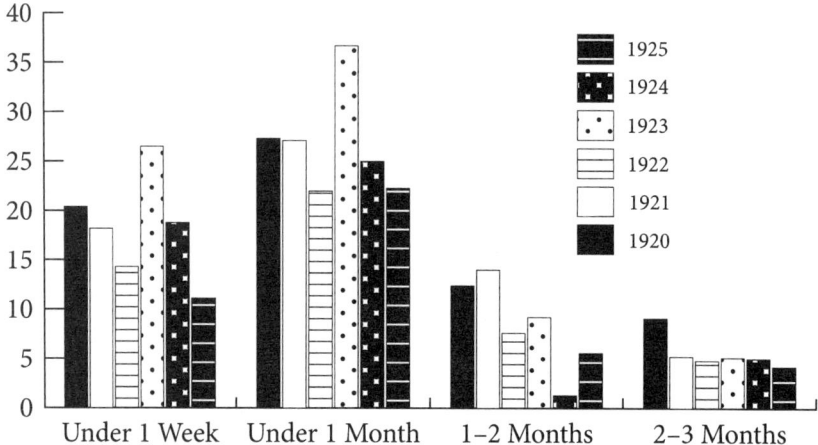

Figure 8.4. Specific age-related infant mortality rates for Mulberry, 1920–1925 rate per 1,000 births. Data taken from "Vital Statistics of Mulberry Health Center; Part IV—Mortality Statistics, c. Infant Mortality Rates," "Table XVI, Summary of Specific Infant Mortality Rates for Mulberry, 1920–1925 (Rate per 1000 Births)," 48.

compilation in 1927. Overall, the Mulberry District's neonatal death rate is significantly lower than the U.S. Birth Registration Area rate (except in 1923). Still, when compared to itself, little changed in terms of a decline in neonatal deaths in Mulberry between 1920 and 1925.[27]

Clearly, perspective is again at work here, as in which data the AICP used to evaluate its success: how the agency evaluated the effectiveness of its prenatal work, reflected in Mulberry's neonatal death rate over time, depended on whether it compared Mulberry to itself or chose to compare Mulberry to the larger scope of the city and nation. In published material and among its peers, the AICP announced that, even with resistance, it was taming midwives, sustaining low maternal mortality rates, and saving neonatal lives—all through its prenatal care program.[28] Privately, however, the AICP voiced concerns freely, questioned data methods, and bemoaned missed opportunities. When the AICP decided to correlate the length of a mother's prenatal care with the survival of her child over its first month of life, it placed itself in a dilemma. The first month of an infant's life is always a critical period. In the Mulberry District, this was especially true, since the standard amount of prenatal care was used to bolster the AICP's argument that there was "clear evidence of a saving of the lives of babies under one month of age."²⁹

The data from figure 8.4 reflects the data that the AICP reported to the public health establishment; the actual infant mortality rates could have been higher because non-resident deaths are not reflected. The data from table 8.1 reflects AICP data that seem very impressive on the surface. However, the 1,990 live births between 1918 and 1922 are those of mothers whose babies were delivered by the AICP. During the same period, however, an estimated 5,660 births in the Mulberry District were reported to the Department of Health; the percentage of total births whose mothers had received *any* amount of prenatal care via the AICP rose from 16 percent in 1918 to a high of 48 percent in 1920 and declined to 41 percent by 1922.³⁰ In other words, although the AICP closely tied neonatal deaths to prenatal care, it attended to a population

TABLE 8.1. Mulberry District: Neonatal Death Rates by Time of Prenatal Care Provided by the AICP / Mulberry Health Center, 1918–1922*

Time period of prenatal care	Total of live reported births	Number of neonatal deaths	Neonatal death rate per live reported births
Inadequate (less than three months)	927	33	35.6
Adequate (three months or more)	1063	21	19.7
Total neonates whose mothers received some period of prenatal care	1,990	54	27.1

* The 1918–1922 time period that I have used is estimated. Although not reflected with the graph in *Protecting the Mother and Child* (8), it is inferred from material in the following from page 5: "Since the work began in May, 1918, and since the report includes only cases delivered prior to October 1ˢᵗ, 1922, comparisons with the total births reported annually is possible for three years only. The fact that in the first eight months, with all the delays attendant on the beginning of such a service, as many as one-eighth of the total births of the year were influenced by the nurses is a remarkable achievement." Later, the AICP admitted that creating a control group of similar numbers of women who had not received any neonatal care had been "impracticable to secure the data for such a study." Between 1916 and 1920, the percentage of neonatal Mulberry deaths for the whole area only exceeded the neonatal death rate percentage of mothers who had received some kind of prenatal care by about 2 percent (29.7 percent overall neonatal death rate, versus 27.1 percent neonatal death rate combined with maternal prenatal care). Nevertheless, the AICP persistently argued that "[t]he difference would undoubtedly have been greater were not the rate for the district influenced by the large proportion of the mothers in the district who had prenatal care," a stance that could never be argued against because the AICP's primary goal had been total control over parturient Mulberry women and their offspring. Hence, contrasting control data had been "impracticable to secure" for the study. According to AICP data, prior to the institution of prenatal care in the Mulberry District in 1916, the neonatal death rate for the area had been 37.1 per 1,000 live births (8).

in which most pregnant women refused prenatal care. No corresponding neonatal death rate reported from the Department of Health was given for a more textured comparison of the efficacy of neonatal work based on the AICP's own standards.[31] The percentages of Italian women who received adequate or inadequate prenatal care may or may not be correct, but unless closely read, the AICP's overall claims and statistics can be misleading. More to the point was the agency's admission that of mothers who had received at least one month of postnatal care, 68 percent had used midwives for home deliveries.

The mothers' use of midwives may have, in fact, saved lives. In *Protecting the Mother and Child*, the AICP had stated that its prenatal program had done nothing to affect the maternal mortality rate from puerperal fever in the area: of the six women who had died under AICP care, five had received more than three months of prenatal care. It is hard to imagine how good prenatal care could prevent deaths occurring from infections due to unsanitary conditions during delivery. In fact, from 1900 to 1935, some studies proved that parturient women were safer delivering with midwives than with physicians; the majority of maternal deaths occurred at the hands of physicians and were attributed to their overzealous interventionism. As a result, puerperal fever could easily come from unsterile forceps and unwashed hands.[32] From 1916 to 1920, Mulberry's maternal mortality rate was 3.7 deaths/1,000 births, compared to almost 5 deaths/1,000 births in New York City, and 8 deaths/1,000 births in the U.S. Death reporting areas.[33] On the other hand, in its own internal study, the AICP revealed that although the Mulberry and New York City maternal mortality rates were quite low compared to that for the nation, since 1921 in the Nursing and Health Demonstration area (which, with sad irony, had focused its work on maternal health care) the number of maternal deaths had risen steadily. Moreover, despite its claims to low overall maternal mortality rates in *Protecting the Mother and Child*, the AICP wrote that "the Mulberry [maternal mortality] rates were markedly high in 1922 and 1923 at the height of the AICP health program in the district with emphasis on prenatal and post natal care," resulting in what they termed as a need for further study.[34]

The only appreciable decline in infant deaths tracked by the AICP occurred in babies between the ages of one and two months: over the six years of its work, the AICP again argued that this marked decrease "was probably one result of prenatal and postnatal instruction." I cannot dispute with confidence using New York City data, however, because the Department of Health had not collected data for every year studied by the AICP in the Mulberry District, and for each age group cohort.[35] Yet one must know and remember an earlier caveat from "Part IV—Mortality Rates, B. Death Rates by Age Group": the 1925 rates for children under the age of four were estimated based on the assumption that "the proportion of children one to four years, for example, bore the same relation" as the area's population rates in the census of 1920.[36] As with the earlier resident/nonresident data debate and the dicey, somewhat misleading data and statements in *Protecting the Mother and Child*, one must approach these statistics with a well-deserved pinch of skepticism, and some of the AICP's claims with an even more critical eye. The decline in the infant mortality rate for babies between the ages of one and two months occurred between 1920 and 1922, when the rate declined dramatically from 20 deaths/1,000 live births to 7.5/1,000. The rate grew slightly by 1924 to about 9/1,000. In 1924–1925, however, the one-to-two-month mortality rate skyrocketed from 9/1,000 to approximately 18/1,000, just shy of its initial 1920 peak. This fluctuation explains the AICP's admission that "[i]t is rather difficult to estimate the amount of success due to our prenatal work in this district for several reasons."[37]

One critical concern voiced by the AICP in its internal study, however, was that the Mulberry District's infant mortality rate for babies between the ages of six months and one year was strikingly higher than that for New York City: twice as high for infants age six to nine months in 1925; three times the mortality rate for those age nine to twelve months.[38] The causes of death were not directly related to tuberculosis, but to other lung- and stomach-related illnesses. Between 1920 and 1925, one-third of the Mulberry District's infant deaths (ages six months to one year) resulted from pneumonia. According to the 1925 data, another third died from enteritis and diarrhea. No equivalent infant mortality causal data exist for New York City by age during the AICP's Mulberry Health Center study period. But the Mulberry mortality data and the AICP's own causal links between infant deaths for these ages groups and corresponding illnesses are equivalent to that for the U.S. Birth Registration Areas (states with the capacity to report morbidity and mortality

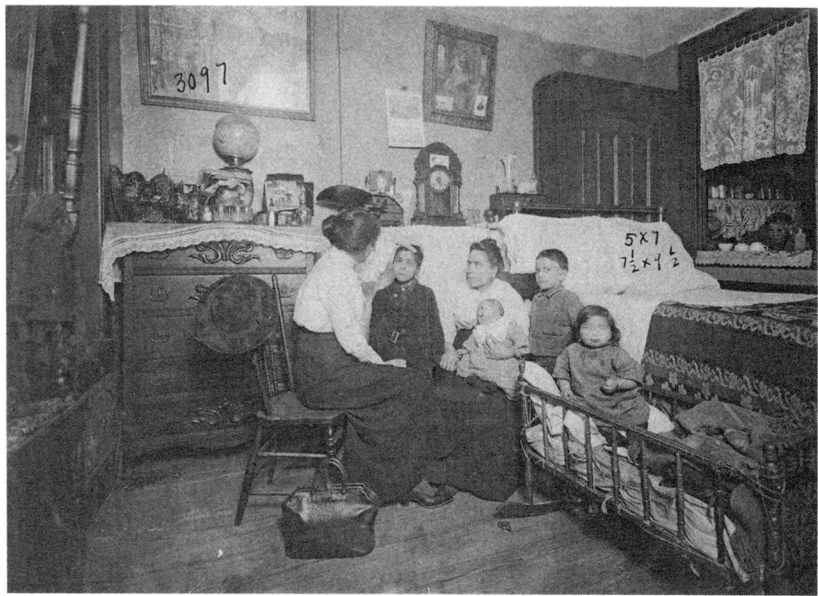

Figure 8.5. Creator unknown, "Mulberry Health Center Album, Prenatal Nurse with Family," circa 1917, Rare Book and Manuscript Library, Columbia University, Community Service Society Collection, http://css.cul.columbia.edu/catalog/rbml_css_0283 (accessed March 2, 2014).

data to the U.S. Public Health Service) for 1924. However, one year later, the Mulberry infant mortality rate from enteritis, pneumonia, and diarrhea was three times worse than that of the U.S. reporting area.[39] And, in 1925, the Mulberry infant death rate for all other diseases of infancy was two and a half times higher than that for the total Birth Registration area.[40] What caused this infant death gap?

First, the AICP admitted that it needed to exert more supervision at the Health Center over mothers with infants in the six-months-to-one-year age cohort. The AICP deemed these babies especially vulnerable because their mothers needed "skilled nutrition and medical advice." Business at the Mulberry Health Center was conducted by age, type of diagnosis, and care needed. The workers gave pre- and postnatal instructions to mothers of children up to two months of age. After that, they referred mothers to baby health stations within the Mulberry Health Center District. Mulberry's nurses picked up the care trail again by visiting the babies at home at ages one and two years. But the plan of passing off mothers and babies from one health nurse to another failed, probably reflected in the fluctuating infant mortality rate. Somehow, while the AICP "presumed" that other agencies and baby health stations were watching the health of babies between the ages of six months and one year, many of these clients may have fallen through the cracks.[41]

Second, considering the resistance to and wariness of the overtures of white public health workers on the part of southern Italian women and their midwives, the result could have been expected. The AICP was ignorant of southern Italian cultural traditions, however. The effects of the AICP studying the Italian six-month-to-one-year mortality problem and its inability to prove statistically that its work had been successful resulted in dismay and angst on its part, as reflected in private departmental records: "Although the population [was] made up of foreign-born, low-income families,"[42] the AICP could not comprehend why Italian mothers had not flocked gratefully to its services. The agency also marveled that, considering that these families could not afford private physicians, they had not reacted favorably to free health care as officials had predicted. In another manifestation of the AICP's limited cultural understanding, it never conceived that southern Italians placed little value on free health services. Accustomed to state-paid physicians in Italy who earned fixed wages and often sported bad reputations, Italians devalued their services because "'when it don't cost anything you might know it is no good.'"[43] This skepticism among the female Italian poor—that free infant health care was worthless, and perhaps dangerous—may have added to the AICP's mounting problems of providing prenatal, postnatal, and early infant care in the Mulberry District. In the end, the AICP concluded that Mulberry's southern Italian mothers needed "more careful health supervision," while admitting that, overall, its infant health plan "ha[d] not worked with any marked success at Mulberry."[44]

So, what AICP health work had been successful in the Mulberry District? With fluctuations in the infant and maternal death rates, and maternal and midwife objections to prenatal care and physician deliveries, the AICP claimed its most successful work had been with younger (preschool-age) children. After beginning its prenatal care, and confident that all children needed educated parents and proper health care throughout their young lives, the AICP purposefully expanded its

TABLE 8.2. Mulberry District: Total Reported Deliveries (1918–1922) versus Deliveries under the Care of the AICP and the Mulberry Health Center

Year	Total reported deliveries	AICP / Mulberry Health Center prenatal cases	Delivery percentage of AICP / Mulberry Health Center prenatal cases
1918	1215	191 (8 months only)	16
1919	1,138	411	36
1920	1,107	533	48
1921	1,100 (estimated)*	521	47
1922	1,100 (estimated)*	453 (9 months only)	41

Data taken from a graph in *Protecting Mother and Child* 5.
* No explanation is given for use of estimates for total reported deliveries in 1921 and 1922.

experiment to include children two through six years old. Arguing that local agencies also covered infants and toddlers and the Department of Health used its nurses to examine school-age children, the AICP said it would shift its focus to the young who languished outside the public health loop, providing protection within their age cohort and preparing them for better health and fewer illnesses after entering school.[45]

As customary, the first infants seen by the AICP during their postnatal period represented a small number of those within the area; only 30 to 50 percent of women who had received prenatal care actually registered their children at infant health stations. From there, the Mulberry Health Center developed its children's health clinic program. Again, progress was slow at first—but this time because neighborhood and surrounding infant clinics and milk stations lacked adequate space and nurses for the number of children the AICP wanted to examine and, as part of the prevention-versus-curative phase that public health itself grappled with, so many mothers brought their children in for cures that no facilities existed for children who were not ill or diseased. In its first year at the New York Diet Kitchen Association, the AICP opened a baby clinic and conducted 604 examinations. By the time the agency had moved, become a community center, and renamed itself the Mulberry Health Center in 1922, it was conducting more than 2,100 examinations, fairly evenly split between first-time and repeat clients.[46]

This bit of success did not stop the AICP from seeing that, as mothers stopped bringing infants to the baby clinic, the numbers of children over the age of two increased. This prompted it to observe that "for a given expenditure of time and money our best contribution to better health of the children in this area lies in providing an intensive service for children of preschool age."[47] The AICP wanted to begin seriously serving the health needs of the estimated four thousand children age six and under within the Mulberry District, and to welcome and pass on the 950 that it imagined would enter at age two or enter school after the age of six and come under the Department of Health's purview. All the agency needed was a plan to isolate these children.

Miss Clara Price, the Mulberry Health Center's supervisor, came up with the idea of forming a consortium or "cooperative experiment" of institutions and agencies that, with their information and efforts consolidated, could provide the AICP with its preschool clients for spring 1923. First, the Department of Health supplied them with the names of

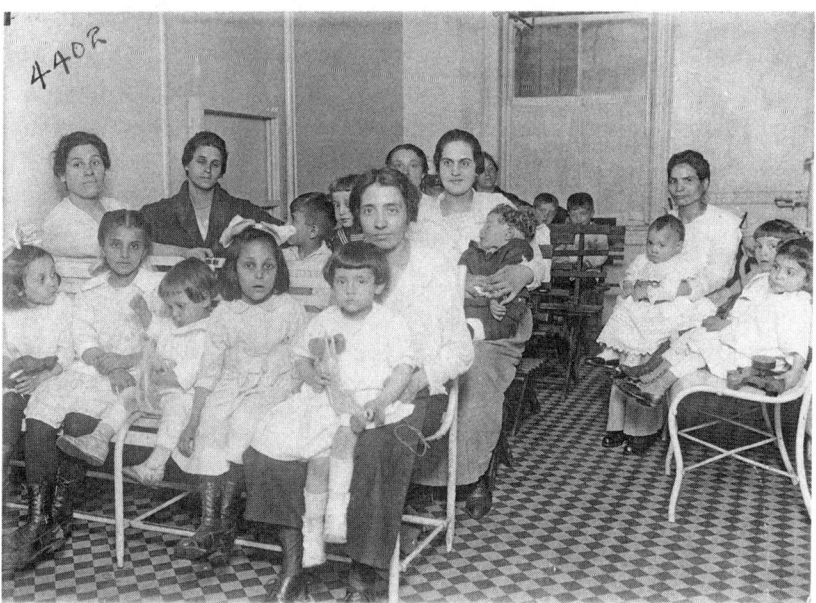

Figure 8.6. Creator unknown, "Mulberry Health Center Album—Mothers and Kiddies Waiting for Care," 1919, Rare Book and Manuscript Library, Columbia University, Community Service Society Collection, http://css.cul.columbia.edu/catalog/rbml_css_0554 (accessed March 2, 2014).

children who had graduated at the age of two from the two publicly funded milk stations in the area. Second, the AICP induced area schools to provide it with a list of preschool-age children whose older siblings attended their institutions. This, along with the children that the AICP already knew about, those encountered by visiting nurses in their rounds, and those whose mothers had received past prenatal care, created a database of seven hundred children, of whom 79 percent received health examinations over the summer.

When *Protecting the Mother and Child* was published, the AICP was restarting the program, expanding the number of children it served, and starting earlier in the year. The agency's examinations and work centered around sound nutrition testing and education, dental hygiene, an anti-rickets campaign, searching for physical defect, such as congenital foot problems, the removal of adenoids and tonsils, lung lesions and breathing capacity, and eye, ear, and skin analyses. Although it missed almost six hundred children who began school in the fall because they had no older brothers and sisters on record for referrals, it considered its first campaign a success. The AICP stated that everyone was happy: the Department of Health because children were being examined who would normally slip between the cracks; the schools because the AICP could examine and refer for treatment or nutrition education those who were ill or malnourished, so that they would enter school on a healthy footing; and the AICP because it had finally found a segment of "neglected" children upon whom it could rivet its focus.[48]

As in Columbus Hill, the AICP used prenatal care as a first step, an entering wedge, toward dealing with the health problems of the Mulberry District. However, between 1920 and 1923, the agency covered only half the total births in the area, and over the five-year period of the report covering the Mulberry Health Center (1918–1923), the AICP's John Gebhart noticed "an alarming mortality among children from pneumonia and among adults from tuberculosis." The agency did experience a reduction in miscarriages and neonatal deaths. But, in fact, the infant and maternal death rates fluctuated and resisted marked change.[49] The second stage, which targeted preschool children, garnered higher success rates in its dental, rickets, and nutrition programs.

The culture, folkways, and worldview of southern Italian women, predicated on their own needs and desires, and those of male and female kin and *paesane*, regulated Italian women's overall rejection of prenatal care and physician deliveries for the work of midwives. However, similar world views and traditions also created a favorable, compliant attitude when it came to Italian mothers and their concerns over the health of their preschool-age children. Thus, what worked for the AICP in one area of health care did not succeed in another. The two programs, offered by the same agencies, met differing levels of resistance and acceptance from southern Italian women, even if their reasons were similar in both cases. In either situation, they refused to let the public health care system manipulate them. Instead, they manipulated it for their own ends.

Despite the rosy picture painted by Gebhart and the AICP in *Protecting the Mother and Child*, had resistance from southern Italian patients and their midwives foiled the efforts of the AICP, the New York City Department of Health, and other agencies? Or had adverse tenement environments and poverty trumped any reasonable efforts of the female clientele and its professional caregivers? Had southern Italian women's assertion of their independence, in challenging native-born whites, actually benefited them and their infants? Or would they have been better off submitting to prenatal and physician care, as they did with preschool care for their older children?

The Mulberry District and Issues of Southern Italian Health: "What Next in Mulberry Bend?"

To review briefly, the New York City Department of Health had invited the AICP in 1917 to institute a public health experiment among Columbus Hill's black community, with a focus on decreasing the neighborhood's ghastly infant and maternal morbidity and mortality rates. In 1918, after one year of success, the AICP found a more racially distinct area in the Mulberry District and began its work there, emphasizing prenatal care and physician/hospital deliveries. This is a pat synopsis; to really see what the AICP thought it had done and why, one must look at the agency's ten-year review as it questioned "What Next in Mulberry Bend?"

This section, contained in "Ten Years in Mulberry Bend," reflects much of the AICP's legacy in Columbus Hill, and even more in the

Mulberry District: optimistic, self-congratulatory, poignant in its missed opportunities and, in internal documents, pained by its failures. The AICP's health work in Columbus Hill and the response of the neighborhood's black mothers had been a roller-coaster ride for the agency: energized by the dramatic decrease in the infant death rate from 1917 to 1918; proud of its initial work and, by the statistics for the first year, justified in narrowing its emphasis to reducing syphilis and congenital syphilis complications in parturient black women and their babies; puzzled at the subsequent increases and decreases in both the maternal and infant death rates; and pained that while making some headway in syphilis testing and treatment, more work existed. The review of ten years of work in the Mulberry District is even harder for one to read because of all the effort, money, and abundance of hospitals, clinics, milk stations, and other health institutions in the area. In short, despite relatively positive public pronouncements in pamphlets on both areas, privately, by 1929, the AICP seemed worn and exasperated.

As the first question in its review—why Mulberry?—the AICP stated that it chose the area because its inhabitants were extremely poor and had not been well served by nearby agencies. This does not reflect Gebhart's earlier 1923 pronouncement that the AICP had wanted to study "this district because it represented a racial grouping."[50] However, the foreword in the 1924 publication, *Protecting the Mother and Child*, does state that the demonstration/experiment was done to coordinate the inadequacies of facilities already in the area, or to create new services that were lacking.[51] As the population decreased over the decade, by 1929 the AICP wondered if the neighborhood now had more than its share of responsive institutions to provide health care, or if its coordinating efforts were still needed.

In a 1924 health study, the AICP had determined that the 15 percent population loss across all ages that had occurred between the 1910 and 1920 census periods reflected a "selective migration," in which families had either earned and saved enough money to return to Italy or had moved to another neighborhood or borough.

The outward movement of Italians from the Mulberry District was also reflected in an overall decline in birthrates and in the numbers of school-age children over the age of fourteen. Thus, families were leaving who were young (either newly married, without children, or

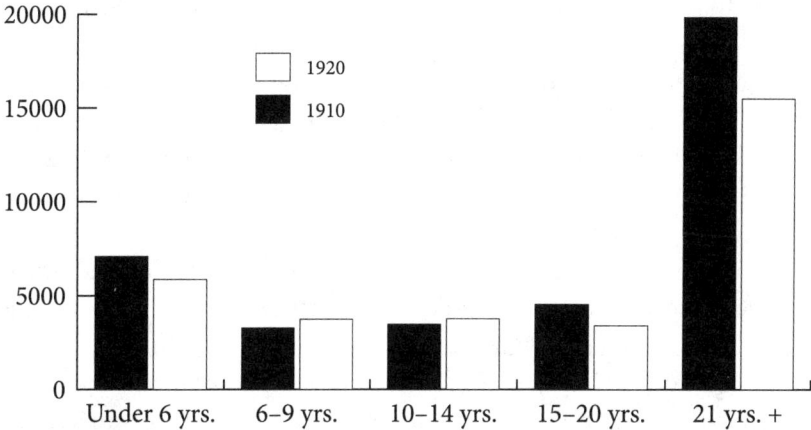

Figure 8.7. 1910 and 1920—Mulberry District comparison of population by age group. From "Population by Age Groups, Mulberry District, New York City, 1910 & 1920 Compared," John C. Gebhart, *The Health of a Neighborhood: A Social Study of the Mulberry District* (New York: New York Association for Improving the Condition of the Poor, 1924), 4.

with children under the age of five) or were older couples who had children age fourteen and over. Literacy rates had increased slightly for those under age twenty-one, with a 50 percent increase in school attendance for six- to nine-year-olds between 1910 and 1920. Moreover, with immigration restrictions during World War I and more permanent restrictions under the revised immigration laws of 1921 and 1924, the numbers of foreign-born southern Italians decreased, and the numbers of first-generation Italian Americans increased. Yet the numbers of males and females who were gainfully employed decreased (from 41.5 percent in 1915 to 35.4 percent in 1922, when the social survey was taken). In addition, the crude death rate for Mulberry's citizens versus that for New Yorkers in general remained high between 1916 and 1920, and in 1922 more than 46 percent of the survey respondents declared themselves suffering from a physical disability. Thus, as the AICP conducted its health demonstration work, even the tenor of its clientele began to change. The number of those left behind who were illiterate in English (or even in Italian) increased, as did periods of unemployment and, from the AICP's perspective, the number of people suffering from ill health. Even with advances in literacy and in the numbers of native-born Italian Americans who were fluent in both English and Italian, Gebhart observed that those who remained in the Mulberry District were "that remnant of the population which has serious economic and educational handicaps."[52] This made the AICP's broad mandate as a coordinator of preventive health care, health education, supervision, dental care, and diagnoses and treatment for pregnant women and their children increasingly difficult.

Southern Italian women and midwives effectively blocked efforts at prenatal care and physician deliveries between 1918 and 1928 to the point that, in 1929, the AICP questioned the logic in continuing its original prenatal focus in the face of such powerful resistance.[53] However, its Mulberry Health Center had successfully served the postnatal and preschool-age children who lived in the area. Upon realizing that baby health stations (already in existence before the AICP opened one in 1919) could effectively monitor babies after six months of supervision by the AICP and other agency nurses, and that the Department of Health's health and hygiene programs monitored children from their first enrollment onward, the AICP targeted children from the ages of two to six for its clinic services.[54]

Thus the AICP's ten-year efforts in Mulberry seemed redeemed. It would not be until the 1930s that appreciable numbers of southern Italian women, whether through circulating more outside their communities and hearing other women speak positively about less traditional modes of childbirth and mothering, having a bad midwifery experience, or approaching the end of their reproductive years and less fearful of peer pressure, would try physicians and hospital deliveries. The choice between home and hospital, midwife and physician, lay in four considerations: what the woman preferred; if her preference was readily available; what her preference cost; and after completion, if she was satisfied by the result.[55] Changes to any or all of these could signal the bed-to-hospital and midwife-to-physician shift, and since midwives were under severe attack, the writing was on the proverbial wall, however faint. By the end of the 1920s, the AICP should have felt redeemed by its preschool health program initiatives. Yet, in May 1929, as it questioned how to proceed, it agreed that its work had declined, being done by other institutions, yet that its work had created greater need for health care in the area. If the latter was valid, they wondered, "How is the center to discharge this obligation to its constituency?"[56]

Conclusion

Somehow, the AICP had produced a questionable reduction in neonatal deaths in the Mulberry District, yet introduced amazingly effective preschool health programs. Had the AICP and the New York City Department of Health given southern Italian women more respect, paid more attention to the cultural identities and traditions in their private lives and to what the women found important for themselves and their children, they might have been more successful in increasing prenatal and postpartum care, lowering the overall infant mortality rate and its corresponding relationships to enteritis and pneumonia, and reducing tuberculosis and respiratory deaths among women. To be sure, the AICP would have needed more help and openness from Mulberry's women. This help and openness gradually expanded by the Great Depression as Italian immigrant women grew more accustomed to doctors, nurses, and hospitals, and as their Italian American daughters explored their new identities as Americans, challenged the centripetal forces of family and community, and replaced the supremacy of maternal and female kinship ideas with those from medical professionals. With more openness, the Mulberry Health Center's nurses and physicians might have diagnosed more pertinent factors that resulted in infant and maternal morbidities and mortalities—evidence of tuberculosis within the family, the effect of cold, dank, airless rooms crowded with family and boarders, the effect of maternal overwork within and outside the home, and the effect of malnourishment resulting from gnawing poverty. Southern Italian women may have kept their identities and their bodies and those of their infants close to their vests, but public and private institutions that funded health care, while ignoring the effects of poverty, kept their monies even tighter. Both parties lost valuable ground in the process.

Comparatively, the health work that occurred in Columbus Hill and the Mulberry District reveals the AICP's successes and failures. As a clearinghouse that merged various private and public agencies to assist the poor and infirm, the AICP valued its public face, perhaps as much as its desire to improve the health of New Yorkers. But how the AICP staff and its allied pool of health care officials, physicians, nurses, and social workers viewed and defined "New Yorkers" shaped its plans and programs. What began as a much-needed health demonstration to show the Department of Health that inordinately high infant and maternal mortality rates in a poor black neighborhood could be addressed and effectively reduced soon moved into a southern Italian neighborhood with lower but still critical levels of infant and maternal deaths. Outcomes differed in both cases—but the differentials cannot be understood in isolation without viewing both neighborhood health experiments through the eyes of its female clientele, and their accompanying stances of accommodation and resistance to the health care they and their children received. While client surveys recording the opinions of African American, British West Indian, or southern Italian women who took part in the health demonstrations were never conducted, the AICP and Department of Health data (even when murky) point to acts of resistance and accommodation that, coupled with attitudes from other sources, albeit songs and plays or migration studies and novels, may draw us closer to their opinions.

The health work done in Columbus Hill and in the Mulberry District may be seen as having ridden the crest of a scientific sea change, one in which germ theory had conclusively eliminated the need for older explanations of disease or health. Racialists had found humoralism and sanitarianism complementary sites from which to link tenets of biological determinism to who should be healthy or diseased and why. Everything was determined by blood; the blood of some was inherently inferior or feeble to the blood of others, even to the point of choosing to live in filthy environments. Germ theory should have taken care of this. Unfortunately, as Nancy Tomes, Troy Duster, and others scholars have shown, even contradictory methods of analysis can become complementary sites of difference when interwoven with prejudices and stigmatizations. While the women and babies of Columbus Hill and the Mulberry District received cutting-edge health care for the time, what they received could have been much more effective if existing social inequalities had not been allowed to shape the experiments—and thus, the outcomes.

NOTES

INTRODUCTION

1. Judith Walzer Leavitt, *Typhoid Mary: Captive to the Public's Health* (Boston: Beacon Press, 1996), 41.

2. William Guilfoy, M.D., and Shirley W. Wynne, M.D., *An Analysis of Mortality Returns of the Sanitary Areas of the Borough of Manhattan for the Year 1915* (New York City Department of Health, 1916), 16–18.

3. Alan M. Kraut, *Silent Travelers: Germs, Genes, and the "Immigrant Menace"* (Baltimore: Johns Hopkins University Press, 1994), 115–127; Nancy Tomes, *The Gospel of Germs: Men, Women, and the Microbe in American Life* (Cambridge, MA: Harvard University Press, 1998), 34–46, 135–164, 183–195. These women also fell under the gaze of native-born middle-class white public health reformers. Black and Southern Italian women responded differently to poverty—a factor that many reformers increasingly perceived as detrimental to adequate health. During the Progressive Era, many public health reformers—regardless of gender—believed that women they perceived as impoverished and possessing a racially gendered inferiority should be educated in proper, middle-class Anglo American modern hygienic methods of health care and mothering in order to protect the health of the native white majority. These measures tended to insure that potentially defective children and adults would not become a financial drain on society, but conform as "Americans" within narrowly defined notions of their proper place in the social order. The health reformers' focus on the "reproductive" nature of women—as sexual, cultural, and civic beings—often ran contrary to how these women viewed themselves and their places within their new societies.

In this book, I use cultural theorist Stuart Hall's definition of "modern" as seen within his description of the development of the "modern state." Hall writes that the concept of the term "modern" is difficult to define and highly contested but, when read through the elements of statehood, connotes issues of power and domination. Briefly, sovereign states have the rights and responsibilities to protect their citizens and, in turn, to command compliance to laws and regulations, to the point of exercising their powers to force adherence because they also have capacities for enforcement. Moreover, even in democracies, sovereign states relate to citizens within hierarchical structures that shape and reflect social inequalities, norms, and dominant cultural mandates. Of course, the state's powers and legitimacy can be challenged, by revolutionary force, or something as nonviolent as citizens using the state's own laws to reign in its powers. I find this conversion of modern and the modern state helpful because the female clientele within my study ultimately dealt with the New York City Department of Health, a governmental entity with powers to protect society even if individual rights and traditions were challenged or even violated in the process. See Stuart Hall, "The State in Question," in *The Idea of the Modern State*, Gregor McLennan, David Held, and Stuart Hall, eds. (Milton Keynes, England: Open University Press, 1984), 14–17.

4. Guilfoy and Wynn, *An Analysis of Mortality Returns of the Sanitary Areas of the Borough of Manhattan for the Year 1915*, 29–31.

5. Stanley Lieberson, *A Piece of the Pie: Blacks and White Immigrants Since 1880* (Berkeley: University of California Press, 1980), 1–15, 250–252.

6. Ibid., xi–xii, 1–15.

7. I reviewed archives for the New York Association for Improving the Condition of the Poor (Columbia University's Butler Library Rare Book and Manuscript Library); the New York City Department of Health (housed at the city's Municipal Archives); daily patient admittance records of the Vanderbilt Clinic and the Sloane Hospital (both were in Columbus Hill), housed at Columbia University's Presbyterian Hospital; the correspondence and records of the Maternity Center Association (Mulberry District) at the Rockefeller University archives in Manhattan (some of the MCA's Mulberry statistical reports are also at Columbia University); and the federal and state census data for New York City (New York City Public Library), and the Schomburg Center for Black Culture. They all have provided rich sources of statistical data.

8. Norman L. Holmes, "Columbus Hill: The Story of a Negro Community." *Opportunity* 1, no. 1 (January 1923): 10.

9. Guilfoy and Wynne, *An Analysis of Mortality Returns*, 16–18.

10. See Allan M. Brandt, *No Magic Bullet: A Social History of Venereal Disease in the United States Since 1880* (New York: Oxford University Press, 1987); Kenneth F. Kiple and Virginia Himmelsteib King, *Another Dimension to the Black Diaspora: Diet, Disease, and Racism* (New York: Cambridge University Press, 1981), Alan M. Kraut, *Silent Travelers: Germs, Genes, and the Immigrant Menace* (Baltimore: Johns Hopkins University Press, 1995); Sandra Opdycke, *No One Was Turned Away: The Role of Public Hospitals in New York City Since 1900* (New York: Oxford University Press: 1999); Katherine Ott, *Fevered Lives: Tuberculosis in American Culture Since 1870* (Cambridge, MA: Harvard University Press, 1996); Sheila M. Rothman, *Living in the Shadow of Death: Tuberculosis and the Social Experience of Illness in American History* (Baltimore: Johns Hopkins University Press, 1994); Naomi Rogers, *Dirt and Disease: Polio Before FDR* (New Brunswick, NJ: Rutgers University Press, 1996); Susan L. Smith, *Sick and Tired of Being Sick and Tired: Black Women's Health Activism in America, 1890–1950* (Philadelphia: University of Pennsylvania Press, 1995).

11. Kraut, *Silent Travelers*, 1–9.

12. The phrase "disease and difference" pertains to an awareness that different cultures respond differently to contagious diseases. For example, upon contact with West African peoples, Europeans noticed increased mortalities from malaria, on their

part, that seemed to bypass Africans or have a diminished effect on them. The supposed African immunity to malaria helped Europeans justify using slave labor in tropical areas of the New World: whites died in much larger numbers, and the European perception of slave immunity meant that Africans were more likely suited to hard, manual labor in the tropics. In reality, West Africans and their descendants did contract the two forms of malaria found in North America: *plasmodia falciparum* and *plasmodia vivax*. Many blacks died if they encountered one type of malaria but had immunity to the other; however, they died in smaller numbers than did previously unexposed Europeans. The resistant antibodies that passed through African mothers who had survived malarial attacks provided the key for their children's survival, but most Europeans racialized this difference. For further discussion, see Todd L. Savitt, "Slave Health and Social Distinctiveness," in *Disease and Distinctiveness in the American South*, Todd L. Savitt and James Harvey Young, eds. (Knoxville: University of Tennessee Press, 1988); Savitt's *Medicine and Slavery: The Diseases and Health Care of Blacks in Antebellum Virginia* (Urbana: University of Illinois Press, paperback reissue, 2002); James O. Breeden, "Disease as a Factor in Southern Distinctiveness," in *Disease and Distinctiveness in the American South*; and Kiple and King, *Another Dimension to the Black Diaspora*. For a discussion of American colonial "seasoning," see Edmund Morgan, *American Slavery, American Freedom* (New York: W. W. Norton, 1975).

13. In theory, "virgin soil" epidemics are those contracted by populations previously unexposed to a new contagion carried by humans with no prior contact (Kraut, *Silent Travelers*, 22). For another perspective on the virgin soil vs. homogenous genetic variability, see Elizabeth A. Fenn, *Pox Americana: The Great Smallpox Epidemic of 1775–1782* (New York: Hill and Wang, 2001).

14. Kraut, *Silent Travelers*, 22–49; Charles E. Rosenberg, *The Cholera Years: The United States in 1832, 1849, and 1866* (Chicago: University of Chicago Press, 1987), 1–9, 175–191.

15. Kraut, *Silent Travelers*, 119–125. Like Dr. William Guilfoy, however, Dr. Stella did agree that Italians were predisposed to having weaker lungs, and thus more susceptible to respiratory diseases resulting from the poor air in urban areas (127).

16. Kraut, *Silent Travelers*, 107–111.

17. See James H. Jones, *Bad Blood: The Tuskegee Syphilis Experiment*, rev. ed. (New York: The Free Press, 1992); Kiple and King, *Another Dimension to the Black Diaspora*; Susan L. Smith, *Sick and Tired of Being Sick and Tired: Black Women's Health Activism in America, 1890–1950* (Philadelphia: University of Pennsylvania Press, 1995).

18. James C. Scott, *Domination and the Arts of Resistance: Hidden Transcripts* (New Haven, CT: Yale University Press, 1990), 1–16.

19. Herbert G. Gutman, *The Black Family in Slavery and Freedom* (New York: Vintage Books, 1977), 453–454. Although Gutman states that the composition of native-born African American and British West Indian households changed over time (both groups accepted more tenants and non-nuclear members), still, the majority of

black families in San Juan Hill (Columbus Hill) and in Central Harlem retained male heads of households between 1905 and 1925.

20. Frances Blascoer, *Colored School Children in New York*, Eleanor Hope Johnson, ed. (New York: Negro Universities Press, 1970; originally published in 1915 by Public Education Association of the City of New York), 81–84; Abram Harris, "Digest of Preliminary Findings in Columbus Hill" (New York, unpublished manuscript, National Urban League, 1922), 2–4.

21. Kraut, *Silent Travelers*, 116–118.

CHAPTER 1. MIGRATION AND THE CITY

1. William Guilfoy, M. D., and Shirley W. Wynne, M. D. *An Analysis of Mortality Returns of the Sanitary Areas of the Borough of Manhattan for the Year 1915* (New York: New York City Department of Health, 1916), 29–31.

2. John Higham, *Send These to Me: Immigrants in Urban America*, rev. ed. (Baltimore: Johns Hopkins University Press, 1984), 20–23; John Higham, *Strangers in the Land: Patterns of American Nativism, 1860–1925* (New Brunswick, NJ: Rutgers University Press, 1994), 110–116; Donna Gabaccia, *From Sicily to Elizabeth Street: Housing and Social Change Among Italian Immigrants, 1880–1930* (Albany: State University of New York Press, 1984), 53–57; Kathie Friedman-Kasaba, *Memories of Migration: Gender, Ethnicity, and Work in the Lives of Jewish and Italian Women in New York, 1870–1924* (Albany: State University of New York Press, 1994), 17–18.

3. Russell Menard reference and quote taken from Rudolph J. Vecoli and Suzanne M. Sinke, eds., *A Century of European Migrations, 1830–1930* (Urbana: University of Illinois Press, 1991), 4.

4. Matthew Frye Jacobson, *Whiteness of a Different Color: European Immigrants and the Alchemy of Race* (Cambridge, MA: Harvard University Press, 1998), 18–19, 116–117, 223–230. Jacobson highlights the "slippery" nature of whiteness, from the mention of the United States offering naturalized citizenship only to "free white persons" in its first 1790 law, to the 1870s, when immigrants of African descent were granted the right to petition for citizen status. The period from the 1870s to the 1920s was also a time when the ambiguity of whiteness hardened as court cases filed by Asians and Mexicans challenged the parameters of "free white persons," and courts created "Caucasian" and whiteness while looking for legal bases for the terms, and thus justified keeping some groups out of the picture.

5. Vecoli and Sinke, *A Century of European Migrations*, 4.

6. Norman A. Holmes, *Preliminary Report of Survey of Colored Population of Columbus Hill and Vicinity* (New York: Lincoln House Committee of the Henry Street Settlement, 1922), 2. Hereafter, this study will be referred to as *Preliminary Report*.

7. Gilbert Osofsky, *Harlem: The Making of a Ghetto: Negro New York, 1890–1930*, 1st ed. (Chicago: Elephant Paperbacks, 1996), 46–52.

8. Norman A. Holmes, "Sociological Survey of the Negro Population of Columbus Hill of New York City" (typescript, Lincoln House Committee on the Henry Street

Settlement, New York, October 14, 1922), 4. Hereafter, this study will be referred to as "Sociological Survey."

9. Holmes, "Sociological Survey," 1. Prior to World War I, Columbus Hill had also been known as San Juan Hill due to the black troops who fought with Theodore Roosevelt on San Juan Hill in the Spanish-American War, and returned back to the area. See Osofsky, *Harlem: The Making of a Ghetto*, 67.

10. Abram L. Harris, "Digest of Preliminary Findings in Columbus Hill" (New York: Lincoln House Committee of the Henry Street Settlement, 1922), photocopy, 3.

11. Holmes, *Preliminary Report*, 2.

12. May 24 meeting minutes of "Mr. Burritt," n.y. (CSS, box 36, folder 132).

13. Holmes, "Sociological Survey," 5–6.

14. Ibid., 6–7.

15. Ibid., 7.

16. Harris, "Digest of Preliminary Findings," 2.

17. Osofsky, *Harlem: The Making of a Ghetto*, 112–113, 123.

18. Bailey B. Burritt letter to Franklin B. Kirkbride, February 5, 1918 (CSS, box 36, folder 132) 4.

19. Nancy Tomes, *The Gospel of Germs: Men, Women, and the Microbe in American Life* (Cambridge, MA: Harvard University Press, 1998), 185.

20. COS Case Record R2036, October 9, 1917 (CSS, box 285), 1. I want to give special thanks to the Community Service Society of New York (CSSNY) for granting me access to the CSSNY archives, located in the Columbia University Rare Book and Manuscript Library. I use pseudonyms to protect the identities of clients, family members, and case workers. The New York City Community Organization Society became known as the Community Service Society in 1939 after merging with the New York City Association for Improving the Condition of the Poor. CSS still plays a critical role in advocating for the city's poor. Unfortunately, there is a large gap in surviving case files between the years 1918 and 1935. According to the COS online finding aid (http://www.columbia.edu/cu/libraries/inside/projects/findingaids/scans/pdfs/ldpd_rbml_4079675.pdf.), the Community Service Society suspects that the original case files were microfilmed, but that these microfilms and many of the original case files were subsequently lost or destroyed. For further information on the Community Service Society, see http://www.cssny.org/pages/our-history, accessed February 24, 2014.

21. COS Case Record R2036, November 1, 1917.

22. COS Case Record R2036, July 30, 1917 and November 1, 1917.

23. COS Case Record R2036, July 26, 1917.

24. COS Case Record R2036, September 11, 1918.

25. COS Case Record R2036, September 11, 1918.

26. Emma Lazarus, "The New Colossus" [titled "Sonnet" in notebook] 1883. Manuscript poem, bound in journal. Courtesy of the American Jewish Historical Society, New York and Newton Centre, Massachusetts (41), http://www.loc.gov/exhibits/haventohome/haven-century.html#obj1, accessed November 12, 2014.

27. Joe William Trotter, ed., *The Great Migration in Historical Perspective: New Dimensions of Race, Class, and Gender* (Bloomington: Indiana University Press, 1991), viii.

28. Darlene Clark Hine, "Black Migration to the Urban Midwest: The Gender Dimension, 1915–1945," in Trotter, *The Great Migration in Historical Perspective*, 127–135.

29. C. Vann Woodward, *Origins of the New South, 187–1913* (Baton Rouge: Louisiana State University Press, 1971), 14, 75. While denouncing use of the term "Bourbon Democrats" to define post-Emancipation whites in Georgia, Woodward states that the label "was a much-abused epithet, with its implications of obstinate adherence to the old loyalties and abhorrence of the new" (14).

30. Jacqueline Jones, *Labor of Love, Labor of Sorrow: Black Women, Work, and the Family, From Slavery to the Present* (New York: Vintage Books, 1995), 153–154, 156.

31. Beverly Guy-Sheftall, "Daughters of Sorrow: Attitudes Toward Black Women, 1880–1920," in *Black Women in United States History*, edited by Darlene Clark Hine (Brooklyn, NY: Carlson Publishing, 1990), 93. See also chapter 2 in Linda Kerber, *No Constitutional Right to be Ladies: Women and the Obligations of Citizenship* (New York: Hill and Wang, 1998).

32. Kerber, *No Constitutional Right to be Ladies*, 50–55

33. Jones, *Labor of Love, Labor of Sorrow*, 58–68.

34. Ibid., 157.

35. Jessie Clark and Gertrude E. McDougald, *A New Day for the Colored Woman Worker* (New York: Consumer's League of the City of New York, 1919), 6–9; Jones, *Labor of Love, Labor of Sorrow*, 153–154. Alice Kessler Harris writes of how women working in factories and stores used race (if needed) to force employers to hire only "whites," and not other European or African American women, or only Polish women, instead of women from other groups. See Harris, *Out to Work: A History of Wage-Earning Women in the United States* (New York: Oxford University Press, 1982), 137–141. I employ "gradations" of whiteness here to describe the ephemeral and socially defined nature of the term, but also its reality as some native-born white women of northern European backgrounds actively discriminated against their southern and eastern European counterparts, to the point of coercing bosses not to hire them. Sadly, in turn, many southern and eastern European women, part of whiteness but not considered fully white by whites, used the same ploys against each other.

36. Osofsky, *Harlem: The Making of a Ghetto*, 57–58. In actuality, women of African descent who worked as domestics in New York City made up less than 3 percent of the total number of domestics; one would be far more likely to see Irish and German women working in the homes of wealthy whites during the period. Also, as home technologies advanced, the need for domestics within the middle classes declined. Also see Carter G. Woodson, *A Century of Negro Migration* (Mineola, NY: Dover, 2002), 172–173.

37. Jones, *Labor of Love, Labor of Sorrow*, 160–162.

38. Trotter, *The Great Migration in Historical Perspective*, "Introduction," 1–14.

39. Farah Jasmine Griffin, *Who Set You Flowin'?: The African-American Migration Narrative* (New York: Oxford University Press, 1995), 10–12.

40. Peter Novick, *That Noble Dream: The "Objectivity Question" and the American Historical Profession* (Cambridge, UK: Cambridge University Press, 1988; reprint, 1996), 1–15.

41. Griffin, *Who Set You Flowin'?*, 13–18.

42. Hazel Carby, "'It Jus' Be's Dat Way Sometime,'" *Radical America* 20, no. 4 (1986): 13.

43. Hine, "Black Migration to the Urban Midwest: The Gender Dimension, 1915–1945," 130–131; Dorothy Roberts, *Protecting the Black Body: Race, Reproduction, and the Meaning of Liberty* (New York: Pantheon Books, 1997), 82, 89; Kevin K. Gaines, *Uplifting the Race: Black Leadership, Politics, and Culture in the Twentieth Century* (Chapel Hill: University of North Carolina Press, 1996), 133–136; Gail Bederman, *Manliness and Civilization: A Cultural History of Gender and Race in the United States, 1880–1917* (Chicago: University of Chicago Press, 1995), 58–60; Glenda Gilmore, *Gender and Jim Crow: Women and the Politics of White Supremacy in North Carolina, 1896–1920* (Chapel Hill: University of North Carolina Press, 1996), 61–89.

44. Gaines, *Uplifting the Race*, 12–13, 72–76, 85–88. Also see Deborah Gray White, *Too Heavy a Load: Black Women in Defense of Themselves, 1894–1994* (New York: W. W. Norton, 1999), 60–66.

45. John F. Matheus, *'Cruiter*, in *Readings from Negro Authors: For Schools and Colleges, with a Bibliography of Negro Literature*, edited by Otelia Cromwell, Lorenzo Dow Turner, and Eva B. Dykes. (New York: Harcourt, Brace and Company, 1931), 162–175. All quotations are taken from this source.

46. Cromwell et al., *Readings from Negro Authors*, 368.

47. CSS Reference Number R2060, COS Case Study Number 173219, letter from the Charity Organization Society to the Superintendent of the City Magistrates' Courts, July 29, 1921 (CSS Case Study, box 286).

48. CSS Reference Number R2060, COS Case Study Number 173219, 1.

49. CSS Reference Number R2060, COS Case Study Number 173219, l; letter from "Registrar" to Miss S., New York Nursery and Child's Hospital, October 28, 1925.

50. CSS Reference Number R2060, COS Case Study Number 173219, letter from the Charity Organization Society to the Superintendent of the City Magistrates' Courts, July 29, 1921.

51. In this book, I use the divisions already accepted by scholars between "Afro-Caribbeans" (largely from non-English-speaking lands) and "West Indians" (from former British colonial holdings), because the bulk of nonnative black migrants of African heritage who came to New York City between the 1880s and the 1930s were, in fact, Jamaican and Barbadian. In terms of Columbus Hill, the 1900, 1905, 1915, and 1925 New York State Census listed persons as "BWI," not by more specific place of origin. Thus Jamaican and Barbadian history, migration, and cultural heritage will be the definition of the term "British West Indian" in this study. See the New York State Census for those particular years, housed at the New York Public Library.

52. Calvin B. Holder, "The Causes and Composition of West Indian Immigration to New York City, 1900–1952," in *Afro-Americans in New York Life and History* 11:2 (January 1987), 9.

53. Miriam Klevan, *The West Indian Americans* (New York: Chelsea House Publishers, 1990), 44.

54. Holder, "The Causes and Composition of West Indian Immigration to New York City, 1900–1952," 10–11. Prior to the 1870s, few West Indians migrated to the United States because transportation links did not exist. With the advent of banana exportation and the acceptance of bananas in the American diet, shipping companies began offering passage. At the end of the nineteenth century, fewer than 4,000 West Indians lived in New York (compared to fewer than 60,000 native-born blacks). Even as the cost of third-class steerage rates increased (from $25 in 1900 to $45 in 1914 and $70 in 1924), the black West Indian population of New York swelled to almost 60,000 by 1930.

Both W. E. B. Du Bois and Carter G. Woodson remarked at the time that most of the African Americans who moved, first from rural areas to southern cities and second from southern cities to large cities in the North, were those who were better educated than those who stayed behind. This was particularly true for African American women. See Du Bois' sociological studies on Philadelphia, Boston, and New York City in *The Black North in 1901: A Social Study* (New York: Arno Press and the New York Times, 1969); Woodson, *A Century of Negro Migration*, 159–164; Clark and McDougald, *A New Day for the Colored Woman Worker*, 9–10. Also see Jones, *Labor of Love, Labor of Sorrow*, in which Jacqueline Jones makes a similar assessment of African American migrant female educational levels.

55. Oscar Handlin, *The Newcomers: Negroes and Puerto Ricans in a Changing Metropolis* (Cambridge, MA: Harvard University Press, 1959), 48–49.

56. Ira De Augustine Reid, *The Negro Immigrant: His Background, Characteristics, and Social Adjustment, 1899–1937* (New York: Columbia University Press, 1939), 24. Much subsequent material not directly quoted is derived from *The Negro Immigrant*.

57. Ibid., 23–25. Here, I use "assimilate" as defined by Paula E. Hyman: a construct and actions more inclusive into the dominant culture than acculturation, or the trading of cultural traditions and symbols for those of the new culture as a means of "fitting in" and taking on new civic status. Instead, assimilation connotes acculturation and absorption: intermarriage and the rejection of endogamy in both ends. See Hyman, *Gender and Assimilation in Modern Jewish History: The Roles and Representation of Women* (Seattle: University of Washington Press, 1995), 13.

58. Edmund Morgan, *American Slavery, American Freedom* (New York: W. W. Norton, 1975), 333–336.

59. Andrew Hacker, *Two Worlds: Black and White, Separate, Hostile, Unequal* (New York: Ballantine Books, 1992), 3–16; Jacobson, *Whiteness of a Different Color*, 7–12, 175–199.

60. Jacobson, *Whiteness of a Different Color*, 158–160, 234–235; Holder, "The Causes and Composition of West Indian Immigration to New York City," 12.

61. Reid, *The Negro Immigrant*, 31–33. The 1924 act also excluded "aliens" deemed ineligible for U.S. citizenship: Chinese, Japanese, (East) Indians, and others who were not "white" or of African descent.

62. Ibid., 33–34.

63. Ibid., 78.

64. Ibid., 83, 85. New York City retained more nonnative-born blacks than any other city by 1930; between 1920 and 1930, blacks shifted in large numbers from the South and Midwest to the North, particularly New York. Their reasons for leaving the South (where almost 40 percent of foreign-born blacks had lived in 1900) were the tightening of racialized discrimination, violence, and prejudice. As a "third-party" population, West Indian blacks felt that both native-born blacks and whites used them unfairly as pawns as they contested power relations within a two-tiered, binary racialized society. Also see Holder, "The Causes and Composition of West Indian Immigration," 11–17.

65. Ibid., 79.

66. Ibid., 80–82.

67. Ibid., 80–82.

68. Ibid., 82–84.

69. Ibid., 84–85.

70. Ibid., 86–87; quotation from 87.

71. Ibid., 88–89.

72. Ibid., 90–91; Handlin, *The Newcomers*, 48–49.

73. Holder, "The Causes and Composition of West Indian Immigration to New York City," 15–19. The higher West Indian literacy levels that Holder asserts may have produced interesting frictions between West Indians and African Americans who competed for housing, jobs, and social status. However, Jacqueline Jones notes that black women who migrated from the South tended to be better educated than those who stayed in the South and had education levels equal to those of their Southern white female counterparts. See Jones, *Labor of Love, Labor of Sorrow*, 152–160.

74. Daniel Patrick Moynihan, *The Negro Family: The Case for National Action* (Washington, DC: U.S. Department of Labor, 1965) 29–45. In his notorious report on urban Negro families, Moynihan made an argument that dogged him until his death: black, female-headed, impoverished households pathologized young black males ("In essence, the Negro community has been forced into a matriarchal structure which, because it is so out of line with the rest of the American society, seriously retards the progress of the group as a whole, and imposes a crushing burden on the Negro male and, in consequence, on a great many Negro women as well"). Unless reproductive-aged African American women became less strident and sexually promiscuous (producing children out of wedlock with men who would not stay as proper male role models), a generation of black males would be lost. Federally funded agencies such as the Job Corps were the answer: structured and defined spaces to teach black male teens how to be responsible men.

75. E. Franklin Frazier, *The Negro Family in the U.S.* (Chicago: University of Chicago Press, 1939), 352–341; Elliot Rudwick, ed., *Black Matriarchy: Myth or Reality?*

(Belmont, CA: Wadsworth, 1971), 14–31; Herbert G. Gutman, *The Black Family in Slavery and Freedom* (New York: Vintage Books, 1977), 444. Gutman's study of the New York City black family between 1900 and 1925 centers on data taken from San Juan Hill, known as Columbus Hill after World War I.

76. Martha Warren Beckwith, *Black Roadways: A Study of Jamaican Folk Life* (Chapel Hill: University of North Carolina Press, 1929), 63.

77. Deborah Gray White, *Ar'n't I a Woman?: Female Slaves in the Plantation South* (New York: W. W. Norton, 1985), 94–107.

78. Paula Giddings quoting Du Bois in *When and Where I Enter: The Impact of Black Women on Race and Sex in America* (New York: Bantam Books, 1984), 137.

79. Gutman, *The Black Family in Slavery and Freedom*, 461–475, 521–530; Stanley Lieberson, *A Piece of the Pie: Blacks and White Immigrants Since 1880* (Berkeley: University of California Press, 1980), 175.

80. Paule Marshall, "Black Immigrant Women in *Brown Girl, Brownstones*," in *Caribbean Life in New York City: Sociocultural Dimensions*, edited by Constance R. Sutton and Elsa M. Chaney. (New York: Center for Migration Studies, 1987), 87.

81. Marshall, "Black Immigrant Women in *Brown Girl, Brownstones*," 88–91.

82. Paule Marshall, *Brown Girl, Brownstones*, 3rd. ed. (Old Westbury, NY: Feminist Press, 1981), 3–10, 30-31.

83. Ibid., 10–11.

84. Ibid., 32–34.

85. Ibid., 24.

86. Thomas Kessner, *The Golden Door: Italian and Jewish Immigrant Mobility in New York City, 1880–1915* (New York: Oxford University Press, 1977), 71–73.

87. CSS Case File Number R1017, COS Case File Number 168649, November 16, 1916, 1–2.

88. CSS Case File Number R1017, COS Case File Number 168649, letter from the Charity Organization Society to Mrs. A., Supervisor, Lower Manhattan District, Department of Public Charities, 1.

89. The absence of women—their voices and their overall perspective—in transmigration literature that usually focuses on only European immigration consists of classics such as Oscar Handlin's *The Uprooted* (1951), John Higham's *Strangers in the Land: Patterns of American Nativism, 1860–1925* (third paperback printing 1994), Kessner, *The Golden Door* (1977), and John Bodnar's *The Transplanted: A History of Immigrants in Urban America* (1985). The gendered masculinity used to undergird migration theories has its roots in the social theories of Robert E. Park and Ernest Burgess of the Chicago School of the 1920s, as seen in publications like *Old World Traits Transplanted*.

90. Friedman-Kasaba, *Memories of Migration*, 7–19.

Migration scholars tended to gender the term "worker" as male. On the other side of the gendered and generational divides were females and children, viewed as non-wage-earning dependents. When women were considered at all, it was within the male framework of wage earner. The latter perception unfortunately distanced women from unpaid, equally important work as carriers of traditions and cultures, childbearers, and child care providers. It made their contributions less visible and also diminished them as intrinsic, critical members within their kinship groups and communities (15–17).

According to Friedman-Kasaba, the "push/pull" and linked assimilationist and human capital models, which lean toward the impact of migration from the perspective of the receiving state, do not work for scholars of women's migration and have been replaced by or reconfigured to incorporate other more inclusive models because:

1. They cannot explicate migration as an individual choice to come to the receiving state; they ignore social and economic relations in the sending state.
2. In push/pull theories, men are motivated by desire to become westernized. This, in effect, leaves out women entirely—what are their motivations?
3. When women's perspectives are considered, they are portrayed as caught between models of cultural uprooting (destruction) or transplantation (continuity).
   a. Uprooting (destruction) cannot explain continued female gender stereotypes in light of migration because they are supposed to have the same desires as their men.
   b. Transplantation (continuity) obscures their hopes for new and better lives, which involves decisions that may run contrary to old traditions (15–19).
4. There is a dualistic trend to brand immigrant women as either saintly victims of migration or social problems awaiting correction.
   a. When push/pull enthusiasts finally look at women and what in their traditional and cultural backgrounds will make their and their families assimilation easier, Friedman Kasaba warns that "contradictory stereotypes of race, gender and class collude. The representation of immigrant women as passive accessories to an overarching process in which they were not fully engaged both reflects and contributes to their continued depiction as 'victims' by researchers, as well as policymakers" (19).
   b. This leads to the saintly vs. harpy stereotype, where social reformers have either focused on their victim state or on how difficult they are when resisting assimilation: "They have been alternately characterized as unproductive, ignorant, crude, brash, and miserly matriarchs who struggled for total control over their households" (19).

Emiliana P. Norther, in "The Silent Half: *Le Contadine del Sud* before the First World War," explains the absence of Italian women from Italian history as the result of past and more recent histories where scholars of the peasantry "studied, recorded, and analyzed the existing societal structure, which was male-directed and male-oriented." Basically, they "read" male and said "male." Also, illiteracy was a problem resulting from "the traditional peasant distrust of education." However, with migration and the war, as males realized they needed literacy in their own language to do well in the United States and as literacy was stressed in the Italian military, male literacy rates increased and female literacy rates declined. This state of illiteracy accounts for the absence or "silence" of southern Italian rural women. More than the muted voices of southern black rural or small-town women, or West Indian women, Italian peasant women, from the unification period through the 1960s, remained silent and largely unheard, except when reflected in governmental statistics. See Betty Boyd Caroli, Robert F. Harney, and Lydio F. Tomasi, eds., *The Italian Immigrant Woman in North America* (Toronto: Multicultural History Society of Ontario, 1978), 3–7.

91. Friedman-Kasaba, *Memories of Migration*, 2–30. For other analyses of gender and migration, see Hasia Diner, *Erin's Daughters in American: Irish Immigrant Women in the Nineteenth Century* (Baltimore: Johns Hopkins University Press, 1983); Nancy Foner, "Sex Roles and Sensibilities: Jamaican Women in New York and London," in *International Migration: The Female Experience*, edited by Rita James Simon and Caroline Brettell (Totowa, NJ: Rowman and Allanheld) 1985; Donna R. Gabaccia, *Seeking Common Ground: Multidisciplinary Studies of Immigrant Women in the United States* (Westport, CT: Greenwood Press, 1992); Pierrette Hondagneu-Sotelo, *Gendered Transitions: Mexican Experiences of Immigration* (Berkeley: University of California Press, 1994); Hyman, *Gender and Assimilation*; Patricia Pessar, "The Role of Gender in Dominican Settlement in the U.S.," in *Women and Change in Latin America*, edited by June Nash and Helen I. Safa (South Hadley, MA: Bergin and Garvey) 1986.

92. Friedman-Kasaba, *Memories of Migration*, 13. For more about how historical and geographical boundaries, and systems of economics, ideas, and politics, change racialized identities over time, see Immanuel Wallerstein, "The Construction of Peoplehood: Racism, Nationalism, Ethnicity," *Sociological Review* 2, no. 2 (Spring 1987): 373–388.

93. Giorgio Bertellini, "Southern Crossings: Italians, Cinema, and Modernity, Italy, 1861—New York, 1920," (PhD diss., New York University, 2001), 15; Alain Locke, "The New Negro," in *The Portable Harlem Renaissance Reader*, edited by David Levering Lewis (New York: Viking Press, 1994), 46–51; Louise Michelle Newman, *White Women's Rights: The Racial Origins of Feminism in the United States* (New York: Oxford University Press, 1999), 3–19. Alain Locke dealt persuasively with the "Negro problem" in the essay "The New Negro" by arguing that times change. As the "Old Negro" had been little more than myth, and as benighted European cities had become recognized as crucial spaces of new, proud identities, Harlem had become "the home of the Negro's Zionism," the axis of the New Negro movement and a space for creativity and racial pride. Louise Newman's discussion of the racialization of the women's rights movement also takes on Bertellini's Italian "Southern problem" and the U.S. "Negro problem." She maintains that white middle-class women overcame the "Woman problem" by racializing their fight for suffrage as a tool to control and subjugate not only black males (and later, black women), but male immigrants with the vote as well. All three "problems," with difference and the control of the dominant culture at their cores, are amazingly similar to *la questione meridionale*.

94. Bertellini, "Southern Crossings," 16. This feminization of race, region, and class is nothing new, of course. It can be seen in American writings of the time, especially those predating the 1860s and the American Civil War. During the 1830s, pro-slavery Southern advocates such as Dr. Josiah Nott wrote voluminous treatises and articles about the inherent inferiority of enslaved African Americans and the "feminine"

nature of the race. According to Reginald Horsman, the debate over the nature of races, the racialization of slavery, and the "woman" question spanned the Atlantic, creating a hothouse environment as scholars in the United States and Europe challenged and informed each others' ideas of inherent superiority and inferiority. In turn, these ideas found their way into the popular culture via newspapers, lectures, sermons, and by word of mouth. They definitely carried over past the Civil War, when some within the Freedman's Bureau counseled black men to become more masculine and manly by taking control over their wives, and thus properly fitting themselves for citizenship, its rights and obligations. For further reading, see Reginald Horsman's *Josiah Nott of Mobile: Southerner, Physician, and Racial Theorist*, and *Race and Manifest Destiny: The Origins of American Racial Anglo-Saxonism*; Amy Dru Stanley, *From Bondage to Contract: Wage Labor, Marriage, and the Market in the Age of Emancipation*; Stephen Jay Gould, *The Mismeasure of Man*, and Bederman, *Manliness and Civilization*.

95. For the late nineteenth and early twentieth century cultural shifts in masculinity, rooted in race, class, and gender fears, see Bederman, *Manliness and Civilization*.

96. Friedman-Kasaba, *Memories of Migration*, 91–104; Bertellini, "Southern Crossings," 20–23. According to Bertellini, this inferior stereotype foisted upon southern Italians by their northern compatriots was accepted by native-born Anglo Americans who, making little distinction between Italians by region, applied the stereotype to all Italians in general. This initially infuriated northern Italians. Later, they and southern Italians accepted this and used it to their advantage by creating the trope of the hardworking, noble, yet illiterate, peasant.

97. Zoe Anderson Norris, *The East Side: Her Magazine*, 1:1 (1909), 10. I presume that Mrs. Norris was twice divorced because she was divorced during the time when she published her magazine. With tongue in cheek, Norris traced her support for the downtrodden back to 1502, when an English lord who sympathized with Scottish rebels was stripped of his titles, and his son, a vicar, ended up making the poor his ministry, and living among them. She also states that, at times, she would "swipe a little souvenir" from tables because another descendant, "a distant renegade Uncle," had purportedly been a pirate (1:4, 7).

98. Norris, *The East Side: Her Magazine*, 1:2 (1909), 4, 10. After bemoaning her little magazine's probable demise without yearly subscribers (at $1/year), by volume 4 of the first year, she proudly admits that she is now read "nearly all over the world; in California; in Honolulu; in England; in Austria; in Hungary." With this success, however, she still had problems convincing the newsboy in the neighborhood that carried her magazine that she could continue its publication without the deep pockets of a financial backer (1:4, 4–5).

I found little information about Mrs. Norris; it seems that no one has written anything about her. She had stories or articles printed in *Everybody's Magazine, The Argosy, The Home Magazine*, and the *10 Story Book*, as well as short pieces in the *New York Times*. During the first year, she began including restaurant and theater reviews toward the end of each edition. In her 1914 obituary, the *New York Times* wrote that

"Mrs. Norris was well known in Bohemian circles and was the promoter of an organization known as the 'Ragged Edge Klub,' composed of writers of radical tendencies and their sympathizers, who met monthly at downtown restaurants." Norris died suddenly at the age of forty-five, survived only by her married daughter (*New York Times* February 14, 1914, 11).

99. Louise C. Odencrantz, *Italian Women in Industry: A Study of Conditions in New York City* (New York: Russell Sage Foundation, 1919), 38–39.

100. Norris, *The East Side: Her Magazine* 1:2, 8–9.

101. Ibid., 12–13.

102. Kessner, *The Golden Door*, 26–32. When Kessner compares the movement of Italian men with that of their Jewish counterparts, he concludes that "[t]he Italian immigration was, by and large, a nonfamily [sic] movement of males in their productive years. These single men came to make some money and go home. . . . Others who did not particularly care about returning to Italy nonetheless did not settle down . . . they moved freely across the city and country, often joining the 'birds of passage' in seeking the most attractive short-range opportunities, ignoring business and enterprise" (31). Between 1880 and 1910, 80 percent of the Italians who migrated to the United States were male (30). With decades of this transatlantic movement, however, I am unaware of any studies that have been done which explore the sexuality of these men, and if they left temporary "wives" and children behind upon emigrating to Italy. Dr. Antonio Stella and Dr. Rocco Brindisi, however, ardently denied the nativist accusation that Italians, like African Americans, were a syphilitic race. Considering that they stated this before the larger influx of Italian women and other family members, and that they may have been referring largely to Italian men (which would fit the focus of social hygienists of the time, preoccupied with married men, prostitutes, and the spread of venereal diseases to "innocents"—wives and unborn children), it is possible that some Italian men may have left American families behind when they returned to their Italian ones. Still, this is speculation only. Future research needs to be done in this area. Also see *No Magic Bullet*, 20–21. For the story of the "white widows" who were left behind in southern Italy, see Linda Reeder, *Widows in White: Migration and the Transformation of Rural Italian Women, Sicily, 1880–1920* (Toronto: University of Toronto Press, 2003), 3–16.

103. Norris, *The East Side: Her Magazine* 1:6 (1909), 16–17. Norris even sees a commonality between the eldest son, himself a boy, who tells her "all the family secrets" the first time they met, and how he and the wife have big eyes and beautiful lashes that remind her of "a certain boy I know and love" (16–17). I do not know who this boy is; at first, I believed her to be referring to her son; but her 1914 obituary states that she was survived by a daughter.

104. Ibid., 20.

105. Ibid., 20–22.

106. Coser, Ankar, and Perrin, *Women of Courage*, 29–30.

107. Norris, *The East Side: Her Magazine*, 1:6, 18.

CHAPTER 2. PROFESSIONALIZATION IN THE CITY

1. Blascoer does not state whether this woman was a native New Yorker, African American, or British West Indian.

2 Frances Blascoer, *Colored School Children in New York* (1915; reprint, New York: Negro Universities Press, 1970), 45.

3. Gerald Leinwand, *1927: High Tide of the Twenties* (New York: Basic Books, 2001), 235. Leinwand quotes Raymond Wolters in a book review characterizing Du Bois as "a fastidious black Brahmin—a connoisseur of the best of Western culture, a devoted chronicler of African contributions to civilization, and also an exhorter urging Negro Americans to make their own special gift to the world. . . . Negroes should be both black and American." See Raymond Wolters, "Personal Connections and the Growth of the NAACP," review of *James Weldon Johnson: Black Leader, Black Voice*, by Eugene Levy (1973), and *J. E. Springarn and the Rise of the NAACP, 1911–1939*, by B. Joyce Ross (1972), in *Reviews in American History* 2, no.1 (March 1974): 140.

4. Robert Ezra Park and Herbert Adolphus Miller, *Old World Traits Transplanted* (New York: Arno Press, 1969), 3–4. Park and Miller define "heritage" as the "fund of attitudes and values which an immigrant groups brings to America." I am expanding this definition to include migrating African Americans as well because, like other groups, they were perceived to be carriers of cultural customs and attitudes that were backward, or certainly not up par with those in modern urban Anglo America.

5. Karla FC Holloway, *Private Bodies, Public Texts: Race, Gender, and a Cultural Bioethics* (Durham, NC: Duke University Press, 2011), 7; 25–66.

6. Charles Rosenberg, *No Other Gods: On Science and American Social Thought*, rev. and expanded ed. (Baltimore: Johns Hopkins University Press, 1997), 1–14. For further readings on the relationships between science and American identity, see Daniel J. Kevles, *In the Name of Eugenics: Genetics and the Uses of Human Heredity* (Berkeley: University of California Press, 1985), 57–69; Sandra Harding, ed., *The "Racial" Economy of Science: Toward a Democratic Future* (Bloomington: University of Indiana Press, 1993), 1–29; Evelyn Nakano Glenn, *Unequal Freedom: How Race and Gender Shaped America Citizenship and Labor* (Cambridge, MA: Harvard University Press, 2002), 1–17; Nayan Shah, *Contagious Divides: Epidemics and Race in San Francisco's Chinatown* (Berkeley: University of California Press, 2001), 1–16.

7. Gwendolyn Mink, *The Wages of Motherhood: Inequality in the Welfare State, 1917–1942* (Ithaca, NY: Cornell University Press, 1999), 3–6.

8. Park and Miller, *Old World Traits Transplanted*, 19–21, 24.

9. Glenda Gilmore, *Who Were the Progressives?* (New York: Bedford/St. Martin's, 2002), 3–4.

10. Seth Koven and Sonya Michel, eds., "Introduction," *Mothers of a New World: Maternalist Politics and the Origins of Welfare States* (New York: Routledge, 1993), 1–42.

11. Mink, *The Wages of Motherhood*, 7.

12. Louise Michelle Newman, *White Women's Rights: The Racial Origins of Feminism in the United States* (New York: Oxford University Press, 1999), 21–55.

13. Alisa Klaus, *Every Child a Lion: The Origins of Maternal and Infant Health Policy in the United States and France, 1890–1920* (Ithaca, NY: Cornell University Press, 1993), 3–5.

14. Quoted in Mary Elizabeth Brown, "Theodore Roosevelt (1858-1919): Race Suicide," in *The Making of Modern Immigration: An Encyclopedia of People and Ideas*, vol. 2, Patrick J. Hayes, ed. (Santa Barbara, CA: ABC-CLIO, 2012), 653; ibid., 31–32, 34; Kevles, *In the Name of Eugenics*, 74.

15. Klaus, *Every Child a Lion*, 16–20, 42.

16. Ibid., 5–13. Linda Gordon, *Pitied But Not Entitled: Single Mothers and the History of Welfare* (Cambridge, MA: Harvard University Press, 1994), 46–47.

17. Tera W. Hunter, *To 'Joy My Freedom: Southern Black Women's Lives and Labors After the Civil War* (Cambridge, MA: Harvard University Press, 1997), 187–218; *Where and When I Enter*, 149.

18. Klaus, *Every Child a Lion*, 13.

19. George Rosen, *A History of Public Health*, expanded ed. (1958; Baltimore: Johns Hopkins University Press, 1993), 270–271, 280–288.

20. Quoted in Alan M. Kraut, introduction, *Silent Travelers: Germs, Genes, and the "Immigrant Menace"* (Baltimore: John Hopkins University Press, 1994), 253. Kraut also uses the term in the subtitle of his book.

21. Nancy Tomes, *The Gospel of Germs: Men, Women, and the Microbe in American Life* (Cambridge, MA: Harvard University Press, 1998), 33; Rosen, *A History of Public Health*, 270–271.

22. Rosen, *A History of Public Health*, 209–211; Tomes, *The Gospel of Germs*, 48–67.

23. Duffy, *A History of Public Health in New York City*, 238–280.

24. Tomes, *The Gospel of Germs*, 46–47.

25. Ibid., 183–195.

26. John Duffy, *From Humors to Medical Science: A History of American Medicine*, 2nd ed. (Urbana: University of Illinois Press, 1993), 7.

27. John Harley Warner, "From Specificity to Universalism in Medical Therapeutics: Transformation in the 19th-Century United States," in *Sickness and Health in American: Readings in the History of Medicine and Public Health*, 3rd rev. ed., edited by Judith Walzer Leavitt and Ronald L. Numbers. (Madison: University of Wisconsin Press, 1997), 87–90.

28. Abraham Flexner, *Medical Education in the United States and Canada: A Report to the Carnegie Foundation for the Advancement of Teaching* (New York: Carnegie Foundation for the Advancement of Teaching, 1910), 6–7.

29. Ronald L. Numbers and John Harley Warner, "The Maturation of American Medical Science," in Walzer and Numbers, *Sickness and Health in America*, 130–132, quote from 136.

30. Ibid., 136.

31. Warner, "From Specificity to Universalism in Medical Therapeutics," 91–98.

32. Numbers and Warner, "The Maturation of American Medical Science," 134–135.

33. Susan Reverby, *Ordered to Care: The Dilemma of American Nursing, 1850–1945* (Melbourne, Australia: Cambridge University Press, 1987), 1–3.

34. Ibid., 11–16.

35. Ibid., 15.

36. Ibid., 43–59.

37. Ibid., 168–179.

38. Darlene Clark Hine, "Opportunity and Fulfillment: Sex, Race, and Class in Health Care Education," *Sage* 2, no. 2 (Fall 1985): 14–16. To be fair, Flexner's report called for the revamping of inferior schools (the majority of medical schools, in his opinion). Many white schools also closed as a result.

39. Hine, "Opportunity and Fulfillment," 15.

40. Darlene Clark Hine, "From Hospital to College: Black Nurse Leaders and the Rise of Collegiate Nursing Schools," *Journal of Negro Educations* 51, no. 3 (Summer 1982): 224.

41. Darlene Clark Hine, *Black Women in White: Racial Conflict and Cooperation in the Nursing Profession, 1890–1950* (Bloomington: Indiana University Press, 1989), xv–xxiii.

CHAPTER 3. WORK IN THE CITY

1. S. Josephine Baker, M. D., *Fighting for Life*, with a historical introduction by Patricia C. Kuszler, M. D., and Charles G. Roland, M. D. (1939; Huntington, NY: Robert E. Krieger, 1980, 42.

2. Ibid., 31–42.

3. Ibid., 48.

4. Ibid., 57–58.

5. Kathryn Kish Sklar, "Protestant Women and Social Justice Activism, 1890–1920" (conference keynote essay presented at the Women and Twentieth-Century Protestantism Conference, Chicago, April 23, 1998). Although Sklar asks why scholars, who try to explain the moral undergirding that fired the maternalist movement, dismiss religion and religious beliefs, it must be noted that in 1993, when Seth Koven and Sonya Michel edited *Mothers of a New World*, which laid the groundwork for historical maternalism and contained an article by Sklar, both they and Sklar acknowledged the decades of religious activism that female reformers had used to introduce the need for social moral responsibility within U.S. culture. See "The Origins of Maternalist Movements" in "Introduction," 10–19; and Sklar's "The Historical Foundation of Women's Power in the Creation of the American Welfare State, 1830–1930," 43–93.

6. Baker, *Fighting for Life*, 20–22.

7. Ibid., 1–2.

8. Ibid., 6–12.

9. John Duffy, *A History of Public Health in New York City, 1866–1966* (New York: Russell Sage Foundation, 1974), 249–264.

10. Baker, *Fighting for Life*, 85–87.

11. Alexis de Toqueville, *Democracy in America*, First published in two volumes, 1835 and 1840. An Electronic Series Publication: http://www2.hn.psu.edu/faculty/jmanis/toqueville/dem-in-america1.pdf, accessed February 25, 2014. The point to which I refer is better stated by Toqueville himself: "As soon as several of the inhabitants of the United States have taken up an opinion or a feeling which they wish to promote in the world, they look out for mutual assistance; and as soon as they have found each other out, they combine. From that moment they are no longer isolated men, but a power seen from afar, whose actions serve for an example, and whose language is listened to" (584).

12. Daniel Walkowitz, *Working with Class: Social Workers and the Politics of Middle-Class Identity* (Chapel Hill: University of North Carolina Press, 1999), 10–18.

13. W. E. Burghardt Du Bois, *The Black North in 1901: A Social Study. A Series of Articles Originally Appearing in The New York Times, November–December 1901* (reprint, New York: Arno Press and the *New York Times*, 1969), 1–2.

14. Ibid., 3–5.

15. Ibid., 5–10.

16. Ibid., 11.

17. Ibid., 12–13.

18. Ibid., 14.

19. Ibid., 15–18.

20. Mary White Ovington, *Black and White Sat Down Together: The Reminiscences of an NAACP Founder*, edited and with a foreword by Ralph E. Luker, and an afterword by Carolyn E. Wedin (New York: Feminist Press at the City University of New York, 1995; first paperback edition, 1996), 4. Ovington's *Reminiscences* were first serially published in the *Baltimore Afro-American* from September 1932 through February 1933.

21. Ovington, *Black and White Sat Down Together*, 5; Carolyn Wedin, *Inheritors of the Spirit: Mary White Ovington and the Founding of the NAACP* (New York: John Wiley and Sons, 1998), 11–12.

22. Wedin, *Inheritors of the Spirit*, 10–11.

23. Ibid., 16, 23–43.

24. Ibid., 47–49.

25. Ibid., 54.

26. Ovington, *Black and White Sat Down Together*, 26.

27. Mary White Ovington, *Half a Man: The Status of the Negro in New York* (1911; New York: Charles Flint Kellogg, 1969), 83–85.

28. Frances Blascoer, *Colored School Children in New York* (New York: Public Education Association of the City of New York, 1915; repr., Negro Universities Press, 1970), 1.

29. Ibid., 1–9, 129–150.

30. Ibid., 176–77.

31. Seth Scheiner, *Negro Mecca: A History of the Negro in New York City, 1865–1920* (New York: New York University Press, 1965), 59.

32. Blascoer, *Colored School Children in New York*, 49–52.
33. Ibid., 34.35.
34. Ibid., 42. Blascoer quotes "Statement by directors."
35. Ibid., 23–25, 40–43.
36. Ibid., 130.
37. Ibid., 129–132.

CHAPTER 4. CULTURE IN THE CITY

1. Hazel V. Carby, *Reconstructing Womanhood: The Emergence of the Afro-American Woman Novelist* (New York: Oxford University Press, 1987), 66.

2. Ibid., 69.

3. Frances E. W. Harper, "Enlightened Womanhood: An Address before the Brooklyn Literary Society, November 15, 1892," http://memory.loc.gov/cgi-bin/query/r?ammem/murray:@field%28DOCID+@lit%28lcrbmrpt1906div0%29%29, accessed November 15, 2014, 2.

4. Ibid., 3–6.

5. The scholarship on these ideas and their corresponding social programs are quite extensive. See Richard Meckel, *Save the Babies: American Public Health Reform and the Prevention of Infant Mortality, 1850–1929* (Baltimore: Johns Hopkins University Press, 1990; Ann Arbor: University of Michigan Press, 1998), and for a comparative look at the effect of racialism on mothers and infant health programs, see Meckel's "Racialism and Infant Health: Late Nineteenth- and Early Twentieth-Century Socio-Medical Discourses on African American Infant Mortality, in *Migrants, Minorities, and Health: Historical and Contemporary Studies*, ed. Lara Marks and Michael Worboys (New York: Routledge, 1997). Also see Rima Apple, "Constructing Mothers: Scientific Motherhood in the Nineteenth and Twentieth Centuries," in *Mothers and Motherhood: Readings in American History*, ed. Rima D. Apple and Janet Golden (Columbus: Ohio State University Press, 1997), 90–110; Georgina D. Feldberg, *Disease and Class: Tuberculosis and the Shaping of Modern North American Society* (New Brunswick, NJ: Rutgers University Press, 1995), 109–124; Loretta J. Ross, "African American Women and Abortions," in Apple and Golden, *Mothers and Motherhood*, 259–276; Sheila M. Rothman, *Living in the Shadow of Death: Tuberculosis and the Social Experience of Illness in American History* (Baltimore: Johns Hopkins University Press, 1994), 86–127; Nayan Shah, *Contagious Divides: Epidemics and Race in San Francisco's Chinatown* (Berkeley: University of California Press, 2001), 205–210, 214–224. Also see Nancy Tomes, *The Gospel of Germs: Men, Women, and the Microbe in American Life* (Cambridge, MA: Harvard University Press, 1998); Alan M. Kraut, *Silent Travelers: Germs, Genes, and the "Immigrant Menace"* (Baltimore: Johns Hopkins University Press, 1994); Dorothy Roberts, *Protecting the Black Body: Race, Reproduction, and the Meaning of Liberty* (New York: Pantheon Books, 1997), to name a few.

6. Meckel, "Racialism and Infant Death," 70–71.

7. Ibid., 70–72, 80–82. I do not agree with Meckel that "race" was appended to the statistics measuring Jews, Italians, or other European migrating groups simply because

reformers and officials were concerned over the havoc their numbers were wreaking on municipal infrastructures. Subsequent to Meckel's essay, scholars have unpacked whiteness and "race" to show that its slipperiness and permeability could indeed embrace official's fears, but the categorization and hierarchialization of Europeans and other nonblack groups had already begun before the era of massive European immigration. For further reading, see Matthew Frye Jacobson, *Whiteness of a Different Color: European Immigrants and the Alchemy of Race* (Cambridge, MA: Harvard University Press, 1998), and Richard Delgado and Jean Stefancic, eds., *Critical White Studies: Looking Behind the Mirror* (Philadelphia: Temple University Press, 1997).

8. Meckel, "Racialism and Infant Death," 72–81.

9. Georgina D. Feldberg, *Disease and Class: Tuberculosis and the Shaping of Modern North American Society* (New Brunswick, NJ: Rutgers University Press, 1995), 11–18, 33. Feldberg discusses the diathetical label given to consumption prior the discovery of the tubercle bacillus, a label that embraced both environmental and hereditary causes with the knowledge that no single cause existed. Thus physicians could tailor causation and therapeutics to the individual and the environment. Also see Sheila M. Rothman, *Living in the Shadow of Death: Tuberculosis and the Social Experience of Illness in American History* (Baltimore: Johns Hopkins University Press, 1994), 179–213, and Barbara Bates, *Bargaining for Life: A Social History of Tuberculosis, 1876–1938* (Philadelphia: University of Pennsylvania Press, 1992), 42–74.

10. Susan Sontag, *Illness as Metaphor* (New York: Farrar, Straus, and Giroux, 1878), 1–39.

11. Helen Barolini, ed., *The Dream Book: An Anthology of Writings by Italian American Women*, rev. ed. (Syracuse, NY: Syracuse University Press, 1985). After searching for writings done by Southern Italian women of the era who spoke on motherhood or mothering, I found nothing. There are interviews done by sociologists (such as Rose Laub Coser, Laura S. Anker, and Andrew J. Perrin's *Women of Courage*) or writings dictated by Italian women to white transcribers (for example, *Rosa*, the life story of Rosa Cavelleri, a northern Italian woman who, as a girl was given to an Italian man in the United States because he had requested a wife). However, as Helen Barolini corroborates, the actual writings of Italian women who migrated to the United States are virtually impossible to find. The vast wealth they gave to this country came through culture and art. Most of the women of southern Italy were not literate in Italian at the time of massive migration (after 1900, Italy began the process of standardizing Italian; the spoken language was rich enough to vary from village to village). Moreover, Barolini argues that Italian men found no interest in the ideas and interests of Italian women, so they were not encouraged to write. "Italian American women did not come from a tradition that considered it valuable for them to narrate their lives as documents of instruction for future generations. They were not given to introspection and the writing of thoughts in diaries," she maintains. "They came from a male-dominant world where their ancillary role" of wife and mother tended to restrict to the *domus* and the family (3–5). See Marie Hall Ets, *Rosa: The Life of an Italian Immigrant* (1970; Madison: University of Wisconsin Press, 1999).

12. Zora Neale Hurston, "Color Struck: A Play in Four Scenes," in *Fire: A Quarterly Devoted to the Younger Negro Audiences*, November 1926, 11.

13. Ibid., 13.

14. Ibid., 14.

15. Angela Davis, *Blues Legacies and Black Feminism: Gertrude "Ma" Rainey, Bessie Smith, and Billie Holiday* (New York: Pantheon, 1998), 10–11.

16. Ivey White Newman, *American Negro Folk-Songs* (Cambridge: Harvard University Press, 1928), 398.

17. Ibid., 313.

18. This reference to "blondes," without the clarification of race, teasingly (boldly, and quite dangerously) crossed early twentieth-century accepted racially gendered boundaries of women's bodies and sexuality. Imagine the work of Ida B. Wells-Barnett, who had successfully campaigned internationally, starting in the 1890s, against lynching as a fallaciously sexualized terrorist tool of economic oppression. Imagine thousands of lynched black men (and women) who, only because they had "gotten out of place" with *any* white person, had been quickly dispatched and lynched on the grounds of getting familiar with or raping white women. Also imagine the later work of Jessie Ames, the female white activist who, revisiting Wells-Barnett's claims during the late 1920s and early 1930s, came to the same conclusion: that lynching was usually a tool of economic, political, and social control, and rarely as retribution for black male sexual license against the vaunted, unquestioned "pure" status of any and all white women. These lyrics upend and call into question both black *and* white male notions of sexual desire, reputation, and power; unfortunately, they simultaneously reinforce the very warped ideas which they attempt to demystify. Perspective, as always, is crucial to the human thoughts and desires behind representations and the variety of acts that encompass human agency. See Barbara Bair, "Remapping the Black/White Body: Sexuality, Nationalism, and Biracial Antimiscegenation Activism in 1920s Virginia," in *Sex, Love, Race: Crossing Boundaries in North American History*, ed. Martha Hodes (New York: New York University Press, 1999), 399–419; Martin Summers, *Manliness and its Discontents: The Black Middle Class and the Transformation of Masculinity, 1900–1930* (Chapel Hill: University of North Carolina Press, 2004); Glenda Elizabeth Gilmore, *Gender and Jim Crow: Women and the Politics of White Supremacy in North Carolina, 1890–1920* (Chapel Hill: University of North Carolina Press, 1996); and Gail Bederman, *Manliness and Civilization: A Cultural History of Gender and Race in the United States, 1880–1917* (Chicago: University of Chicago Press, 1995).

19. Newman, *American Negro Folk Songs*, 316.

20. Ibid., 394.

21. Ibid., 329.

22. Darlene Clark Hine, "Rape and the Inner Lives of Black Women in the Middle West," *Signs* 14, no. 4 (Summer 1989): 912–913.

23. Ibid., 915–916. Hine argues that some middle-class African American women have been actors in a racially gendered world that gave them no space on the pedestal

of womanhood. Negative, sexualized stereotypes of black womanhood filled the silence that occurred when they kept their inner lives and thoughts hidden in an attempt to control any hint of illicit behavior that would support negative stereotypes.

24. In 1998, while attending the University of California, Los Angeles, I had the privilege of being a teaching assistant for Robert Hill as he taught African American nationalism using autobiographies. He highlighted black male preoccupations with reputation during the lecture. During discussion sections, I incorporated his ideas into Hazel Carby's argument in "'It Jus Be's Dat Way Sometime,'" in which she notes that black female blues singers understood the unequal landscape of the United States more adroitly than middle- and upper-class black women. They understood the parameters of race, class, gender, and sexuality and found the pretentions of white respectability—for the sake of gaining white respect and inclusion—preposterous and a waste of time. Building on these foundations, I argue that African American blueswomen went one crucial step further. As black female entertainers, they shamelessly embraced the sexualized reputations that had been reserved for black men and thus demanded respect from everyone.

25. Deborah Gray White, *Too Heavy a Load: Black Women in Defense of Themselves, 1894–1994* (New York: W. W. Norton, 1999), 52–66; Gilmore, *Gender and Jim Crow*, 147–176; Rosalyn Terborg-Penn, *African American Women in the Struggle for the Vote, 1850–1920* (Bloomington: Indiana University Press, 1998), 54–80; Kevin K. Gaines, *Uplifting the Race: Black Leadership, Politics, and Culture in the Twentieth Century* (Chapel Hill: University of North Carolina Press, 1996), 34–46; for the "culture of dissemblance" see Hines, "Rape and the Inner Lives of Black Women in the Middle West," 912–920.

26. Since the 1990s, some scholars of the women of the Harlem Renaissance have revisited the writings of Jessie Redmon Fauset and argued for a revised reading of her four novels, maintaining that she actually critiqued and turned the black bourgeoisie on its head in *There is Confusion* (New York: Boni and Liveright, 1924). For variations on the debate, see Carol Allen, *Black Women Intellectuals: Strategies of Nation, Family, and Neighborhood in the Works of Pauline Hopkins, Jessie Fauset, and Marita* Bonner (New York: Garland Publications, 1998); Carol J. Batker, *Reforming Fictions: Native, African, and Jewish American Women's Literature and Journalism in the Progressive Era* (New York: Columbia University Press, 2000); Licia Morrow Calloway, *Black Family (Dys)function in Novels by Jessie Fauset, Nella Larsen, and Fannie Hurst* (New York: P. Lang, 2003); Hazel V. Carby, *Reconstructing Womanhood: The Emergence of the Afro-American Woman Novelist* (New York: Oxford University Press, 1987); Sharon L. Jones, *Rereading the Harlem Renaissance: Race, Class, and Gender in the Fiction of Jessie Fauset, Zora Neale Hurston, and Dorothy West* (Westport, CT: Greenwood Press, 2002); David Levering Lewis, ed., *The Portable Harlem Renaissance Reader* (New York: Penguin Books, 1995); Jacquelyn Y. McClendon, *The Politics of Color in the Fiction of Jessie Fauset and Nella Larsen* (Charlottesville: University Press of Virginia, 1995); Cheryl Wall, *Women of the Harlem Renaissance* (Bloomington: Indiana University

Press, 1995); Carolyn Wedin Sylvander, *Jessie Redmon Fauset: Black American Writer* (Troy, NY: Whitston Publishing Company, 1981); Harriet E. Wilson et al, *The Soul of a Woman* (London: The X Press, 1996).

27. Carby, "'It Jus Be's Dat Way Sometime,'" 11–12.

28. Ibid., 11–14; Davis, *Blues Legacies and Black Feminism*, 3–41.

29. Paul Garon and Beth Garon, *Woman with Guitar: Memphis Minnie's Blues* (San Francisco: City Light Books, 2014), 264–265.

30. Ibid., 265.

31. Ibid.; Eric Sackheim, comp., *The Blues Line: A Collection of Blues Lyrics* (New York: Grossman Publishers, 1969), 57.

32. Davis, *Blues Legacies and Black Feminism*, 214.

33. Sackheim, *The Blues Line*, 44.

34. Davis, *Blues Legacies and Black Feminism*, 264–265.

35. Irma Watkins-Owens, *Blood Relations: Caribbean Immigrants and the Harlem Community, 1900–1930* (Bloomington: Indiana University Press, 1996), 11–22.

36. Tom Redcam, "O Little Green Island Far Over the Sea," in *A Treasury of Jamaican Poetry*, edited J. E. Clare McFarlane (London: University of London Press, 1949), 15–16.

37. Claude McKay, "Flame-Heart" in McFarlane, *A Treasury of Jamaican Poetry*, 67.

38. *Treasure of Jamaican Poetry* 16.

39. G. Llewellyn Watson, *Jamaican Sayings: With Notes on Folklore, Aesthetics, and Social Control* (Tallahassee: Florida A&M University Press, 1991), 1–3.

40. Ibid., 3–10.

41. Ibid., 151, number 188.

42. Ibid., 151, number 190.

43. Ibid., 151–152, number 191.

44. Ibid., 152, number 193.

45. Ibid., 150, number 185.

46. Ibid., 150–151, number 187.

47. Ibid., 248, number 65.

48. Ibid., 250, number 87.

49. Ibid., 249, number 82.

50. Izett Anderson, M. D., and Frank Cundall, F. S. A. *Jamaica Negro Proverbs and Sayings: Collected and Classified According to Subjects* (London: West India Committee for the Institute of Jamaica, 1927), 14–15, numbers 7 and 8, 14.

51. Ibid., 29, number 194.

52. Ibid., 47, number 440.

53. Olive Lewin, *Rock It Come Over: The Folk Music of Jamaica* (Kingston, Jamaica: University of the West Indies Press, 2000), 23–24.

54. Ibid., 56–58. Lewin maintains that had white masters or overseers paid attention to the words of the song, they would have bristled at its "social commentary" on miscegenation, the unequal sexualized power relations between slave women and white men, and between female field slaves and house slaves.

CHAPTER 5. BIRTHING IN THE CITY: COLUMBUS HILL

1. Community Service Society [CSS], "Introductory Statement Prepared for the Amsterdam News," Columbia University, New York City, box 36, folder 132, 1–2 n.d. In this press release on the Columbus Hill Health Center (presumably dated after October 1, 1929, the latest date mentioned), the study of the health experiment that began in the area in 1917 was instigated by Burritt at Emerson's request.

2. Bailey B. Burritt to Franklin B. Kirkbride, January 13, 1917, CSS, box 36, folder 132.

3. Bailey B. Burritt to Franklin B. Kirkbride, February 5, 1918, CSS, box 36, folder 132, 2. The AICP's work in Columbus Hill began in April, 1917. Less than one year later, Burritt advised Kirkbride that, according to Miss Price, the nurse hired to work with Columbus Hill's blacks, all pregnant mothers were now given Wassermann testing for syphilis.

4. John C. Gebhart, *Health Work for Mothers and Children in a Colored Community* (New York: New York Association for Improving the Condition of the Poor, 1924), 3–4.

5. Abbie Roberts Weaver et al., "Report on a Study of Caroline Rest [Home], Made During March and April, 1933" (unpublished manuscript, New York Association for Improving the Condition of the Poor, May 1, 1933), 6.

6. Burritt to Kirkbride, January 13, 1917, CSS, box 36, folder 132.

7. Kirkbride to Burritt, March 16, 1917, CSS, box 36, folder 132. While not used in this letter, I have used the term "experiment" because, in later minutes, that is what the AICP itself termed its Columbus Hill work. See May 24 meeting notes of "Mr. Burritt," n.y., CSS, box 36, folder 132, 1.

8. Alfred Crosby, *The Forgotten Pandemic: The Influenza of 1918*, 2nd ed. (New York: Cambridge University Press, 2003). Neither Crosby nor John M. Barry can explain why, with a history of black mortality rates that run twice as high or higher than those for whites, regardless of disease, chronic illness, or injury, the black influenza rates for 1918–1919 were half that of whites. Nationwide, problems existed with reporting areas and data (twenty-two states could not report mortality data by 1920; most were in the South where, coincidentally, the overwhelming majority of African Americans still lived). Nevertheless, the switch in mortality rates from influenza-related deaths held strongly among New York City's black populations. Also see John M. Barry, *The Great Influenza: The Epic Story of the Deadliest Plague in History* (New York: Viking Books, 2004).

9. Burritt to Kirkbride, January 13, 1917.

10. Robert E. Chaddock, PhD, "Sanitary Districts in the Analysis of Municipal Mortality and Morbidity Data," *American Journal of Public Health* 6, no. 6 (June 1916): 533–535.

11. Ibid., 534–535.

12. John Duffy, *A History of Public Health in New York City, 1866–1966* (New York: Russell Sage Foundation, 1974), 107.

13. Chaddock, "Sanitary Districts in the Analysis of Municipal Mortality and Morbidity Data," 536.

14. John Snow, *On the Mode of Communication of Cholera* (London: John Churchill, New Burlington Street, England, 1855).

15. Dr. David. V. Cohn, "The Life and Times of Louis Pasteur," http://www.founders ofscience.net/interest1.htm, accessed February 26, 2014.

16. Frank M. Snowden, *Naples in the Time of Cholera: 1884–1911* (Cambridge, UK: Cambridge University Press, 1995), 67–69. When von Pettenkofer, assured of his correctness, tried to infect himself with a large dose of the *vibrio cholerae* mixed in water, his less-certain assistants, without his knowledge, greatly diluted the dosage so that he would not die from the disease. When Koch finally replicated the bacteria in his laboratory (no small feat: cholera is highly fragile and hard to reproduce in vitro), and the scientific community largely accepted cholera as an infectious bacterium borne through the oral/fecal route, von Pettenkofer committed suicide. Suicide is always unfortunate, and it was even more so with the death of von Pettenkofer, whose insistence on sanitary measures to combat the spread of cholera was correct, even though he had gotten the etiology all wrong.

17. Chaddock, "Sanitary Districts in the Analysis of Municipal Mortality and Morbidity Data," 537.

18. Duffy, *A History of Public Health in New York City, 1866–1966*, 105–106.

19. Chaddock, "Sanitary Districts in the Analysis of Municipal Mortality and Morbidity Data," 538.

20. William Guilfoy, M.D., and Shirley W. Wynne, M.D., *An Analysis of Mortality Returns of the Sanitary Areas of the Borough of Manhattan for the Year 1915* (New York City Department of Health, 1916), 4.

21. Guilfoy and Wynne, *An Analysis of Mortality Returns*, 3–4.

22. Norman L. Holmes, "Columbus Hill: The Story of a Negro Community," *Opportunity* 1, no. 1 (April 1923): 10.

23. Guilfoy and Wynne, *An Analysis of Mortality Returns*, 15–17. The area of Columbus Hill where the infant mortality rate was highest should also include residents from West 60th through West 62nd Streets between Columbus and Amsterdam Avenues, in the 113th Sanitary District, where one-sixth of the inhabitants were black. The haphazard methodology of identifying and categorizing sanitary districts by race made for suspect overall morbidity and mortality statistics. For example, since the AICP chose to work with people of African descent within "Columbus Hill" (also known earlier as San Juan Hill, which Guilfoy and Wynne stated was contained in the 119th District), the actual area encompassed parts of three sanitary districts, which did not always result in "clean" statistics.

24. Ibid., 16–18.

25. Burritt to Kirkbride, February 5, 1918. Burritt advised Kirkbride that, according to Miss Price, the AICP nurse hired to work with Columbus Hill's blacks, all pregnant mothers were given Wassermann testing for syphilis. "You will be interested in this connection to know that in nearly 50 per cent of the families we are finding positive Wassermanns," Burritt wrote.

26. Quoted in James H. Jones, *Bad Blood: The Tuskegee Syphilis Experiment* (1981; New York: The Free Press, 1993), 27.

27. David Mc Bride, *From TB to AIDS: Epidemics Among Urban Blacks Since 1900* (Albany: State University of New York Press, 1991), 17–19.

28. Jones, *Bad Blood*, 29.

29. Ibid., 41.

30. Dr. Frank M. Snowden, lecture on the Paris School of medicine, Yale University, February 5, 2004.

31. Katherine Ott, *Fevered Lives: Tuberculosis in American Culture Since 1870* (Cambridge, MA: Harvard University Press, 1996), 56–57; Charles E. Rosenberg, *The Cholera Years: The United States in 1832, 1849, and 1866* (Chicago: University of Chicago Press, 1987), 1–9, 175–191.

32. Snowden, *Naples in the Time of Cholera*, 99–154.

33. Naomi Rogers, *Dirt and Disease: Polio Before FDR* (New Brunswick, NJ: Rutgers University Press, 1996), 30–71. The New York City polio outbreak of 1916 is an excellent example. Despite epidemiological proof, physicians and public health officials targeted the immigrant poor, and especially Italians, as the source of the disease. No amount of proof that polio inflicted its heaviest damage among native middle-class white children who lived in areas with good sanitation could dissuade officials from mounting massive sanitation and health education campaigns among the poor.

34. Nancy Leys Stepan, "Race and Gender: The Role of Analogy in Science," in *The "Racial" Economy of Science: Toward a Democratic Future*, ed. Sandra Harding (Bloomington: Indiana University Press, 1993), 360, 364–367; Gail Bederman, *Manliness and Civilization: A Cultural History of Gender and Race in the United States, 1880–1917* (Chicago: University of Chicago Press, 1995), 5–23; Daniel J. Kevles, *In the Name of Eugenics: Genetics and the Uses of Human Heredity* (Berkeley: University of California Press, 1985), 45–49.

35. Stephen Jay Gould, *The Mismeasure of Man* (New York: W. W. Norton, 1981) 30–72, 146–232; Reginald Horsman, *Race and Manifest Destiny: The Origins of American Racial Anglo-Saxonism*. Cambridge, MA: Harvard University Press, 1981), 43–61; Matthew Frye Jacobson, *Whiteness of a Different Color: European Immigrants and the Alchemy of Race* (Cambridge, MA: Harvard University Press, 1998), 6–10; Ott, *Fevered Lives*, 100–110; Nancy Tomes, *The Gospel of Germs: Men, Women, and the Microbe in American Life* (Cambridge, MA: Harvard University Press, 1998), 184.

36. Susan Moeller, "The Cultural Construction of Urban Poverty: Images of Poverty in New York City, 1890–1917," *Journal of American Culture* 18, no. 4 (1995): 1–3. Also see Dawn Greeley, "Beyond Benevolence: Gender, Class, and the Development of Scientific Charity in New York City, 1882, 1935" (PhD diss., State University of New York, Stony Brook, 1995); Nancy Weiss, "Save the Children: the History of the Children's Bureau, 1903–1918" (PhD diss., University of California, Los Angeles, 1974), 192–193; Louis I. Dublin, "The Mortality of Early Infancy," in *Transactions of the Thirteenth-Annual Meeting of the American Child Hygiene Association, Washington, D.C., October 12–14, 1922* (Albany, NY: J. B. Lyon Company, Printers, 1923), 1. Dublin

argued that, along with teaching mothers how to correctly feed their children, to put a dent in preventable neonatal deaths and stillbirths, mothering had to be understood as a job, one as vital as those held by men who received remuneration for their labor. Unfortunately, even with Mother's Pensions, which paid little and shifted female dependency from the deceased, divorced, or absent husband, women as heads of household now became dependent on the state, and little helpful attention was focused on the alleviation of poverty as an environmental hazard to prenatal, neonatal, and infant health. Also see Linda Gordon, *Pitied But Not Entitled: Single Mothers and the History of Welfare, 1890–1935* (Cambridge: Harvard University Press, 1994), 129, 141; Gwendolyn Mink, "The Lady and the Tramp: Gender, Race, and the Origins of the American Welfare State," in *Women, the State, and Welfare*, ed. Linda Gordon (Madison: University of Wisconsin Press, 1990), 106–111.

37. John C. Gebhart, *Health Work for Mothers and Children in a Colored Community* (New York: Association for Improving the Condition of the Poor, 1924), 4, 6. Gebhart, "Syphilis as a Prenatal Problem," *Journal of Social Hygiene* 10, no. 4 (August 1924): 208; *Annual Report of the Department of Health of the City of New York for the Calendar Year 1918* (New York: New York City Department of Health, 1918), 139; *Annual Report of the Department of Health of the City of New York for the Calendar Year 1919* (New York: New York City Department of Health, 1919), 133.

38. May 24 meeting notes of "Mr. Burritt," CSS, box 36, folder 132, 1. Although this document has no year, I believe it is the transcript of a meeting held at the home of Mrs. Arthur Holden on May 20, 1924, which was called to address the need for the continuation of health work in Columbus Hill, its direction, and its funding. Taken from "Minutes of the Meeting: Held at the Residence of Mrs. Arthur Holden, 67 East 92nd St., May 20, 1924 to Consider a Health Program for the Columbus Hill District," CSS, box 36, folder 132, 1. Also, the speakers' names and the order of the comments in the May 24 meeting notes match those of the May 20, 1924 minutes.

The terms "experiment" and "demonstration" were used interchangeably by privately funded public health concerns at the time, who would propose health work within a particular area to the Department of Health, carry out the work and show health department officials how it could be done, and, if accepted, continue the work—now with a percentage of public funding, of course. See Karen Buhler-Wilkerson, "False Dawn: The Rise and Fall of Public Health Nursing, 1900–1930" (PhD diss., University of Pennsylvania, 1984), 108–111.

39. Burritt to Kirkbride, February 5, 1918, 2.

40. May 24 meeting notes of "Mr. Burritt," 1–3; Columbia University College of Physicians and Surgeons, *Report of the Dean for the Academic Year ending June 30, 1924* (published in 1925), 11–23.

41. May 24 meeting notes of "Mr. Burritt," 1–2.

42. May 24 meeting notes of "Mr. Burritt," 6. Dr, Blumenthal stated that the infant mortality rate had been 130/1,000 in Columbus Hill, compared to 70/1,000 for the city; the maternal mortality rate had been 26/1,000 in Columbus Hill, compared to "5 or 6, so that the necessity for doing work in this area is quite evident."

43. Gebhart, *Health Work for Mothers and Children in a Colored Community*, 3. At the beginning of the pamphlet, Gebhart states, "It is generally recognized that syphilitic infection is one of the most fruitful cases of still-births, miscarriages, and early death of infants. A prenatal service which makes no provision for detecting syphilitic infection in prospective mothers and which fails to provide continuous treatment for those found to be infected will therefore fail to accomplish optimum results in the saving of lives of mothers and babies. This again is one of the striking problems of this district. Syphilis is particularly prevalent among the colored mothers of this area and to have neglected this phase of the problem would have been an inexcusable oversight in our prenatal service" (3–4).

44. May 24 meeting notes of "Mr. Burritt," 13.

45. Gebhart, *Health Work for Mothers and Children in a Colored Community*, 5; May 24 meeting notes of "Mr. Burritt," 4. A Mr. Hubert, the New York City Urban League Secretary who was also in attendance at the meeting, revealed that with a "foreign element [that] is more that 50% of the population" of Columbus Hill, when the "substantial citizens of that district move out, to Harlem and elsewhere," the area's need for outside assistance increases (8)

46. May 24 meeting notes of "Mr. Burritt," 3–4.

47. Allan M. Brandt, *No Magic Bullet: A Social History of Venereal Disease in the United States Since 1880* (New York: Oxford University Press, 1985), 149. In 1916, Dr J. Whitridge Williams, an obstetrician at Johns Hopkins Hospital, revealed that 26 percent of 700 fetal deaths occurred from congenital syphilis. He required Wassermann tests for all pregnant women who came for the services of his prenatal clinic.

48. Jones, *Bad Blood*, 16–17.

49. Ibid., 18.

50. Kenneth F. Kiple and Virginia Himmelsteib King, *Another Dimension to the Black Diaspora: Diet, Disease, and Racism* (New York: Cambridge University Press, 1981), 43–44, 62; Susan L. Smith, *Sick and Tired of Being Sick and Tired: Black Women's Health Activism in America, 1890–1950* (Philadelphia: University of Pennsylvania Press, 1995), 5.

51. Smith, *Sick and Tired of Being Sick and Tired*, 17–19.

52. Rogers, *Dirt and Disease*, 70; Vanessa Northington Gamble, M.D., *Germs Have no Color Line: Blacks and American Medicine, 1900–1940* (New York: Garland, 1989), 1. Gamble took the title of her book from a 1929 Chicago hospital funding campaign of the same name. Its purpose was to raise money for a black medical training facility within Provident Hospital. Also see David Mc Bride, *From TB to AIDS: Epidemics Among Urban Blacks Since 1900* (Albany: State University of New York Press, 1991).

53. Jones, *Bad Blood*, 40. In chapter 2 of *Bad Blood*, James Jones's review of Progressive Era medical journal articles about black health and the debate over race versus environment shows how easily physicians slide between both categories. While Jones explains the period as one in which "[p]ublic health officials believed more in the power of science than the weakness of any race," he also maintains that "[h]ealth

officials persisted in the belief that racial differences existed in susceptibility, severity, and complications of diseases" (36, 40). My research has unearthed the same subtle shift that Jones saw within his analysis. However, these physicians and officials worked during what has been termed the "nadir" of black existence in the United States. Thus, I do not find it problematic that they often collapsed environmental causes of poor health into behavioralism—and rooted unhealthy behavior, or susceptibility to disease, within a racialistic paradigm. Clearly, "race," as perceived in the late nineteenth and early twentieth centuries, was large and amorphous enough to easily contain warring ideologies.

54. Loyd Thompson, M.D., and Lyle. B. Kingery, M.D., "Syphilis in the Negro," *American Journal of Syphilis* 3 (1919): 393–394.

55. Ibid., 385.

56. Alisa Klaus, *Every Child a Lion: The Origins of Maternal and Infant Health Policy in the United States and France, 1890–1920* (Ithaca, NY: Cornell University Press, 1993), 35–36; Edward H. Beardsley, *A History of Neglect: Health Care for Blacks and Mill Workers in the Twentieth-Century South* (Knoxville: University of Tennessee Press, 1987), 23–24.

57. L. C. Allen, M.D., "The Negro Health Problem," *American Journal of Public Health* 5, no. 3 (March 1915): 194; A. G. Fort, Ph.B., M.D., "The Negro Health Problem in Rural Communities," *American Journal of Public Health* 5, no. 3 (March 1915): 192.

58. C. E. Terry, M.D., "The Negro, a Public Health Problem," *Southern Medical Journal* 7 (June, 1914): 458–459.

59 Brandt, *No Magic Bullet*, 19–23; Antonio Stella, M.D., *Some Aspects of Italian Immigration to the United States: Statistical Data and General Considerations Based Chiefly Upon the United States Censuses and Other Official Publications* (New York: G. P. Putnam, 1924), 69–71; Klaus, *Every Child a Lion*, 123.

60. Bederman, *Manliness and Civilization*, 20–31; Brandt, *No Magic Bullet*, 19–21; *White Women's Rights*, 39–42.

61. Brandt, *No Magic Bullet*, 8; Klaus, *Every Child a Lion*, 34–35, 277–278.

62. Brandt, *No Magic Bullet*, 16–17, 31–35.

63. Charles M. Whitney, M.D., "The Impossibility of Curing Syphilis by Salvarsan Alone and the Dangers Arising From Insufficient Treatment," *Interstate Medical Journal* 23 (1916): 83.

64. Brandt, *No Magic Bullet*, 40–41. Salvarsan, a generic term for arsphenamine and other arsenic-based compounds, was also called "606" because it was the 606th chemical compound that finally worked in his experiments. Because salvarsan was highly toxic, Ehrlich invented Neosalvarsan or "914" in 1912. It was widely used by U.S. physicians by 1915, though its worldwide acceptance did not occur during the 1920s. Mercury treatments were still used in conjunction with arsenigens.

65. Brandt, *No Magic Bullet*, 40; Jones, *Bad Blood*, 45.

66. Brandt, *No Magic Bullet*, 40; Jones, *Bad Blood*, 7. In a retrospective on the efficacy of salvarsan and neosalvarsan (arsphenamine and neoarsphenamine) issued in

1972 because of the public uproar over the Tuskegee Experiment, Dr. Donald W. Prinz of the U.S. Center for Disease Control argued that "the drugs [had] offered 'more potential harm for the patient than potential benefit'" (243, n.12).

67. Lewis W. Elias, M.D., "The Intravenous Administration of Salvarsan in Babies," *Southern Medical Journal* 7, no. 9 (September 1914): 708–710. According to Elias, the method used to administer salvarsan treatments to infants "[was] the result of evolution." At first, physicians required the anesthetization of the infant and the removal of an arm vein by dissection. Then, salvarsan was instituted within the arm via a "fine glass canula." Since infant veins were so small and fragile, a second, "external jugular" method was devised. A doctor would inject salvarsan through the child's skin and into the jugular vein. However, this would not work on so-called "fat babies," and led physicians to resort to the first method. The third and final method consisted of injecting salvarsan into scalp veins. Elias stated, "When the child cried the veins swelled out prominently, and owing to the fibrous and bony attachments it was very easy to enter [the vein]." This method became the last and best way to administer salvarsan and, according to Elias's 1914 article, had resulted in only one case of scalp discoloration, which had disappeared in a few days.

68. Wilhelm Wechselmann, M.D., "Reports of Salvarsan Fatalities," *Urologic and Cutaneous Review* 17 (1913): 649–651.

69. Walter G. Baetz, M.D., "Syphilis in Colored Canal Laborers: A Resume of 500 Consecutive Medical Cases," *New York Medical Journal* (1914): 820.

70. H. H. Hazen, M.D., "Practical Observations on Syphilis, VI," *American Journal of Syphilis* 7, no. 3 (July 1923): 417.

71. E. Meyer, "Clinical and Experimental Research on the Action of Salvarsan Upon Congenital Syphilis of the Foetus Through Treatment of the Mother," *Journal of Cutaneous Diseases* 33 (1915): 418–419. Using his own test results and those from another physician, Meyer stated that he was "convinced that the combined mercury-salvarsan treatment far excels the mercury or mercury-oxide treatment." He further argued that although salvarsan could not permeate a "healthy" placenta, it would if the woman was infected with syphilis. "The action of antisyphilitic treatment during pregnancy is primarily upon the maternal infection, thus preventing infection of the placenta. Salvarsan is well borne by the pregnant. No abortions or haemorrhages or foetal [sic] deaths were seen after the intravenous injections." In addition, Meyer advocated administering salvarsan to children borne of syphilitic mothers "even though [the children] show no signs of the disease" (418).

72. Brandt, *No Magic Bullet*, 44, 149; Walter E. Welz, M.D., and Alfred E. Van Nest, M.D., "Observations on the Treatment of Syphilis in Pregnancy in the Department of Health in Detroit," *American Journal of Obstetrics and Gynecology* 4 (1922): 174–177. Prior to describing their work to reduce premature infant deaths and stillbirths in Detroit, the doctors paid homage to Williams's study.

73. Louis I. Dublin, M.D., "The Mortality of Early Infancy," 92–93.

74. Brandt, *No Magic Bullet*, 44; 149.

CHAPTER 6. HEALTH IN COLUMBUS HILL

1. Bailey B. Burritt to Franklin B. Kirkbride, April 11, 1917, CSS box 36, folder 132,1. Burritt told Kirkbride that Price had made a "careful study of the distribution of the colored population of the West side with reference to the infant mortality among that group" and, based on this research, had determined to limit her focus to Sanitary Districts 115 and 119. He realized that "a scattered colored population" existed in two other census districts but decided to not include them because their health problems were "not nearly so acute . . . and it seemed wise to use, at least in the beginning of the work, to confine our efforts to the 115th district and then if we find that we can take on more, to include the 119th district."

This noted, the area of Columbus Hill where the infant mortality rate was highest *should have also included* black residents from West 60th through West 62nd Streets between Columbus and Amsterdam Avenues, in the 113th Sanitary District. There, one-sixth of the inhabitants were black. If the infant mortality rate for the 113th Sanitary District is included with that of districts 115 and 119, the 1915 black IMR soars from about 33 percent to almost 45 percent. The haphazard methodology of identifying and categorizing sanitary districts by race made for suspect overall morbidity and mortality statistics. For example, since the AICP chose to work with people of African descent within "Columbus Hill" (also known earlier as "San Juan Hill," which Guilfoy and Wynne stated was contained in the 119th District), the actual area encompassed parts of three sanitary districts, which did not always result in "clean" statistics. See William Guilfoy, M.D., and Shirley W. Wynne, M.D., *An Analysis of Mortality Returns of the Sanitary Areas of the Borough of Manhattan for the Year 1915* (New York: New York City Department of Health, 1916), 15–17; Norman A. Holmes, "Sociological Survey of the Negro Population of Columbus Hill of New York City" (typescript, Lincoln House Committee on the Henry Street Settlement, New York, October 14, 1922), 1 2, 8–9.

2. Bailey B. Burritt to Franklin B. Kirkbride, February 5, 1918, CSS, box 32, folder 132. Although Burritt's admission that "[t]he practice of giving Wassermann tests has been extended to all expectant mothers. This was formerly given only to in-door (in-patient) cases" does not specifically note black women, the letter reports only the status of health work performed for Columbus Hill's blacks. Taken within this context, it would seem illogical to infer that Burritt was suddenly referring to native-born white or European women, along with black women, as "all expectant mothers."

3. May 24 meeting notes of "Mr. Burritt," n.d., CSS, box 36, folder 132, 3. A Miss Phillips, presumably an AICP nurse or nursing supervisor, stated that the AICP carried "over 95% of the expectant mothers in that district."

4. "Colored Prenatal" report, October 1, 1918 to September 30, 1919, CSS, box 67, folder 132, 1.

5. "Colored Prenatal" report, 1. Out of the remaining non-syphilitic stillbirths during the period, two resulted from mothers with pneumonia, one was a breech birth performed by a private physician, one set of twins was born prematurely, and one

death resulted from a midwife's case, where the woman refused to give further information. Of the four remaining neonatal deaths, one resulted from a cerebral hemorrhage ("Wass. Negative)," one from pneumonia, one "prematurity (mother had pneumonia)," and one infant died from a congenital defect (cleft palate). The report covered 523 families, out of which 492 were listed as "under observation." Over 2,000 persons lived in these families. Out of 294 women given prenatal care, almost 24 percent were diagnosed as syphilitic. (I cannot determine with certainty where the 294 number originated because of conflicting statistics.)

6. May 24 meeting notes of "Mr. Burritt," 9.

7. Ibid. 9–10.

8. H. H. Hazen, M.D., "Practical Observations on Syphilis, VI," *American Journal of Syphilis* 7, no. 3 (July 1923): 422.

9. Ibid., 422–424; Allan M. Brandt, *No Magic Bullet: A Social History of Venereal Disease in the United States Since 1880* (New York: Oxford University Press, 1985), 130. Dr. Henry H. Hazen operated a syphilis clinic at the Freedman's Bureau Hospital in Washington, DC, and taught at Georgetown University. In 1923, he outlined steps that physicians should follow if they saw positive physical signs of syphilis in a patient, and yet received a negative Wassermann reaction from the laboratory.

10. Burritt to Kirkbride, February 5, 1918, 2; May 24 meeting notes of "Mr. Burritt," 12.

11. Holmes, "Sociological Survey," 11. For the most part, Dr. Henry H. Hazen reflected on the fact that, among the hundreds of cases of black syphilitics he treated at the Freedman's Bureau Hospital in Washington, DC, most responded to treatments and returned for follow-up care as well as whites. In fact, Hazen declared, that " 'The secret of treating blacks is to show them that you are taking an interest in them, and also that you mean just what you say.' " His proof was that " 'a number of cases have been coming in regularly for two or three years.' " Quoted in James H. Jones, *Bad Blood: The Tuskegee Syphilis Experiment* (1981; New York: The Free Press, 1993), 46.

12. Charles M. Whitney, M.D., "The Impossibility of Curing Syphilis by Salvarsan Alone and the Dangers Arising From Insufficient Treatment," *Interstate Medical Journal* 23 (1916): 80.

13. Ibid., 81–83.

14. Ibid., 85–86.

15. Nancy Schrom Dye, "Modern Obstetrics and Working-Class Women: The New York Midwifery Dispensary, 1890–1920," *Journal of Social History* 20 (1987): 550.

16. Sandra Opdycke, *No One Was Turned Away: The Role of Public Hospitals in New York City Since 1900* (Cambridge, UK: Oxford University Press, 1999). Opdycke's study compares the parallel missions of charity service that categorized Bellevue and New York Hospital in the early twentieth century, and rapidly diverged during the 1920s. Her first two chapters give excellent coverage of the funding controversies faced by both private and public hospitals, and the choice of whether to align with teaching universities or remain separate.

17. "History of the College of Physicians and Surgeons," http://ps.columbia.edu/about-ps/history-college-physicians-and-surgeons, February 26, 2014.

18. Adele Lerner, archivist, Medical Archives of New York Weill-Cornell Center of New York Presbyterian Hospital, discussion with the author, April 27, 1999.

19. Columbia University College of Physicians and Surgeons, *Report of the Dean for the Academic Year Ending June 30, 1924* (Annual Report of the Dean, P & S [1909–1924], loose copy box 1/2), 23–24.

20. Jones, *Bad Blood*, 49–50. During the 1920s, federal funding for syphilis research plummeted because the war, and the threat posed by public airing of high numbers of diseased service men, ceased to be a relevant public health hazard in the eyes of Congress.

21. Brandt, *No Magic Bullet*, 116. The white rate of venereal disease was believed to be 10%.

22. Ibid., 25–27.

23. Columbia University College of Physicians and Surgeons, *Report of the Dean for the Academic Year Ending June 16, 1916* (Annual Report of the Dean, P & S [1909–1923], loose copy box 1/2), 13.

24. Columbia Alumni News-Alumni Federation of Columbia University, Inc., 13:15 (January 27, 1922); *Report of the Dean for the Academic Year Ending June 30, 1921* (Annual Report of the Dean, P & S [1909–1923], loose copy box 1/2), 11.

25. Columbia University College of Physicians and Surgeons, *Report of the Dean for the Academic Year Ending June 30, 1923* (Annual Report of the Dean, P & S [1909–1923], loose copy box 1/2), 17–19.

26. Columbia University College of Physicians and Surgeons, *Report of the Dean for the Academic Year Ending June 30, 1924*, 11–16.

27. John C. Gebhart, *Health Work for Mothers and Children in a Colored Community* (New York: New York Association for Improving the Condition of the Poor, 1924), 7–11; John C. Gebhart, "Syphilis as a Prenatal Problem," *Journal of Social Hygiene* 10, no. 4 (August 1924): 208. I use, but question, the veracity of the AICP's statistics because of problems between data reflected in internal vs. external reports.

28. Louis I. Dublin, M.D., "The Mortality of Early Infancy," in *Transactions of the Thirteenth Annual Meeting of the American Child Hygiene Association, Washington, D.C., October 12-14, 1922* (Albany, NY: J. B. Lyon Company, Printers, 1923), 83–88.

29. Ibid., 91.

30. Todd L. Savitt, "Slave Health and Social Distinctiveness," in *Disease and Distinctiveness in the American South*, ed. Todd L. Savitt and James Harvey Young (Knoxville: University of Tennessee Press, 1988), 120–123.

31. Ibid., 123–126. For colonial American whites and seasoning, see Edmund Morgan, *American Slavery, American Freedom* (New York: W. W. Norton, 1975).

32. Savitt, "Slave Health and Social Distinctiveness," 126, 128.

33. Todd L. Savitt, *Medicine and Slavery: The Diseases and Health Care of Blacks in Antebellum Virginia* (Urbana: University of Illinois Press, 2002), 41–45.

34. Savitt, "Slave Health and Social Distinctiveness," 126–127. For the debate over "virgin soil" vs. a lack of genetic variability among Native Americans that left them highly vulnerable to the ravaged of small pox, see Elizabeth A. Fenn, *Pox Americana: The Great Smallpox Epidemic of 1775–1782* (New York: Hill and Wang, 2001), 25–27.

35. James O. Breeden, "Disease as a Factor in Southern Distinctiveness," in Savitt and Young, *Disease and Distinctiveness in the American South*, 4–6.

36. David McBride, *From TB to AIDS: Epidemics Among Urban Blacks Since 1900* (Albany: State University of New York Press, 1991), 15–19.

37. Katherine Ott, *Fevered Lives: Tuberculosis in American Culture Since 1870* (Cambridge, MA: Harvard University Press, 1996), 13–16.

38. Ibid., 53–68.

39. McBride, *From TB to AIDS*, 15–19.

40. Alan M. Kraut, *Silent Travelers: Germs, Genes, and the "Immigrant Menace"* (Baltimore: Johns Hopkins University Press, 1994), 115–127; Nancy Tomes, *The Gospel of Germs: Men, Women, and the Microbe in American Life* (Cambridge, MA: Harvard University Press, 1998), 34–46, 135–164, 183–195.

41. Kenneth F. Kiple and Virginia Himmelsteib King, *Another Dimension to the Black Diaspora: Diet, Disease, and Racism* (New York: Cambridge University Press, 1981), 140–141.

42. Ibid., 139–141. The authors also agreed with Todd Savitt that scrofula, or the "great scourge" of nineteenth-century blacks, was probably a genetically distinctive form of tuberculosis that largely affected only Africans and their descendants. Tuberculosis was a European disease which, upon close white/Indian contact, struck Native Americans with incredible ferocity. White contacts in Western Africa remained largely confined to coastal areas. Thus, as in a "balkanized" area, tuberculosis spread more slowly to West Africans. Many of those who were kidnapped and enslaved had little prior contact with the disease. Some died, but many overcame the infection. What is commonly known today as scrofula is a bovine tubercular disease—hardly one that blacks, with characteristically higher levels of lactose intolerance, would actually have contracted from infected milk. Kiple and Himmelsteib King argue that scrofula, a rampant disease among antebellum and post-Emancipation blacks, was a form of miliary tuberculosis and thus a misnomer resulting from blatant white misdiagnoses of "black" diseases (142–143).

43. Marie Oleatha Pitts Moseley, "A History of Black Leaders in Nursing: The Influence of Four Black Community Health Nurses on the Establishment, Growth, and Practice of Public Health Nursing in New York City, 1900–1930" (PhD diss., Columbia University Teachers College, 1992), 43. The AICP also realized, at least on paper, that a black nurse was important in securing help for Columbus Hill's black residents. In Burritt's first letter to Kirkbride requesting financial help to fund a nurse in Columbus Hill, he revealed that "it would be better, I believe, to have a colored person" trained to handle "family social problems" as the AICP's first visiting nurse. However, he lamented that none could be found, and hired Miss Price, a white woman. By the late

1920s, all of the nurses and nurse supervisors covering Columbus Hill's black community were black. See Burritt letters to Kirkbride dated January 13, 1917, and March 30, 1917, and an "Introductory Statement" prepared for the *Amsterdam News* (CSS, box 36, folder 132). For black/white cooperation in tuberculosis campaigns and tuberculosis as a "negro disease," see Tera Hunter, *To Joy My Freedom: Southern Black Women's Lives and Labors after the Civil War* (Cambridge, MA: Harvard University Press, 1997), 195–218; and Tomes, *The Gospel of Germs*, 220–233.

44. Moseley, "A History of Black Leaders in Nursing," 75, 88.

45. Ibid., 89–90.

46. Ibid., 91–94. Jessie Sleet, "Tuberculosis Among Negroes," was printed in *The Third Annual Report of the Committee on the Prevention of Tuberculosis of the Charity Organization Society of the City of New York, for the Year 1904–1905*. Marie Oleatha Pitts Moseley reprinted this article in its entirety in her dissertation. I quote Sleet from this source.

47. Moseley, "A History of Black Leaders in Nursing," 94–95.

48. Tanya Hart, "Constructing Syphilis and Black Motherhood: Maternal Health Care for Women of African Descent in New York's Columbus Hill, 1915–30," *Women, Gender and Families of Color* 1, no. 1 (Spring 2013): 33–58. Samuel Kelton Roberts Jr.'s excellent work, *Infectious Fear*, chronicles African Americans and tuberculosis in early twentieth century Baltimore. He writes that whites termed blacks who resisted tuberculosis testing and treatment as "incorrigible consumptives," reflecting the mistrust, fear of stigmatization, and resistance that blacks levied against being defined as tubercular. I have found no such resistance from black women against syphilis testing and treatment in my research. I think this largely stems from the nature of venereal diseases which, from the public eye, are largely invisible, while anyone coughing during early twentieth century anti-spitting and other tuberculosis information campaigns might have been stigmatized as tubercular, rightly or wrongly, by family and friends, coworkers, and strangers. See Samuel Kelton Roberts Jr., *Infectious Fear: Politics, Disease, and the Health Effects of Segregation* (Chapel Hill: University of North Carolina Press, 2009), 142–148.

49. Guilfoy and Wynne, *An Analysis of Mortality Returns*, 15–18.

50. Sheila M. Rothman, *Living in the Shadow of Death: Tuberculosis and the Social Experience of Illness in American History* (Baltimore: Johns Hopkins University Press, 1994), 179–193. For more on the racial, class, and gendered subjectivities that lay beneath forced confinements in New York City, see Judith Walzer Leavitt, *Typhoid Mary: Captive to the Public's Health* (Boston: Beacon Press, 1996).

51. May 24 meeting notes of "Mr. Burritt," 12.

52. Ott, *Fevered Lives*, 140–141.

53. Holmes, "Sociological Survey," 10. One of the areas, Sanitary District 31, was a "downtown business section" with a tuberculosis death rate of 1,113/100,000, but a population of 621. The other area, Sanitary District 109, incorporated part of the Tenderloin, an equally impoverished neighborhood. There, the tuberculosis mortality

was slightly higher than that of Columbus Hill: 606/100,000, and the population slightly over 4,700 in 1922.

54. Bailey B. Burritt to Franklin B. Kirkbride, April 16, 1918, CSS, box 36, folder 132.

CHAPTER 7. BIRTHING IN THE CITY: THE MULBERRY DISTRICT

1. Quoted in William Guilfoy, M.D., and Shirley W. Wynne, M.D., *An Analysis of Mortality Returns of the Sanitary Areas of the Borough of Manhattan for the Year 1915* (New York: New York City Department of Health, 1916), 29. In part of Guilfoy and Wynne's "Recommendations" from the aftermath of the 1915 morbidity and mortality data, they stated, "Deaths should be tabulated in all Boroughs by sanitary areas in order to enable the Department to pick out the sore spots in the Boroughs and, having picked them out, to concentrate their efforts in them rather than scattering their forces throughout the Borough with the result that in favorable districts there is little to be done and too many employes [sic] to do it, while in the unfavorable districts the force is not sufficient to more than scratch the surface" (30).

2. Ibid., 29–31.

3. John C. Gebhart, "Five-Years' Experience With a Community Health Program: A Report on Mulberry Health Center" (New York: New York Association for Improving the Condition of the Poor, 1923), CSS, box 61, folder 367, 11, 4.

4. Guilfoy and Wynne, *An Analysis of Mortality*, 28–29. Guilfoy and Wynne focused on the 113th, 115th, 119th, and 153rd sanitary districts in their section entitled "The Mortality in the Negro Districts" (the 115th and part of the 113th contained the black population of Columbus Hill, as well as the southern border, W. 62nd Street, from Amsterdam to the River, in the 119th District). However, both agreed that "there is dire need of health work in all the negro [sic] districts."

5. Tukufu Zuberi and Eduardo Bonilla-Silva, eds., *White Logic, White Methods: Racism and Methodology* (New York: Rowman and Littlefield, 2008).

6. Gebhart, "Five Year's Experience with a Community Health Program," 1.

7. "Mulberry Health Center Survey" (New York City: New York Association for Improving the Condition of the Poor, 1923), CSS, box 61, folder 367, 11, 2. In the 1922–1923 survey of the Mulberry District, the AICP reported that out of the more than 13,000 adults, 12,000 had been born in Italy; 5,000 in Campagna, 4,500 in Sicily (both regions considered part of southern Italy), and 2,600 from four other regions. Since the majority originated from southern Italian regions, I use the terms "Italian" and "southern Italian" interchangeably.

8. See Gebhart, "Five Year's Experience with a Community Health Program"; "Ten Years in Mulberry Bend" (New York: New York Association for Improving the Condition of the Poor Statistical Bureau, May 1929) CSS, box 61, folder 367, 8; "Mulberry Health Center Survey," 1-4; Elizabeth C. Tandy, "Report to the Executive Secretary on the Mulberry Community Sickness Study" (prepared for the Committee on Dispensary Development, New York, May 1, 1923), CSS, box 61, folder 367, 11; "Vital Statistics of Mulberry Health Center, 1915–1925" (New York: New York Association for Improving the Condition of the Poor Statistics Bureau, 1927), CSS, box 61, folder 367, 11.

9. Guilfoy and Wynne, *An Analysis of Mortality Returns*, 22–29.

10. Reginald Horsman, *Race and Manifest Destiny: The Origins of American Racial Anglo-Saxonism*. Cambridge, MA: Harvard University Press, 1981), 139–186; Matthew Frye Jacobson, *Whiteness of a Different Color: European Immigrants and the Alchemy of Race* (Cambridge, MA: Harvard University Press, 1998), 39–90.

11 Oxford Dictionary, http://www.oxforddictionaries.com/us/definition/american_english/contadino, accessed December 1, 2014.

12. Alan M. Kraut, *Silent Travelers: Germs, Genes, and the "Immigrant Menace"* (Baltimore: John Hopkins University Press, 1994), 107–109; Jacobson, *Whiteness of a Different Color*, 80; Alisa Klaus, *Every Child a Lion: The Origins of Maternal and Infant Health Policy in the United States and France, 1890–1920* (Ithaca, NY: Cornell University Press, 1993), 34–38; Gwendolyn Mink, "The Lady and the Tramp: Gender, Race, and the Origins of the American Welfare State," *Women, Welfare, and the State* (Madison: University of Wisconsin Press, 1990), 92–98.

13. Ross quoted in Kraut, *Silent Travelers*, 109.

14. "Ten Years in Mulberry Bend," 14.

15. Jacobson, *Whiteness of a Different Color*, 92–96.

16. Antonio Stella, M.D., "Tuberculosis and the Italians in the United States," in *Charities* 12:18 (May 1904): 486–489; Louis I. Dublin, M.D., "The Mortality of Foreign Race Stocks: A Contribution to the Quantitative Study of the Vigor of the Racial Elements in the Population of the United States," in *Scientific Monthly* 14:1 (January 1922), 95–101.

17. Kraut, *Silent Travelers*, 123. Antonio Stella branded accusations that Italians brought syphilis with them as salacious. Just as for the claims that Italians were rampant tuberculosis carriers, Stella maintained again that Italians contracted far more diseases in the United States than they had brought from their homeland.

18. Kraut, *Silent Travelers*, 115.

19. Ibid., 115–117; Phyllis H. Williams, *Southern Italian Folkways in Europe and America, a Handbook for Social Workers, Visiting Nurses, School Teachers, and Physicians* (New Haven, CT: Yale University Press, 1938), 166.

20. Regarding the spotty dependability of laboratory testing during the Progressive Era, the occurrence of false positive and false negative tests proliferated, depending on the laboratory used and who conducted the tests. To read more about the difficulties of laboratory testing and the power of the public health community to intern suspected carriers at will, see Judith Walzer Leavitt, *Typhoid Mary: Captive to the Public's Health* (Boston: Beacon Press, 1996).

21. Kraut, *Silent Travelers* 51–53, 66–67, 76. The USPHS presence in Ellis Island began in 1891, when the federal government passed a health act that affected all prospective immigrants: they had to undergo health inspections before departing from or arriving in the United States. Steamship companies bore the cost of the health inspection—and the detainment and housing costs when immigrants were deemed to ill to travel. These costs, however, were easily offset by the tremendous windfall in profits made by transporting immigrant populations to the U.S.

By 1893, persons entering the U.S. through Ellis Island were subjected to extensive questions regarding their medical histories. However, people leaving Italy were checked for illnesses by American health officials prior to boarding. The Italian government went further; in 1908, they began conducting their own pre-embarkment health inspections. Those lucky enough to pass Italian health exams, yet destined for steerage, received the most intensive testing upon arrival in New York City. Wealthy Italians were detained for only a few minutes.

22. Tandy, "Report to the Executive Secretary on the Mulberry Community Sickness Study," 8–9.

23. Stella, "Tuberculosis and the Italians in the United States," 486.

24. Ibid., 487. Stella characterized the racialized tuberculosis statistics coming from the New York City Department of Health as data from "a recent table" with no specific date, but the tuberculosis mortality rates he reported are: for Negroes, 548.4/10,000; for Irish, 428/10,000; and for Italians, 149.9/10,000. Also, as was common for the era, Stella alternates usage between tuberculosis and consumption, even twenty years after the discovery of the *tubercle bacillus*. The difference, of course, is dramatic, even for the sometimes questionable laboratory means of the time. Tuberculosis could be accurately diagnosed because its distinctive shape had been discovered earlier by laboratory isolation. Consumption, an older, amorphous term, may or may not have been tuberculosis prior to Koch's 1882 discovery of the tubercle bacillus because of physician subjectivity. Without laboratory testing and identification methods, a doctor's reason of "death as resulting from consumption" could have meant any (and any combination of) breathing-related complications. Even with the discovery of microbes and the establishment of the field of bacteriology and laboratory access, physicians still clung to older explanations of tuberculosis that co-mingled the disease with nineteenth-century consumption, while gradually embracing the new scientific methods and etiologies. The transformation from older methods to the acceptance of germ theory and bacteriology came grudgingly over time, and scientists, physicians, and health officials and reformers often clung to amalgams of contrary yet complementary views. Thus, consumption—the traditional name, however outmoded and incorrect—remained popular into the early twentieth century and was used contemporaneously with biomedically defined tuberculosis. Even with the supposed objectivity of new medical enhancements, public health officials and workers, and physicians themselves, still subjectively stigmatized individuals and groups as carriers of certain diseases because of their race and country of origin, and their gender. See Georgina D. Feldberg, *Disease and Class: Tuberculosis and the Shaping of Modern North American Society* (New Brunswick, NJ: Rutgers University Press, 1995), 36–38; Katherine Ott, *Fevered Lives: Tuberculosis in American Culture Since 1870* (Cambridge, MA: Harvard University Press, 1996), 3–4, 7; Naomi Rogers, *Dirt and Disease: Polio Before FDR* (New Brunswick, NJ: Rutgers University Press, 1996), 66–71; Sheila M. Rothman, *Living in the Shadow of Death: Tuberculosis and the Social Experience of Illness in American History* (Baltimore: Johns Hopkins University Press, 1994), 15–16; Nancy Tomes, *The*

Gospel of Germs: Men, Women, and the Microbe in American Life (Cambridge, MA: Harvard University Press, 1998), 28–47. For a complete social history of tuberculosis, see Barbara Bates, *Bargaining for Life: A Social History of Tuberculosis, 1878–1938* (Philadelphia: University of Pennsylvania Press, 1992).

25. Stella, "Tuberculosis and the Italians in the United States," 487.
26. Ibid.
27. Ibid., 488.
28. Jessie Sleet, "Tuberculosis Among Negroes," *The Third Annual Report of the Committee on the Prevention of Tuberculosis of the Charity Organization Society of the City of New York, for the Year 1904–1905*. Marie Oleatha Pitts Moseley reprinted this article in its entirety her dissertation, from which I have taken this information. See "A History of Black Leaders in Nursing: The Influence of Four Black Community Health Nurses on the Establishment, Growth, and Practice of Public Health Nursing in New York City, 1900–1930" (PhD diss., Columbia University Teachers College, 1992), 91–94.
29. Stella, "Tuberculosis and the Italians in the United States" 487.
30. Dublin, "The Mortality of Foreign Race Stocks," 95.
31. Ibid., 94-96.
32. Ibid., 93–95.
33. Ibid., 95–99.
34. Mae M. Ngai, *Impossible Subjects: Illegal Aliens and the Making of Modern America* (Princeton: Princeton University Press, 2014), 3.
35. Stella, "Tuberculosis and the Italians in the United States," 488.
36. Tandy, "Report to the Executive Secretary on the Mulberry Community Sickness Study," 6–7
37. Stella, "Tuberculosis and the Italians in the United States," 488–489.
38. Dorothy C. Wertz, "What Birth Has Done for Doctors: A Historical View," in *The Medicalization of Obstetrics: Personnel, Practice, and Instruments*, ed. Philip K. Wilson (New York: Garland, 1996) 3–9; Judith Pence Rooks, *Midwifery and Childbirth in America* (Philadelphia: Temple University Press, 1997), 1–2; 15.
39. Deborah Gray White, *Ar'n't I a Woman?: Female Slaves in the Plantation South* (New York: W. W. Norton, 1985), 114–116; Sharla M. Fett, *Working Cures: Healing, Health, and Power on Southern Slave Plantations* (Chapel Hill: University of North Carolina Press, 2002), 51–58; 129–130.
40. Rooks, *Midwifery and Childbirth in America*, 17–20.
41. Ibid., 19–20; Wertz, "What Birth Has Done For Doctors: A Historical View," 5–6.
42. Rooks, *Midwifery and Childbirth in America*, 15–20. Also see other midwifery and obstetrical works, such as Charlotte G. Borst, *Catching Babies: The Professionalization of Childbirth, 1870–1920* (Cambridge, MA: Harvard University Press, 1995); Judith Walzer Leavitt, *Brought to Bed: Childbearing in America, 1750–1950* (New York: Oxford University Press, 1987; Dorothy C. Wertz and Richard W. Wertz, *Lying In: A History of Childbirth in America* (New York: Schocken Books, 1979).

43. Angela Danzi, *From Home to Hospital: Jewish and Italian American Women and Childbirth, 1920–1940* (Lanham, MD: University Press of America, 1997), 33–46.

44. Rosalie Bell, M.D., "The Supervision of Midwives in the City of New York," *Monthly Bulletin of the Department of Health of the City of New York*, 4, no. 7 (July 1914): 166.

45. Ibid., 166–169.

46. Helen M. Wallace, M.D., Curtis L. Mendelsohn, M.D., Leona Baumgartner, M.D., and Ruth Rothmayer, R.N., "The Practice of Midwives in New York City," *New York State Journal of Medicine* 48, no. 1 (January 1, 1948): 67.

47. Bell, "The Supervision of Midwives in the City of New York," 166.

48. Rose Mary Murphy Tyndall, "A History of the Bellevue School for Midwives: 1911–1936" (PhD diss., Columbia University Teachers College, 1978), 66.

49. Ibid., 66.

50. Bell, "The Supervision of Midwives in the City of New York," 169. According to New York City Department of Health statistics for the year 1913, slightly less than 10 percent of New York's licensed midwives listed the United States as their place of birth. The United States ranked fifth; rounding out the top five places were: Austria (21 percent), Italy (26 percent), Germany (23 percent), and Russia (15 percent).

51. Tyndall, "A History of the Bellevue School for Midwives: 1911–1936," 66.

52. Danzi, *From Home to Hospital*, 34, 47–74. Also see Valerie Lee, *Granny Midwives and Black Women Writers: Double-Dutched Readings* (New York: Routledge, 1996); Onnie Lee Logan and Katherine Clark, *Motherwit: An Alabama Midwife's Story* (New York: E. P. Dutton, 1989); Gertrude Jacinta Fraser, *African American Midwifery in the South: Dialogues of Birth, Race, and Memory* (Cambridge, MA: Harvard University Press, 1998). Italian American women remained some of the most stalwart supporters of midwives, with the exception of rural southern African American women who, by necessity as much as rebellion, kept the tradition alive until the 1940s. The ascendancy and training of midwives would not occur again until the second wave of feminism in the 1970s.

53. Richard A. Meckel, *Save the Babies: American Public Health Reform and the Prevention of Infant Mortality, 1850–1929* (Baltimore: Johns Hopkins University, 1990), 159–160.

54. Ibid., 160–161.

55. Ibid., 41–45; Tomes, *The Gospel of Germs*, 101–103.

56. Quoted in Meckel, *Save the Babies*, 45–48.

57. Ibid., 48–49.

58. Molly Ladd Taylor, *Mother-Work: Women, Child Welfare, and the State, 1890–1930* (Urbana: University of Illinois Press, 1994), 177–184.

59. Louis I. Dublin, M.D., "The Mortality of Early Infancy," in *Transactions of the Thirteenth-Annual Meeting of the American Child Hygiene Association, Washington, D.C., October 12-14, 1922* (Albany, NY: J. B. Lyon Company, Printers, 1923), 83-84; Taylor, *Mother-Work*, 190.

60. Dublin, "The Mortality of Early Infancy," 84.

61. Ibid. The combination of the neonatal mortality rates from tuberculosis and other infectious diseases would not include those from pneumonia and influenza, however.
62. Ibid., 85-87.
63. Quoted in Dublin, "The Mortality of Early Infancy," 85.
64. Ibid., 85-86.
65. Ibid., 87-88.
66. Ibid., 89, and Rooks, *Midwifery and Childbirth in America*, 20.
67. Preeclampsia affects one out of every ten parturient women and has no etiology. It damages the mother's placenta, which can lead to high blood pressure, protein in the urine (albuminuria), and swelling. In babies, preeclampsia in the mother can retard growth, and cause oxygen deprivation (https://www.preeclampsia.org/signs-and-symptoms, February 27, 2014). Eclampsia can follow preeclampsia. Under the old definition, eclampsia was toxemia, a very common disease of pregnancy which also has no known etiology. Eclampsia was mostly an antepartum (before birth) disease that could result in seizures, comas, or "intracranial hemorrhage." It usually occurred after the twentieth week of pregnancy, but could also result after birth (http://www.webmd.com/hypertension-high-blood-pressure/guide/understanding-preeclampsia-eclampsia-basic-information, February 27, 2014). Albuminuria occurs when a damaged kidney leaks albumin (a type of protein) into the urine. A positive albuminuria urine test means that the individual has diabetic kidney disease. Albuminuria can also mask a propensity for heart disease (http://www.kidney.org/atoz/content/albuminuria.cfm, accessed February 27, 2014). It may also signal hypertension (http://www.kidney.org/atoz/content/albuminuria.cfm, accessed February 27, 2014).
68. http://www.kidney.org/atoz/content/albuminuria.cfm, accessed February 27, 2014; http://my.diabetovalens.com/complications/art15-tp3.asp, accessed December 1, 2014.
69. https://www.preeclampsia.org/signs-and-symptoms, accessed February 27, 2014.
70. Dublin, "The Mortality of Early Infancy," 6–7. When Dublin stated that "[t]he mortality from eclampsia was reduced to about one-third of the proportion that usually occurs in the general population from this cause," he gave no other data to support his assertion.
71. Dystocia literally means "difficult labor" or the "abnormally slow progress of labor," resulting from one or only a combination of weak or uncoordinated uterine contractions that do not adequately open the uterus; the misalignment of the baby in the birth canal; a narrow pelvis that will not allow the baby to pass through into the birth canal; or problems within the birth canal itself. Most often, however, dystocia results from a small pelvis that does not allow the baby easy passage into the birth canal, or weak, ineffectual, uncoordinated contractions (http://emedicine.medscape.com/article/273053-overview, accessed February 27, 2014).
72. Dublin, "The Mortality of Early Infancy," 9. Dublin offered no difference between what he termed a "congenital malformation" or "congenital debility."
73. Ibid., 9–10.

74. http://emedicine.medscape.com/article/273053-overview, accessed February 27, 2014.

75. Dublin, "The Mortality of Early Infancy," 11.

CHAPTER 8. HEALTH IN THE MULBERRY DISTRICT

1. John C. Gebhart, *Protecting the Mother and Child* (New York: New York Association for Improving the Condition of the Poor, 1924), 3.

2. See Richard Meckel, *Save the Babies: American Public Health Reform and the Prevention of Infant Mortality, 1850–1929* (Baltimore: Johns Hopkins University Press, 1990; Ann Arbor: University of Michigan Press, 1998); George W. Lowis and Peter G. McCaffery, "Sociological Factors Affecting the Medicalization of Midwifery," in *Midwifery and the Medicalization of Childbirth: Comparative Perspectives*, ed. Edwin Van Teijlingen, George Lowis, Peter McCaffery, and Maureen Porter (Huntington, NY: Nova Science Publishers, 2000), 21–24.

3. "Ten Years in Mulberry Bend" (New York: New York Association for Improving the Condition of the Poor Statistical Bureau, May 1929), 31. In 1927 alone, the AICP revealed that future prenatal work in the Mulberry District seemed doomed because of the continued use of midwives.

4. Angela D. Danzi, *From Home to Hospital: Jewish and Italian American Women and Childbirth, 1920–1940* (Lanham, MD: University Press of America, 1997), 54.

5. "Ten Years in Mulberry Bend," 31. The AICP blamed midwives for fostering "a definite sentiment against pre-natal care," and the natural occurrence of a declining birthrate as Italians who could afford to leave moved to better areas.

6. Gebhart, *Protecting the Mother and Child*, 9–18

7. Alan M. Kraut, *Silent Travelers: Germs, Genes, and the "Immigrant Menace"* (Baltimore: John Hopkins University Press, 1994), 110–115.

8. Gebhart, *Protecting the Mother and Child*, 3.

9. Ibid., 10–12. See also "Ten Years in Mulberry Bend," 4–7, for the complete 1918–1928 AICP timeline in the Mulberry District.

10. Gebhart, *Protecting Mother and Child*, foreword, 3, 5, 11–12.

11. "Ten Years in Mulberry Bend," 4–8; Bailey B. Burritt to Franklin B. Kirkbride, February 5, 1918, CSS, box 36, folder 132, 2. Although the AICP stated that its problems began in 1922, when shrinking monies and an expanding nurse caseload resulted in "the decline in numbers of patients attending clinics and receiving examinations," the Health Center received almost five hundred thousand dollars for operations between 1918 and 1928. In addition, the nursing division had seen almost 250,000 cases (9).

12. Gebhart, *Protecting the Mother and Child*, 3–4.

13. Ibid., 4.

14. John C. Gebhart, *Health Work for Mothers and Children in a Colored Community* (New York: New York Association for Improving the Condition of the Poor, 1924), 6. Between 1917 and 1923, the AICP supervised 1,224 births in Columbus Hill; by 1923, it proudly claimed to have provided prenatal care for 98 percent of the area's black

female parturient population; out of 1,204 prenatal cases seen by the AICP, only 22 had a midwife delivery, and one additional woman used a "Bellevue" midwife.

15. Quoting Robert Higham in Robert Orsi, "The Religious Boundaries of an Inbetween People: Street *Feste* and the Problem of the Dark-Skinned Other in Italian Harlem, 1920–1990," *American Quarterly* 44, no. 3 (September 1992): 314–319.

16. "Ten Years in Mulberry Bend," 31.

17. Gebhart, *Protecting the Mother and Child*, 4.

18. Ibid., 5–6.

19. "Ten Years in Mulberry Bend," 31.

20. To be fair, while I have not seen the effect of nonresidents on AICP data in its Mulberry publications, John Gebhart does mention it in *Health Work for Mothers and Children in a Colored Community*. He states that while black women were "unusually willing to avail themselves of the excellent medical services provided by hospitals and dispensaries of the area," word-of-mouth recommendations had resulted in "lodgers," or pregnant women of African descent who would temporarily move to the area for free prenatal care and deliveries, then move back to their own neighborhoods. Gebhart adds that area hospitals had decided to refuse these women services (5).

21. "Vital Statistics of Mulberry Health Center, 1915–1925; Part IV—Mortality Rates, B. Death Rates by Age Groups," (New York: New York Association for Improving the Condition of the Poor, 1927), CSS, box 61, folder 367, 11, 31–33.

22. Columbus Hill experienced the same "nonresident" problem, which, if its data reflects too many infant births/1,000 of the population versus too many infant deaths/1,000 live births, also calls its data into question. See "Minutes of meeting with Mr. Burritt," n.y. (CSS, box 36, folder 132), 4.

23. "Vital Statistics of Mulberry Health Center, 1915–1925; Part IV—Mortality Statistics, C. Infant Mortality Rates" (New York: New York Association for Improving the Condition of the Poor, 1927), CSS, box 61, folder 367, 11, 40.

24. "Vital Statistics of the Mulberry Health Center; Part V—Comparative Statement of Vital Statistics of Mulberry, Bellevue-Yorkville, East Harlem Health Center District (Total). East Harlem Nursing and Health Demonstration Area, Manhattan Borough, New York City, and the United States Registration Areas, 1920–1925" (New York: New York Association for Improving the Condition of the Poor, 1927), CSS, box 61, folder 367, 11, 95. The actual national birth registration area was not created until 1915 and consisted of only ten states that, surprisingly, included 31 percent of the nation's population. By 1927, almost 77 percent of the country was reported in the data from thirty-five states. Prior to 1915, and with no national databank to collect or record birth data, individual states reported their birth statistics decennially to the Bureau of the Census in the years between 1850 and 1900.

25. "Vital Statistics of Mulberry Health Center, 1915–1925; Part IV—Mortality Statistics, C. Infant Mortality Rates," 40.

26. Gebhart, *Protecting the Mother and Child*, 7. The actual quote reads "There is, however, clear evidence of a saving of the lives of babies under one month of age."

27. "Vital Statistics of Mulberry Health Center, 1915–1925; Part IV—Mortality Rates, B. Death Rates by Age Group," 49–52.

28. Gebhart, *Protecting the Mother and Child*, 4–7. I will discuss the maternal mortality discrepancies later.

29. Ibid., 7.

30. Ibid., 4–5. In *Protecting the Mother and Child*, Table III, page 5 gives the number of Mulberry deliveries under "Mulberry Prenatal Service Compared With The Total Births Reported For the District" as 5,660 for the years 1918–1922. Estimated figures of 1,100 are given for both 1921 and 1922. By comparison, in "Vital Statistics of Mulberry Health Center, 1915–1925; Part III—Comparison of Birth Rates for Mulberry and New York City, 1915–1925," Table VI reports that in 1920, 1,207 women delivered under the care of the Mulberry Health Center (instead of the 1,107 reported in *Protecting the Mother and Child*, Table III, 5), and 1,145 and 1,046 actual deliveries occurred in the years 1921 and 1922, respectively. See Table VI—"Birth Rates for Mulberry Health Center, 1915–1925," 14, in "Vital Statistics."

31. Gebhart, *Protecting the Mother and Child*, 4–8.

32. Judith Pence Rooks, *Midwifery and Childbearing in America* (Philadephia: Temple University Press, 1997), 18–20.

33. Gebhart, *Protecting the Mother and Child*, 7.

34. "Vital Statistics of the Mulberry Health Center; Part V—Comparative Statement of Vital Statistics of Mulberry, Bellevue-Yorkville, East Harlem Health Center District (Total). East Harlem Nursing and Health Demonstration Area, Manhattan Borough, New York City, and the United States Registration Areas, 1920–1925," 105–106.

35. "Vital Statistics of Mulberry Health Center, 1915–1925; Part IV—Mortality Statistics, C. Infant Mortality Rates," 40–42.

36. "Vital Statistics of Mulberry Health Center, 1915–1925; Part IV—Mortality Rates, B. Death Rates by Age Groups," 33.

37. "Vital Statistics of Mulberry Health Center, 1915–1925; Part IV—Mortality Statistics, C. Infant Mortality Rates," 41, 43b.

38. Ibid., 42.

39. "Vital Statistics of Mulberry Health Center, 1915–1925; Part IV—Mortality Statistics, D. Causes of Infant Mortality, by Age Groups" (New York: New York Association for Improving the Condition of the Poor, 1927), CSS, box 61, folder 367, 11, 53. As with the spike in 1924–1925 infant deaths from one to two months, the AICP gives no reasons why this year resulted in so many more infant deaths than those that occurred in 1925–1926.

40. Ibid., 53.

41. Ibid., 54.

42. Ibid., 55.

43. Ibid., 53–55; quoted in Phyllis H. Williams, *South Italian Folkways in Europe and America: A Handbook for Social Workers, Visiting Nurses, School Teachers, and Physicians* (New Haven, CT: Yale University Press, 1938), 160.

44. "Vital Statistics of the Mulberry Health Center, 1915–1925: Part IV—Mortality Statistics, D. Causes of Infant Mortality, by Age Groups," 53–55.

45. John C. Gebhart, "Five Year's Experience with a Community Health Program: A Report on Mulberry Health Center" (New York: The Association for Improving the Condition of the Poor, 1923) CSS, box 61, folder 367:11, 1.

46. Gebhart, *Protecting the Mother and Child*, 9–10.

47. Ibid., 11–12.

48. Ibid., 12–17.

49. Gebhart, "Five Year's Experience with a Community Health Program," 1, 5.

50. Ibid., 1.

51. Gebhart, *Protecting the Mother and Child*, 2.

52. John C. Gebhart, *The Health of a Neighborhood: A Social Study of the Mulberry District* (New York: New York Association for Improving the Condition of the Poor, 1924), 5–15.

53. "Ten Years in Mulberry Bend," 21.

54. Gebhart, *Protecting the Mother and Child*, 9–10. In 1919, the AICP opened its child examination space in the New York Diet Kitchen Association's building. Like other dispensaries and clinics whose nurses were prepared to care for and diagnose sick infants and children, the Diet Kitchen Association did not have staff trained for well children who only needed examinations. The AICP filled this void, later moving its well-baby clinic to the Mulberry Community House, which became the Mulberry Health Center in 1922. See "Ten Years in Mulberry Bend," 54–55.

55. Danzi, *From Home to Hospital*, 48.

56. "Ten Years in Mulberry Bend," 30–32.

BIBLIOGRAPHY

NEW YORK CITY MANUSCRIPT COLLECTIONS

Charity Organization Society (COS). Community Service Society Archives. Rare Book and Manuscript Library. Columbia University.

Columbia College of Physicians and Surgeons Archive. Columbia University Presbyterian Hospital.

Community Service Society Archives. Rare Book and Manuscript Library. Columbia University.

James Weldon Johnson Manuscript Collection. Beinecke Library. Yale University.

Maternity Center Association Archive. Rockefeller University. New York City.

New York Association for Improving the Condition of the Poor (AICP). Community Service Society Archives. Rare Book and Manuscript Library. Columbia University.

New York City Department of Health Archive. Municipal Archives. New York City.

New York Nursery and Child's Hospital Archive. Medical Center Archives. New York Presbyterian/Weill Cornell Hospital. New York City.

Schomburg Center for Research in Black Culture. New York Public Library. New York City.

Sloane Hospital for Women Archive. Augustus C. Long Health Sciences Library. Columbia University Medical Center.

Vanderbilt Clinic Archive. Augustus C. Long Health Sciences Library. Columbia University Medical Center.

NEWSPAPERS

Amsterdam News (New York, New York)
Baltimore Afro-American (Baltimore, Maryland)
Chicago Defender (Chicago, Illinois)
New York Times (New York, New York)
New York Age (New York, New York)

PRIMARY SOURCES

American Child Hygiene Association. *Transactions of the Eleventh Annual Meeting, St. Louis, Mo., October 11–13, 1920*. Baltimore: Franklin Printing Company, 1921.

Annual Report of the Department of Health of the City of New York for the Calendar Year 1918. New York: New York City Department of Health, 1918.

Annual Report of the Department of Health of the City of New York for the Calendar Year 1919. New York: New York City Department of Health, 1919

Clark, Jessie and Gertrude E. Mc Dougald. *A New Day for the Colored Woman Worker.* New York: Consumer's League of the City of New York, 1919.

Dublin, Louis I., M.D. "The Mortality of Early Infancy." In *Transactions of the Thirteenth Annual Meeting of the American Child Hygiene Association, Washington, D.C., October 12-14, 1922.* Albany, NY: J. B. Lyon Company, Printers, 1923.

Du Bois, W. E. Burghardt, ed. *The Health and Physique of the Negro American: Report of a Social Study made under the Direction of Atlanta University; Together with the Proceedings of the Eleventh Conference for the Study of the Negro Problems, Held at Atlanta University, on May the 29th, 1906.* Atlanta: Atlanta University Press, 1906.

Gebhart, John C. "Five-Years' Experience With a Community Health Program: A Report on Mulberry Health Center." Photocopy. New York: New York Association for Improving the Condition of the Poor, 1923.

———. *The Health of a Neighborhood: A Social Study of the Mulberry District.* New York: New York Association for Improving the Condition of the Poor, 1924.

———. *Health Work for Mothers and Children in a Colored Community.* New York: New York Association for Improving the Condition of the Poor, 1924.

———. *Protecting the Mother and Child.* New York: New York Association for Improving the Condition of the Poor, 1924.

Guilfoy, William, M.D. and Shirley W. Wynne, M. D. *An Analysis of Mortality Returns of the Sanitary Areas of the Borough of Manhattan for the Year 1915.* New York: New York City Department of Health, 1916.

Harper, Frances E. W. "Enlightened Motherhood: An Address Before the Brooklyn Literary Society, November 15th, 1892." Library of Congress. http://lcweb2.loc.gov/cgi-bin/query/r?ammem/murray:@field%28DOCID+@lit%28lcrbmrpt1906div0%29%29. Accessed February 22, 2014.

Harris, Abram L. "Digest of Preliminary Findings in Columbus Hill." Photocopy. New York: Lincoln House Committee of the Henry Street Settlement, 1922.

Holmes, Norman A. "Preliminary Report of Survey of Colored Population of Columbus Hill and Vicinity." Photocopy. New York: Lincoln House Committee of the Henry Street Settlement, 1922.

———. "Sociological Survey of the Negro Population of Columbus Hill of New York City." Photocopy. New York: Lincoln House Committee of the Henry Street Settlement, 1922.

Hurston, Zora Neale. "Color Struck: A Play in Four Scenes." In *Fire: A Quarterly Devoted to the Younger Negro Audiences* (November 1926): 7–14.

Matheus, John F. 'Cruiter. In *Readings from Negro Authors: For Schools and Colleges, with a Bibliography of Negro Literature*, edited by Otelia Cromwell, Lorenzo Dow Turner, and Eva B. Dykes. New York: Harcourt, Brace, 1931.

McFarlane, J. E. Clare, ed. *A Treasury of Jamaican Poetry.* London: University of London Press, 1949.

McKay, Claude. "Flame-Heart." In *A Treasury of Jamaican Poetry*, edited by J. E. Clare McFarlane. London: University of London Press, 1949.

Moynihan, Daniel Patrick. *The Negro Family: The Case for National Action*. Washington, DC: United States Department of Labor, 1965.
"Mulberry Health Center Survey." Photocopy. New York City: New York Association for Improving the Condition of the Poor, 1923.
Norris, Zoe Anderson. *The East Side: Her Magazine*. 4 volumes. New York: Zoe Anderson Norris, 1909–1913.
Redcam, Tom. "O Little Green Island Far Over the Sea." In *A Treasury of Jamaican Poetry*, edited by J. E. Clare McFarlane. London: University of London Press, 1949.
"Ten Years in Mulberry Bend." Photocopy. New York: New York Association for Improving the Condition of the Poor Statistics Bureau, 1929.
Tandy Elizabeth C. "Report to the Executive Secretary on the Mulberry Community Sickness Study." Photocopy. New York City: Committee on Dispensary Development, May 1, 1923.
"Vital Statistics of Mulberry Health Center, 1915–1925." Photocopy. New York: New York Association for Improving the Condition of the Poor Statistics Bureau, 1927.
Weaver, Abbie Roberts, et al. "Report on a Study of Caroline Rest, Made During March and April, 1933." Unpublished manuscript. New York: New York Association for Improving the Condition of the Poor, May 1, 1933.
Wood, Clement, ed. *Negro Songs: An Anthology*. Girard, KS: Haldeman Julius, 1924.
Woolston, Eliza Y. "The Harlem Birth Control Clinic: The Intersection of Race and Class in Depression Era Harlem." Senior essay in the Department of History, Yale University. April 14, 1997.

SECONDARY SOURCES

Abel, Emily. *Tuberculosis and the Politics of Exclusion: A History of Public Health and Migration to Los Angeles*. New Brunswick, NJ: Rutgers University Press, 2007.
Agamben, Giorgio. *Homo Sacer: Sovereign Power and Bare Life*. Translated by Daniel Heller-Roazen. Stanford, CA: Stanford University Press, 1998.
Aleandri, Emelise. *The Italian-American Immigrant Theatre of New York City*. Charleston, SC: Arcadia, 1999.
———. *Little Italy*. Charleston, SC: Arcadia, 2002.
Allen, Carol. *Black Women Intellectuals: Strategies of Nation, Family, and Neighborhood in the Works of Pauline Hopkins, Jessie Fauset, and Marita Bonner*. New York: Garland, 1998.
Allen, L. C., M.D. "The Negro Health Problem." *American Journal of Public Health* 5, no.3 (March 1915): 194–203.
Anderson, Izett, M.D., and Frank Cundall, F.S.A. *Jamaica Negro Proverbs and Sayings: Collected and Classified According to Subjects*. London: West India Committee for the Institute of Jamaica, 1927.
Apple, Rima D. "Constructing Mothers: Scientific Motherhood in the Nineteenth and Twentieth Centuries." In *Mothers and Motherhood: Readings in American History*, 90–110, edited by Rima D. Apple and Janet Golden. Columbus: Ohio State University Press, 1997.

Apple, Rima D. *Mothers and Medicine: A Social History of Infant Feeding, 1890–1950.* Madison: University of Wisconsin Press, 1987.

———, ed. *Women, Health, and Medicine in America: A Historical Handbook.* New York: Garland, 1990.

———, and Janet Golden, eds. *Mothers and Motherhood: Readings in American History.* Columbus: Ohio State University Press, 1997.

Askhyk, Dan, Fred L. Gardaphe, and Anthony Julian Tamburri, eds. *Shades of Black and White: Selected Essays from the 30th Annual Conference of the American Italian Historical Association, November 1997, Cleveland, Ohio.* American Italian Historical Association, 1999.

Baer, Hans A., and Merrill Singer. *African-American Religion in the Twentieth Century: Varieties of Protest and Accommodation.* Knoxville: University of Tennessee Press, 1992.

Baetz, Walter G., M.D. "Syphilis in Colored Canal Laborers: A Resume of 500 Consecutive Medical Cases." *New York Medical Journal* 100 (1914): 820–837.

Bair, Barbara. "Remapping the Black/White Body: Sexuality, Nationalism, and Biracial Antimiscegenation Activism in 1920s Virginia." In *Sex, Love, Race: Crossing Boundaries in North American History*, edited by Martha Hodes. New York: New York University Press, 1999.

Baker, S. Josephine, M. D. *Fighting for Life.* 1939. Historical introduction by Patricia C. Kuszler, M. D. and Charles G. Roland, M.D. Huntington, NY: Robert E. Krieger, 1980.

Barolini, Helen, ed. *The Dream Book: An Anthology of Writings by Italian American Women.* 1985. Rev. ed. Syracuse, NY: Syracuse University Press, 2001.

Barry, John M. *The Great Influenza: The Epic Story of the Deadliest Plague in History.* New York: Viking, 2004.

Barry, Jonathan, and Colin Jones, eds. *Medicine and Charity Before the Welfare State.* London: Routledge, 1991.

Bates, Barbara. *Bargaining for Life: A Social History of Tuberculosis, 1876–1938.* Philadelphia: University of Pennsylvania Press, 1992.

Batker, Carol J. *Reforming Fictions: Native, African, and Jewish American Women's Literature and Journalism in the Progressive Era.* New York: Columbia University Press, 2000.

Beardsley, Edward H. "Race as a Factor in Health." In *Women, Health, and Medicine in America: A Historical Handbook*, edited by Rima D. Apple. New York: Garland, 1990.

Beckwith, Martha Warren. *Black Roadways: A Study of Jamaican Folk Life.* Chapel Hill: University of North Carolina Press, 1929.

Bederman, Gail. *Manliness and Civilization: A Cultural History of Gender and Race in the United States, 1880–1917.* Chicago: University of Chicago Press, 1995.

Bell, Rosalie, M.D. "The Supervision of Midwives in the City of New York." *Monthly Bulletin of the Department of Health of the City of New York* 4, no. 7 (July 1914): 166–172.

Belmonte, Frances R. *Women and Health: An Annotated Bibliography*. Lanham, MD: Scarecrow Press, 1997.

Bendroth, Margaret Lamberts, and Virginia Lieson Brereton, eds. *Women and Twentieth-Century Protestantism*. Urbana: University of Illinois Press, 2002.

Billingsley, Andrew. *Mighty Like a River: The Black Church and Social Reform*. New York: Oxford University Press, 1999.

Bertellini, Giorgio. "Southern Crossings: Italians, Cinema, and Modernity (Italy, 1861– New York, 1920)." PhD diss., New York University, 2001.

Bisodol Company. *Vomiting of Pregnancy: A Symposium of the Current Literature*. New Haven, CT: Bisodol Company, 1932.

Blascoer, Frances. *Colored School Children in New York*. 1915. Reprint. New York: Negro Universities Press, 1970.

Blight, David W. *Race and Reunion: The Civil War in American Memory*. Cambridge, MA: Belknap Press of Harvard University Press, 2001.

Bodnar, John. *The Transplanted: A History of Immigrants in Urban America*. 1985. Reprint. Bloomington: Indiana University Press, 1987.

Bogdan, Janet Carlisle. "Childbirth in America, 1650–1990." In *Women, Health, and Medicine in America: A Historical Handbook*, edited by Rima D. Apple. New York: Garland, 1990.

Boris, Eileen. "The Power of Motherhood: Black and White Activist Women Redefine the 'Political.'" In *Mothers of a New World: Maternalist Politics and the Origins of Welfare States*, edited by Seth Koven and Sonya Michel. New York: Routledge, 1993.

———, and Jennifer Klein. *Caring for America: Home Health Workers in the Shadow of the Welfare State*. New York: Oxford University Press, 2012.

Borst, Charlotte G. *Catching Babies: The Professionalization of Childbirth, 1870–1920*. Cambridge, MA: Harvard University Press, 1995.

Brandt, Allan M. *No Magic Bullet: A Social History of Venereal Disease in the United States Since 1880*. New York: Oxford University Press, 1985.

Breeden, James O. "Disease as a Factor in Southern Distinctiveness." In *Disease and Distinctiveness in the American South*, edited by Todd L. Savitt and James Harvey Young. Knoxville: University of Tennessee Press, 1988.

Brindisi, Rocco, M. D. "The Italian and Public Health." In *The Italian in America: The Progressive View, 1891–1914*, edited by Lydio F. Tomasi. New York: Center for Migration Studies, 1972.

Brown, Mary Elizabeth. " 'The Adoption of the Tactics of the Enemy': The Care of Italian Immigrant Youth in the Archdiocese of New York during the Progressive Era." In *Immigration to New York*, edited by Selma Cantor Berrol, William Pencak, and Randall M. Miller. New York: Balch Institute for Ethnic Studies, 1991: 109–125.

———. "Theodore Roosevelt (1858-1919): Race Suicide." In *The Making of Modern Immigration: An Encyclopedia of People and Ideas*. Vol. 2, edited by Patrick J. Hayes. Santa Barbara, CA: ABC-CLIO, 2012: 651–662.

Buhler-Wilkerson, Karen. "False Dawn: The Rise and Fall of Public Health Nursing, 1900–1930." PhD diss., University of Pennsylvania, 1984.

Buhler-Wilkerson, Karen. "Left Carrying the Bag: Experiments in Visiting Nursing, 1877–1909." *Nursing Research* 36, no. 1 (January/February 1987): 42–47.

Butler, Josephine E. *Personal Reminiscences of a Great Crusade*. Westport, CT: Hyperion Press, 1911.

Byrd, W. Michael, M.D., and Linda A. Clayton, M.D. *An American Health Dilemma: Race, Medicine, and Health Care in the United States*. 2 vols. New York: Routledge, 2001.

Calhoon, Claudia Marie. "Tuberculosis, Race, and the Delivery of Health Care in Harlem, 1922–1939." *Radical History Review* 80 (Spring 2001): 101–119.

Calloway, Licia Morrow. *Black Family (Dys)function in Novels by Jessie Fauset, Nella Larsen, and Fannie Hurst*. New York: P. Lang, 2003.

Cannistraro, Philip V., ed. *The Italians of New York: Five Centuries of Struggle and Achievement*. New York: New-York Historical Society and the John D. Calandra Italian American Institute, 2000.

Carby, Hazel V. " 'It Jus Be's Dat Way Sometime': The Sexual Politics of Women's Blues." In *Unequal Sisters: A Multicultural Reader in U. S. Women's History*, edited by Vicki L. Ruiz and Ellen Carol Du Bois. New York: Routledge, 1994.

———. " 'On the Threshold of Woman's Era': Lynching, Empire, and Sexuality in Black Feminist Theory." *Critical Inquiry* 12 (Autumn 1985): 262–277.

———. *Reconstructing Womanhood: The Emergence of the Afro-American Woman Novelist*. New York: Oxford University Press, 1987.

Caroli, Betty Boyd, Robert F. Harney, and Lydio F. Tomasi, eds. *The Italian Immigrant Woman in North America*. Toronto: Multicultural History Society of Ontario, 1978.

Cash, Floris Barnett. "Radicals or Realists: African American Women and the Settlement House Spirit in New York City." *Afro-Americans in New York Life and History* 15, no. 1:7–17.

Chaddock, Robert E., Ph.D. "Sanitary Districts in the Analysis of Municipal Mortality and Morbidity Data." *American Journal of Public Health* 6, no. 6 (June 1916): 533–544.

Clark, Jessie, and Gertrude E. McDougald. *A New Day for the Colored Woman Worker*. New York: Consumer's League of the City of New York, 1919.

Cohen, Miriam. *From Workshop to Office: Two Generations of Italian Women in New York City, 1900–1950*. Ithaca, NY: Cornell University Press, 1992.

Collins, Patricia Hill. *Black Feminist Thought: Knowledge, Consciousness, and the Politics of Empowerment*. New York: Routledge, 2008.

Correnti, Santi. *Proverbi e Modi di Dire Siciliani di Ieri e di Oggi*. Rome: Newton and Compton, 1995.

Coser, Rose Laub, Laura S. Anker, and Andrew J. Perrin. *Women of Courage: Jewish and Italian Immigrant Women in New York*. Westport, CT: Greenwood Press, 1999.

Cote, James E., and Charles G. Levine. *Identity Formation, Agency, and Culture: A Social Psychological Synthesis*. Mahwah, NJ: Lawrence Erlbaum Associates, 2002.

Craddock, Susan. *City of Plagues: Disease, Discovery, and Deviance in San Francisco*. Minneapolis: University of Minneapolis Press, 2000.

Cromwell, Otelia, Lorenzo Dow Turner, and Eva B. Dykes, eds. *Readings from Negro Authors: For Schools and Colleges, with a Bibliography of Negro Literature.* New York: Harcourt, Brace, 1931.
Crosby, Alfred. *The Forgotten Pandemic: The Influenza of 1918.* 2nd ed. New York: Cambridge University Press, 2003.
Danzi, Angela D. *From Home to Hospital: Jewish and Italian American Women and Childbirth, 1920–1940.* Lanham, MD: University Press of America, 1997.
Davis, Angela. *Blues Legacies and Black Feminism: Gertrude "Ma" Rainey, Bessie Smith, and Billie Holiday.* New York: Pantheon, 1998.
Delgado, Richard, and Jean Stefancic, eds. *Critical White Studies: Looking Behind the Mirror.* Philadelphia: Temple University Press, 1997.
De Piero, Antonio. *L'Isola Della Quarantina: Le Avventure di un Manovale Friulano nei Primi Decenni Grandi Emigrazioni.* Florence, Italy: Giunti Gruppo Editoriale, 1994.
Di Donato, Pietro. *Christ in Concrete: A Novel.* Indianapolis: Bobbs–Merrill, 1939.
Dill, Bonnie Thornton. "Across the Boundaries of Race and Class: An Exploration of the Relationship between Work and Family among Black Female Domestic Servants." PhD diss., New York University, 1979.
Diner, Hasia. *Erin's Daughters in America: Irish Immigrant Women in the Nineteenth Century.* Baltimore: Johns Hopkins University Press, 1983.
Dodson, Howard, Christopher Moore, and Roberta Yancy. *The Black New Yorkers: The Schomburg Illustrated Chronology, 400 Years of African American History.* New York: John Wiley and Sons, 2000.
Dreiser, Theodore. *The Color of a Great City.* New York: Boni and Liveright, 1923.
Dublin, Louis I., M.D. "The Mortality of Foreign Race Stocks: A Contribution to the Quantitative Study of the Vigor of the Racial Elements in the Population of the United States." *Scientific Monthly* 14, no. 1 (January 1922): 94–104.
———, and Alfred J. Lotes, D. Sc. *The Money Value of a Man.* New York: Ronald Press, 1930. New York: Ronald Press, 1946.
Du Bois, Florence. *A Guide to Statistics of Social Welfare in New York City.* New York: Welfare Council of New York City, 1930.
Du Bois, W. E. Burghardt. *The Black North in 1901: A Social Study. A Series of Articles Originally Appearing in The New York Times, November-December 1901.* Reprint, New York: Arno Press and New York Times, 1969.
Dubos, Rene, and Jean Dubos. *The White Plague: Tuberculosis, Man and Society.* Boston: Little, Brown, 1952.
Duffy, John. *From Humors to Medical Science: A History of American Medicine.* 2nd ed. Urbana: University of Illinois Press, 1993.
———. *A History of Public Health in New York City, 1866–1966.* New York: Russell Sage Foundation, 1974.
———. *The Sanitarians: A History of American Public Health.* Reprint. Urbana: University of Illinois, 1992.
Duster, Troy. *Backdoor to Eugenics.* 2nd ed. New York: Routledge, 2003.

Dye, Nancy Schrom. "Modern Obstetrics and Working-Class Women: The New York Midwifery Dispensary, 1890–1920." *Journal of Social History* 20, no. 3 (1987): 549–564.

Elias, Lewis W., M.D. "The Intravenous Administration of Salvarsan in Babies." *Southern Medical Journal* 7, no. 9 (September 1914): 708–709.

Ets, Marie Hall. *Rosa: The Life of an Italian Immigrant*. University of Minnesota Press, 1970. Madison: University of Wisconsin Press, 1999.

Ettinger, Laura E. *Nurse-Midwifery: The Birth of a New American Profession*. Columbus: Ohio State University Press, 2006.

Fauset, Jessie Redmon. *There is Confusion*. New York: Boni and Liveright, 1924.

Feldberg, Georgina D. *Disease and Class: Tuberculosis and the Shaping of Modern North American Society*. New Brunswick, NJ: Rutgers University Press, 1995.

Fenn, Elizabeth A. *Pox Americana: The Great Smallpox Epidemic of 1775–1782*. New York: Hill and Wang, 2001.

Fessenden, Tracy, Nicholas F. Radel, and Magdelena J. Zaborowska. *The Puritan Origins of American Sex: Religion, Sexuality, and National Identity in American Literature*. New York: Routledge, 2001.

Flexner, Abraham. *Medical Education in the United States and Canada: A Report to the Carnegie Foundation for the Advancement of Teaching*. New York: Carnegie Foundation for the Advancement of Teaching, 1910.

Foner, Nancy. *In a New Land: A Comparative View of Immigration*. New York: New York University Press, 2005.

———. *Islands in the City: West Indian Migration to New York*. Berkeley: University of California Press, 2001.

———. "Sex Roles and Sensibilities: Jamaican Women in New York and London." In *International Migration: The Female Experience*, edited by Rita James Simon and Caroline B. Brettell. Totowa, NJ: Rowman and Allanheld, 1985.

———, and George M. Fredrickson, eds. *Not Just Black and White: Historical and Contemporary Perspectives on Immigration, Race, and Ethnicity in the United States*. New York: Russell Sage Foundation, 2004.

Fordyce, John A., M.D., Isadore Rosen, M.D., and C. N. Meyers, M.D. "Quantitative Studies in Syphilis from a Clinical and Biologic Point of View." *American Journal of the Medical Sciences* 164, no. 4 (1922): 492–513.

Fort, A. G., Ph.B., M.D. "The Negro Health Problem in Rural Communities." *American Journal of Public Health* 5, no.3 (March 1915): 191–193.

Fraser, Gertrude Jacinta. *African American Midwifery in the South: Dialogues of Birth, Race, and Memory*. Cambridge, MA: Harvard University Press, 1998.

Frazier, E. Franklin. *The Negro Family in the U. S.* Chicago: University of Chicago Press, 1939.

Friedman-Kasaba, Kathi. *Memories of Migration: Gender, Ethnicity, and Work in the Lives of Jewish and Italian Women in New York, 1870–1924*. Albany: State University of New York Press, 1994.

Gabaccia, Donna. *From the Other Side: Women, Gender, and Immigrant Life in the U.S., 1820–1990*. Bloomington: Indiana University Press, 1994.

———. *From Sicily to Elizabeth Street: Housing and Social Change Among Italian Immigrants, 1880–1930.* Albany: State University of New York Press, 1984.
Gaines, Kevin K. *Uplifting the Race: Black Leadership, Politics, and Culture in the Twentieth Century.* Chapel Hill: University of North Carolina Press, 1996.
Gamble, Vanessa Northington, M.D. *Germs Have No Color Line: Blacks and American Medicine, 1900–1940.* (New York: Garland, 1989.
———. *Making a Place for Ourselves: The Black Hospital Movement, 1920–1945.* New York: Oxford University Press, 1995.
Garon, Paul, and Beth Garon. *Woman with Guitar: Memphis Minnie's Blues.* New York: Da Capo Press, 1992.
Gates, Henry Louis, and Nellie Y. McKay, eds. *The Norton Anthology of African American Literature.* New York: W. W. Norton, 1997.
Gebhart, John. "Syphilis as a Prenatal Problem." *Journal of Social Hygiene* 10, no. 4 (August 1924): 208–217.
Giddings, Paula. *When and Where I Enter: The Impact of Black Women on Race and Sex in America.* New York: Bantam Books, 1984.
Gilmore, Glenda Elizabeth. *Gender and Jim Crow: Women and the Politics of White Supremacy in North Carolina, 1890–1920.* Chapel Hill: University of North Carolina Press, 1996.
———. *Who Were the Progressives?* Boston: Bedford/St. Martins, 2002.
Ginzberg, Eli, Howard Berliner, and Miriam Ostow. *Improving Health Care of the Poor: The New York City Experience.* New Brunswick, NJ: Transaction Publishers, 1997.
Glenn, Evelyn Nakano. *Unequal Freedom: How Race and Gender Shaped American Citizenship and Labor.* Cambridge, MA: Harvard University Press, 2002.
Goldberg, David Theo. "The Social Formation of Racist Discourse." In *Anatomy of Racism*, edited by David Theo Goldberg. Minneapolis: University of Minnesota Press, 1990.
Goodwin, E. Marvin. *Black Migration in America from 1915 to 1960: An Uneasy Exodus.* Lewiston, NY: Edwin Mellon Press, 1990.
Gordon, Linda. *Pitied, But Not Entitled: Single Mothers and the History of Welfare, 1890–1935.* Cambridge, MA: Harvard University Press, 1995.
———, ed. *Women, the State, and Welfare.* Madison: University of Wisconsin Press, 1990.
Gottlieb, Peter. "Rethinking the Great Migration: A Perspective from Pittsburgh." In *The Great Migration in Historical Perspective: New Dimensions of Race, Class, and Gender*, edited by Joe William Trotter. Bloomington: Indiana University Press, 1991.
Gould, Stephen Jay. *The Mismeasure of Man.* New York: W. W. Norton, 1981.
Grasso, Mario. *Lingua Delle Madri: Voce e Pensiero dei Siciliani nel Tempo.* Catania, Italy: Prova d'Autore, 1994.
Greeley, Dawn. "Beyond Benevolence: Gender, Class, and the Development of Scientific Charity in New York City, 1882, 1935." PhD diss., State University of New York, Stony Brook, 1995.
Green, Dan S. and Edwin D. Driver, eds. *W. E. B. Du Bois on Sociology and the Black Community.* Chicago: University of Chicago Press, 1978.

Green, Howard Whipple. *Infant Mortality and Economic Status: Cleveland Five City Area, 1919–1937*. Cleveland: Cleveland Health Council, 1939.
Griffin, Farah Jasmine. *Who Set You Flowin'? The African-American Migration Narrative*. New York: Oxford University Press, 1995.
Grim, David S., M.D. "Treatment of Syphilis as Carried out in the Vanderbilt Clinic, New York City." *Procedures of the Medical Association Isthmian Canal Zone* 11 (1918): 64–69.
Gross, Kali N. *Colored Amazons: Crime, Violence, and Black Women in the City of Brotherly Love, 1880–1910*. Durham, NC: Duke University Press, 2006.
Grossman, James R. *Land of Hope: Chicago, Black Southerners, and the Great Migration*. Chicago: University of Chicago Press, 1989.
Gutman, Herbert G. *The Black Family in Slavery and Freedom*. New York: Vintage Books, 1977.
Guy-Sheftall, Beverly. "Daughters of Sorrow: Attitudes Toward Black Women, 1880–1920." In *Black Women in United States History*, edited by Darlene Clark Hine. Brooklyn, NY: Carlson, 1990.
Hacker, Andrew. *Two Worlds: Black and White, Separate, Hostile, Unequal*. New York: Ballantine Books, 1992.
Hajo, Cathy Moran. *Birth Control on Main Street: Organizing Clinics in the United States, 1916–1939*. Urbana: University of Illinois Press, 2010.
Hall, Stuart. "The Emergence of Cultural Studies in the Humanities." *October* 53, The Humanities as Social Technology (Summer 1990): 11–23.
———. "The State in Question." In *The Idea of the Modern State*, edited by Gregor McLennan, David Held, and Stuart Hall. Milton Keynes, UK: Open University Press, 1984.
Hammonds, Evelynn. *Childhood's Deadly Scourge: The Campaign to Control Diphtheria in New York City, 1880–1930*. Baltimore: Johns Hopkins University Press, 1999.
Handlin, Oscar. *The Newcomers: Negroes and Puerto Ricans in a Changing Metropolis*. Cambridge, MA: Harvard University Press, 1959.
Harding, Sandra. *Science and Social Inequality: Feminist and Postcolonial Issues*. Urbana: University of Illinois Press, 2006.
———. *The "Racial" Economy of Science: Toward a Democratic Future*. Bloomington: University of Indiana Press, 1993.
Harley, Sharon. "For the Good of Family and Race: Gender, Work, and Domestic Roles in the Black Community, 1880–1930." *Signs: Journal of Women and Culture in Society* 15, no. 2 (Winter 1990): 338–349.
Harris, Alice Kessler. *In Pursuit of Equity: Women, Men, and the Quest for Economic Citizenship in 20th-Century America*. New York: Oxford University Press, 2001.
———. *Out to Work: a History of Wage-Earning Women in the United States*. New York: Oxford University Press, 1982.
Harrison, Shelby M., and Allen Eaton. *Welfare Problems in New York City: Which Have Been Studies and Reported Upon During the Period from 1915 through 1925*. New York: Welfare Council of New York City, 1926.

Hayes, Patrick J., ed. *The Making of Modern Immigration: An Encyclopedia of People and Ideas.* Vol. 2. Santa Barbara, CA: ABC-CLIO, 2012.

Hazen, H. H., M.D. "Practical Observations on Syphilis, VI." *American Journal of Syphilis* 7, no. 3 (July 1923): 417–426.

Hibbs, Henry H., Jr. *Infant Mortality: Its Relation to Social and Industrial Conditions.* New York: Department of Child-Helping, Russell Sage Foundation, 1916.

Hicks, Cheryl D. *Talk With You Like A Woman: African American Women, Justice, and Reform in New York, 1890–1935.* Chapel Hill: University of North Carolina Press, 2010.

Higginbotham, Evelyn Brooks. *Righteous Discontent: The Women's Movement in the Black Baptist Church, 1880–1920.* Cambridge, MA: Harvard University Press, 1994.

Higham, John. *Send These to Me: Immigrants in Urban America.* Atheneum, 1975. Baltimore: Johns Hopkins University Press, 1984.

———. *Strangers in the Land: Patterns of American Nativism, 1860–1925.* Greenwood Press, 1981. New Brunswick, NJ: Rutgers University Press, 1994.

Hine, Darlene Clark. "Black Migration to the Urban Midwest: The Gender Dimension, 1915–1945." In *The Great Migration in Historical Perspective: New Dimensions of Race, Class, and Gender*, edited by Joe William Trotter Jr. Bloomington: Indiana University Press, 1991.

———. *Black Women in United States History.* Brooklyn, NY: Carlson, 1990.

———. *Black Women in White: Racial Conflict and Cooperation in the Nursing Profession, 1890–1950.* Bloomington: University of Indiana Press, 1989.

———. "The Ethel Johns Report: Black Women in the Nursing Profession, 1925." *Journal of Negro History* 67, no. 3 (Autumn 1982): 212–228.

———. "From Hospital to College: Black Nurse Leaders and the Rise of Collegiate Nursing Schools." *Journal of Negro Education* 51, no. 3 (Summer 1982): 222–237.

———. "Opportunity and Fulfillment: Sex, Race, and Class in Health Care Education." *Sage* 2, no. 2 (Fall 1985): 14–17.

———. "Rape and the Inner Lives of Black Women in the Middle West." *Signs.* 14, no. 4 (Summer 1989): 912–920.

———, and Kathleen Thompson. *A Shining Thread of Hope: The History of Black Women in America.* New York: Broadway Books, 1998.

Hodes, Martha, ed. *Sex, Love, Race: Crossing Boundaries in North American History.* New York: New York University Press, 1999.

Holder, Calvin B. "The Causes and Composition of West Indian Immigration to New York City, 1900–1952." *Afro-Americans in New York Life and History* 11:1 (January 1987): 7–27.

Holloway, Karla FC. *Private Bodies, Public Texts: Race, Gender, and a Cultural Bioethics.* Durham, NC: Duke University Press, 2011.

Holmes, Norman L. "Columbus Hill: The Story of a Negro Community." *Opportunity* 1, no. 2 (February 1923): 10–11.

Hondagneu-Sotelo, Pierrette. *Gendered Transitions: Mexican Experiences of Immigration.* Berkeley: University of California Press, 1994.

Horsman, Reginald. *Josiah Nott of Mobile: Southerner, Physician, and Racial Theorist.* Baton Rouge: Louisiana State University Press, 1987.

——. *Race and Manifest Destiny: The Origins of American Racial Anglo-Saxonism.* Cambridge, MA: Harvard University Press, 1981.

Horwood, Murray P., M.S., Ph.D. *Public Health Surveys: What They Are, How to Make Them, How to Use Them.* New York: John Wiley and Sons, 1921.

Huggins, Nathan. *Harlem Renaissance.* New York: Oxford University Press, 1971.

Hunter, Tera. *To 'Joy My Freedom: Southern Black Women's Lives and Labors after the Civil War.* Cambridge, MA: Harvard University Press, 1997.

Hurston, Zora Neale. *The Complete Stories: Introduction by Henry Louis Gates, Jr. and Sieglinde Lemke.* New York: Harper Collins Publishers, 1995.

——. *The Sanctified Church.* Berkeley: Turtle Island Foundation, 1981.

Hyman, Paula E. *Gender and Assimilation in Modern Jewish History: The Roles and Representation of Women.* Seattle: University of Washington Press, 1995.

Jacobson, Matthew Frye. *Whiteness of a Different Color: European Immigrants and the Alchemy of Race.* Cambridge, MA: Harvard University Press, 1998.

Jarrett, Mary C. *Chronic Illness in New York City, Volume I: The Problems of Chronic Illness.* New York: Columbia University Press for the Welfare Council of New York City, 1933.

Jones, Eugene Kinckle. "Negro Migration in New York State." *Opportunity* 3, no. 1 (January 1926): 7–11.

Jones, Jacqueline. *Labor of Love, Labor of Sorrow: Black Women, Work, and the Family, from Slavery to the Present.* New York: Vintage Books, 1995.

Jones, James H. *Bad Blood: The Tuskegee Syphilis Experiment.* Chicago: Free Press, 1993.

Jones, R. Frank, and Kline A. Price. "The Incidence of Gonorrhea Among Negroes." *Journal of Negro Education* 6, no. 3 (July 1937): 364–376.

Jones, Sharon L. *Rereading the Harlem Renaissance: Race, Class, and Gender in the Fiction of Jessie Fauset, Zora Neale Hurston, and Dorothy West.* Westport, CT: Greenwood Press, 2002.

Jones, Woodrow Jr., and Mitchell F. Rice, eds. *Health Care Issues in Black America: Policies, Problems, and Prospects.* Westport, CT: Greenwood Press, 1987.

Katzman, David. *Seven Days a Week: Women and Domestic Service in Industrializing America.* New York: Oxford University Press, 1978.

Kelley, Robin D. G. *Yo' Mama's Disfunktional! Fighting the Culture Wars in Urban America.* Boston: Beacon Press, 1997.

Kerber, Linda K. *No Constitutional Right to Be Ladies: Women and the Obligations of Citizenship.* New York: Hill and Wang, 1998.

Kessner, Thomas. *The Golden Door: Italian and Jewish Immigrant Mobility in New York City, 1880–1915.* New York: Oxford University Press, 1977.

Kevles, Daniel J. *In the Name of Eugenics: Genetics and the Uses of Human Heredity.* Berkeley: University of California Press, 1985.

Kimball, Solon T. "An Alabama Town Surveys its Health Needs." In *Health, Culture and Community: Case Studies of Public Reactions to Health Programs,* edited by Benjamin D. Paul and Walter B. Miller. New York: Russell Sage Foundation, 1955.

Kiple, Kenneth F., and Virginia Himmelsteib King. *Another Dimension to the Black Diaspora: Diet, Disease, and Racism*. New York: Cambridge University Press, 1981.

Kiser, Clyde Vernon. *Sea Island to City: A Study of St. Helena Islanders in Harlem and Other Urban Centers*. Columbia University thesis, 1932. New York: Atheneum, 1969.

Klaus, Alisa. *Every Child a Lion: The Origins of Maternal and Infant Health Policy in the United States and France, 1890–1920*. Ithaca, NY: Cornell University Press, 1993.

Klevan, Miriam. *The West Indian Americans*. New York: Chelsea House, 1990.

Kline, Wendy. *Building a Better Race: Gender, Sexuality, and Eugenics from the Turn of the Century to the Baby Boom*. Berkeley: University of California Press, 2001.

Knopf, S. Adolphus, M.D. *A History of the National Tuberculosis Association: The Anti-Tuberculosis Movement in the United States*. New York: National Tuberculosis Association, 1922.

Knox, J. H. Mason Jr., M.D., and Paul Zentai, M.D. "The Health Problem of the Negro Child." *American Journal of Public Health* 16, no. 8 (1926): 805–809.

Knupfer, Anna Meis. *Toward a Tenderer Humanity and a Nobler Womanhood: African American Women's Clubs in Turn-of-the-Century Chicago*. New York: New York University Press, 1996.

Koven, Seth, and Sonya Michel, eds. *Mothers of a New World: Maternalist Politics and the Origins of Welfare States*. New York: Routledge, 1993.

Kraut, Alan M. *Silent Travelers: Germs, Genes, and the "Immigrant Menace."* Baltimore: John Hopkins University Press, 1994.

Ladd-Taylor, Molly. *Mother-Work: Women, Child Welfare, and the State, 1890–1930*. Urbana: University of Illinois Press, 1994.

———. "My Work Came out of Agony and Grief: Mothers and the Making of the Sheppard-Towner Act." In *Mothers of a New World: Maternalist Politics and the Origins of Welfare States*, edited by Seth Koven and Sonya Michel. New York: Routledge, 1993.

Laidlaw, Walter, ed. *Statistical Sources for Demographic Studies of Greater New York, 1910*. New York: New York Federation of Churches, 1913.

———, ed. *Statistical Sources for Demographic Studies of Greater New York, 1920*. New York: New York 1920 Census Committee, 1922.

Larson, Edward J. *Sex, Race, and Science: Eugenics in the Deep South*. Baltimore: Johns Hopkins University Press, 1996.

La Sorte, Michael. *La Merica: Images of Italian Greenhorn Experience*. Philadelphia: Temple University Press, 1985.

Leavitt, Judith Walzer. *Typhoid Mary: Captive to the Public's Health*. Boston: Beacon Press, 1996.

———, and Ronald L. Numbers, eds. *Sickness and Health in America: Readings in the History of Medicine and Public Health*. 3rd rev. ed. Madison: University of Wisconsin Press, 1997.

Lederer, Susan. *Subjected to Science: Human Experimentation in America Before the Second World War*. Baltimore: Johns Hopkins University Press, 1995.

Leinwand, Gerald. *1927: High Tide of the 1920s*. New York: Basic Books, 2001.

Levine, Lawrence W. *Black Culture and Black Consciousness: Afro-American Folk Thought From Slavery to Freedom*. New York: Oxford University Press, 1977.

Lewin, Olive. *Rock It Come Over: The Folk Music of Jamaica*. Kingston, Jamaica: University of the West Indies Press, 2000.

Lewis, Earl. "Expectation, Economic Opportunities, and Life in the Industrial Age: Black Migration to Norfolk, Virginia, 1910–1945." In *The Great Migration in Historical Perspective: New Dimensions of Race, Class, and Gender*, edited by Joe William Trotter. Bloomington: Indiana University Press, 1991.

Lewis, David Levering, ed. *The Portable Harlem Renaissance Reader*. New York: Viking Press, 1994.

Lewis, Earl. *In Their Own Interests: Race, Class, and Power in Twentieth Century Norfolk, Virginia*. Berkeley: University of California Press, 1991.

Lieberson, Stanley. *A Piece of the Pie: Blacks and White Immigrants Since 1880*. Berkeley: University of California Press, 1980.

Litoff, Judy Barrett. *The American Midwife Debate: A Sourcebook on its Modern Origins*. Westport, CT: Greenwood Press, 1986.

Litt, Jacquelyn S. *Medicalized Motherhood: Perspectives from the Lives of African-American and Jewish Women*. New Brunswick, NJ: Rutgers University Press, 2000.

Locke, Alain, ed. *The New Negro*. Introduction by Arnold Rampersad. New York: Atheneum, 1992.

Logan, Onnie Lee, and Katherine Clark. *Motherwit: An Alabama Midwife's Story*. New York: E. P. Dutton, 1989.

Lowis, George W., and Peter G. Mc Caffery. "Sociological Factors Affecting the Medicalization of Midwifery." In *Midwifery and the Medicalization of Childbirth: Comparative Perspectives*, edited by Edward Van Teijlingen, George W. Lowis, Peter G. McCaffery, and Maureen Porter. Huntington, NY: Nova Science Publishers, 2000.

Marks, Harry. "Epidemiologists Explain Pellagra: Gender, Race, and Political Economy in the Work of Edgar Sydenstricker." *Journal of the History of Medicine and Allied Sciences* 58, no. 1 (January 2003): 34–55.

Marks, Lara, and Michael Worboys, eds. *Migrants, Minorities, and Health: Historical and Contemporary Studies*. New York: Routledge, 1997.

Marshall, Paule. "Black Immigrant Women in *Brown Girl, Brownstones*." *Caribbean Life in New York City: Sociocultural Dimensions*. Center for Migration Studies, Special Issue 7:1 (January 1989): 79–85.

———. *Brown Girl, Brownstones*. 3rd ed. First published by Chatham Bookseller, 1972. Old Westbury, NY: Feminist Press, 1981.

McBride, David. *From TB to AIDS: Epidemics Among Urban Blacks Since 1900*. Albany: State University of New York Press, 1991.

———. "The Black-White Mortality Differential in New York State, 1900–1950." *Afro-Americans in New York Life and History* 14, no. 2 (July 1990): 71–89.

McCall, Emmanuel L., compiler. *Black Church Lifestyles*. Nashville, TN: Broadman Press, 1986.

McClendon, Jacquelyn Y. *The Politics of Color in the Fiction of Jessie Fauset and Nella Larsen*. Charlottesville: University Press of Virginia, 1995.

McLennan, Gregor, David Held, and Stuart Hall, eds. *The Idea of the Modern State*. Milton Keynes, UK: Open University Press, 1984.

Meckel, Richard. "Racialism and Infant Death: Late Nineteenth- and Early Twentieth-Century Socio-Medical Discourses on African American Infant Mortality." In *Migrants, Minorities, and Health: Historical and Contemporary Studies*, edited by Lara Marks and Michael Worboys. New York: Routledge, 1997.

———. *Save the Babies: American Public Health Reform and the Prevention of Infant Mortality, 1850–1929*. Ann Arbor: University of Michigan Press, 1998. First published by Johns Hopkins University Press, 1990.

Medaglia, Azadeh. *Patriarchal Structures and Ethnicity in the Italian Community in Britain*. Aldershot, UK: Ashgate, 1992.

Melvin, Patricia Mooney. "Milk to Motherhood: The New York Milk Committee and the Beginning of Well-Child Programs." *Mid-America: An Historical Review* 65, no. 3 (October 1983): 111–134.

Menard, Russell. Quotation taken from *A Century of European Migrations, 1830–1930*, edited by Rudolph J. Vecoli and Suzanne M. Sinke. Urbana: University of Illinois Press, 1991.

Messikomer, Carla M., with Judith P. Swazey and Allen Glickman, eds. *Society and Medicine: Essays in Honor of Renee C. Fox*. New Brunswick, NJ: Transaction Publishers, 2003.

Meyer, E. "Clinical and Experimental Research on the Action of Salvarsan upon Congenital Syphilis of the Foetus Through Treatment of the Mother." *Journal of Cutaneous Diseases* 33 (1915): 418.

Michel, Sonja. *Children's Interests/Mother's Rights: The Shaping of American's Child Care Policy*. New Haven, CT: Yale University Press, 1999.

———. "The Limits of Maternalism: Policies Toward American Wage-Earning Mothers During the Progressive Era." In *Mothers of a New World: Maternalist Politics and the Origins of Welfare States*, edited by Seth Koven and Sonya Michel. New York: Routledge, 1993.

Mink, Gwendolyn. "The Lady and the Tramp: Gender, Race, and the Origins of the American Welfare State." In *Women, the State, and Welfare*, edited by Linda Gordon. Madison: University of Wisconsin Press, 1990.

———. *The Wages of Motherhood: Inequality in the Welfare State, 1917–1942*. Ithaca, NY: Cornell University Press, 1996.

———, and Rickie Solinger, eds. *Welfare: A Documentary History of U.S. Policy and Politics*. With a foreword by Frances Fox Piven. New York: New York University Press, 2003.

Mitchell, Michele. *Righteous Propagation: African Americans and the Politics of Racial Destiny after Reconstruction*. Chapel Hill: University of North Carolina Press, 2004.

Model, Suzanne. "Mode of Job Entry and the Ethnic Composition of Firms: Early Twentieth-Century Migrants to New York City." *Sociological Forum* 3, no. 1 (1988): 110–127.

Moeller, Susan. "The Cultural Construction of Urban Poverty: Images of Poverty in New York City, 1890–1917." *Journal of American Culture* 18, no. 4 (1995): 1–16

Morantz-Sanchez, Regina. *Sympathy and Science: Women Physicians in American Medicine.* Chapel Hill: University of North Carolina Press, 2000.

Morgan, Edmund S. *American Slavery, American Freedom: The Ordeal of Colonial Virginia.* Reprint. New York: W. W. Norton, 1995.

Morse, Dean. W. *Pride Against Prejudice: Work in the Lives of Older Blacks and Young Puerto Ricans.* Montclair, NJ: Allanheld, Osmun, 1980.

Moynihan, Daniel Patrick. *The Negro Family: The Case for National Action.* Washington, DC: U. S. Department of Labor, 1965.

Muhammad, Khalil Gibran. *The Condemnation of Blackness: Race, Crime, and the Making of Modern Urban America.* Cambridge, MA: Harvard University Press, 2011.

National Tuberculosis Association. *A Directory of Sanatoria, Hospitals, Day Camps and Preventoria for the Treatment of Tuberculosis in the United States.* New York: National Tuberculosis Association, 1931.

Newman, Louise Michelle. *White Women's Rights: The Racial Origins of Feminism in the United States.* New York: Oxford University Press, 1999.

Ngai, Mae M. *Impossible Subjects: Illegal Aliens and the Making of Modern America.* Princeton, NJ: Princeton University Press, 2014.

Norther, Emiliana P. "The Silent Half: *Le Contadine del Sud* Before the First World War." In *The Italian Immigrant Woman in North America*, edited by Betty Boyd Caroli, Robert F. Harney, and Lydio F. Tomasi. Toronto: Multicultural History Society of Ontario, 1978.

Novick, Peter. *That Noble Dream: The "Objectivity Question" and the American Historical Profession.* Cambridge University Press, 1988. Reprint. Cambridge, UK: Cambridge University Press, 1996.

Numbers, Ronald L., and John Harley Warner. "The Maturation of American Medical Science." In *Sickness and Health in America: Readings in the History of Medicine*, edited by Judith Walzer Leavitt and Ronald L. Numbers. 3rd ed. Madison: University of Wisconsin Press, 1997.

Odencrantz, Louise C. *Italian Women in Industry: A Study of Conditions in New York City.* New York: Russell Sage Foundation, 1919.

Omi, Michael, and Howard Winant. *Racial Formation in the United States: From the 1960s to the 1990s.* 2nd ed. New York: Routledge, 1994.

Opdycke. Sandra. *No One Was Turned Away: The Role of Public Hospitals in New York City Since 1900.* New York: Oxford University Press, 1999.

Orsi, Robert. "The Religious Boundaries of an Inbetween People: Street *Feste* and the Problem of the Dark-Skinned Other in Italian Harlem, 1920–1990." *American Quarterly* 44, no. 3 (September 1992): 313–347.

Osofsky, Gilbert. *Harlem: The Making of a Ghetto, Negro New York, 1890–1930*. New York: Harper and Row, 1966. 2nd ed. Chicago: Elephant Paperbacks, 1996.

Ott, Katherine. *Fevered Lives: Tuberculosis in American Culture Since 1870*. Cambridge, MA: Harvard University Press, 1996.

Ovington, Mary White. *Black and White Sat Down Together: The Reminiscences of an NAACP Founder*. Edited and with a foreword by Ralph E. Luker. Afterword by Carolyn E. Wedin. New York: Feminist Press at the City University of New York, 1996.

———. *Half a Man: The Status of the Negro in New York*. Longmans, Green and Company, 1911. New York: Charles Flint Kellogg, 1969.

———. *Hazel*. New York: Crisis, 1913.

Painter, Nell Irwin. *Exodusters: Black Migration to Kansas after Reconstruction*. New York: Alfred A. Knopf, 1977.

———. Foreword. In *The Great Migration in Historical Perspective: New Dimensions of Race, Class, and Gender*, edited by Joe William Trotter. Bloomington: Indiana University Press, 1991.

———. *Southern History Across the Color Line*. Chapel Hill: University of North Carolina Press, 2002.

———. *Standing at Armageddon: The United States, 1877–1919*. New York: W. W. Norton, 1987.

Parascandola, James. *Sex, Sin, and Science: A History of Syphilis in America*. Westport, CT: Praeger, 2008.

Park, Robert Ezra. *Old World Traits Transplanted*. New York: Harper and Brothers, 1921. New York: Arno Press, 1969.

———, and Ernest W. Burgess. *Introduction to the Science of Sociology, Including the Original Index to Basic Sociological Concepts*. 1921. 3rd ed., rev. Chicago: University of Chicago Press, 1969.

———, and Herbert Adolphus Miller. *Old World Traits Transplanted*. 1921. New York: Arno Press and the New York Times, 1969.

Park, Roswell, M.D., L.L.D. *The Evil Eye Thanatology and Other Essays*. Boston: Richard G. Badger, 1912.

Paul, Benjamin D., and Walter B. Miller, eds. *Health, Culture and Community: Case Studies of Public Reactions to Health Programs*. New York: Russell Sage Foundation, 1955.

Pearl, Raymond, Ph.D. "Variation in the Rate of Infant Mortality in the United States Birth Registration Area." In *Transactions of the Eleventh Annual Meeting, St. Louis, Mo., October 11–13. 1920, American Child Hygiene Association*. Baltimore: Franklin Printing Company (1921): 213–29.

Pencak, William, Selma Berrol, and Randall M. Miller, eds. *Immigration to New York*. New York: New-York Historical Society, 1991.

Pernick, Martin S. *The Black Stork: Eugenics and the Death of "Defective" Babies in American Medicine and Motion Pictures Since 1915*. New York: Oxford University Press, 1999.

Pessar, Patricia. "The Role of Gender in Dominican Settlement in the U.S." In *Women and Change in Latin America*, edited by June Nash and Helen I. Safa. South Hadley, MA: Bergin and Garvey, 1986.

Pitts Moseley, Marie Oleatha. "A History of Black Leaders in Nursing: The Influence of Four Black Community Health Nurses on the Establishment, Growth, and Practice of Public Health Nursing in New York City, 1900–1930." PhD diss., Columbia University Teachers College, 1992.

Pivar, David. J. *Purity and Hygiene: Women, Prostitution, and the "American Plan," 1900–1930.* Westport, CT: Greenwood Press, 2002.

Plunz, Richard. *A History of Housing in New York City: Dwelling Type and Social Change in the American Metropolis.* New York: Columbia University Press, 1990.

Rawlins, E. Elliott, M.D. "Wanted: A Negro Hospital in New York City." *Colored American Magazine* 4, no. 16 (April 1909): 221–222.

Reeder, Linda. *Widows in White: Migration and the Transformation of Rural Italian Women, Sicily, 1880–1920.* Toronto: University of Toronto Press, 2003.

Reid, Ira De Augustine. *The Negro Immigrant: His Background, Characteristics, and Social Adjustment, 1899–1937.* New York: Columbia University Press, 1939.

Reverby, Susan M. *Ordered to Care: The Dilemma of American Nursing, 1850–1945.* Melbourne: Cambridge University Press, 1987.

Roberts, Dorothy. *Protecting the Black Body: Race, Reproduction, and the Meaning of Liberty.* New York: Pantheon Books, 1997.

Roberts, Samuel Kelton, Jr. *Infectious Fear: Politics, Disease, and the Health Effects of Segregation.* Chapel Hill: University of North Carolina Press, 2009.

Rogers, Naomi. *Dirt and Disease: Polio Before FDR.* New Brunswick, NJ: Rutgers University Press, 1996.

Rogers, Wyatt M., Jr. *Christianity and Womanhood: Evolving Roles and Responsibilities.* Westport, CT: Praeger, 2002.

Rooks, Judith Pence. *Midwifery and Childbirth in America.* Philadelphia: Temple University Press, 1997.

Rosen, George. *A History of Public Health.* 1958. Expanded ed. Baltimore: Johns Hopkins University Press, 1993.

Rosenberg, Charles E. *The Cholera Years: The United States in 1832, 1849, and 1866.* Chicago: University of Chicago Press, 1987.

———. *No Other Gods: On Science and American Social Thought.* Rev. and expanded ed. Baltimore: Johns Hopkins University Press, 1997.

Ross, Loretta J. "African American Women and Abortions." In *Mothers and Motherhood: Readings in American History*, edited by Rima D. Apple and Janet Golden. Columbus: Ohio State University Press, 1997.

Rothman, Sheila M. *Living in the Shadow of Death: Tuberculosis and the Social Experience of Illness in American History.* Baltimore: Johns Hopkins University Press, 1994.

Rudwick, Elliot, ed. *Black Matriarchy: Myth or Reality?* Belmont, CA: Wadsworth, 1971.

Sackheim, Eric, compiler. *The Blues Line: A Collection of Blues Lyrics*. New York: Grossman, 1969.

Sacks, Marcy S. *Before Harlem: The Black Experience in New York City before World War I*. Philadelphia: University of Pennsylvania Press, 2006.

Samuels, Adah B. "Lincoln Home and Hospital." *Colored American Magazine* 1, no. 17 (July 1909): 24–26.

Savitt, Todd L. *Medicine and Slavery: The Diseases and Health Care of Blacks in Antebellum Virginia*. 1978. Urbana: University of Illinois Press, 2002.

———. "Slave Health and Social Distinctiveness." In *Disease and Distinctiveness in the American South*, edited by Todd L. Savitt and James Harvey Young. Knoxville: University of Tennessee Press, 1988.

———, and James Harvey Young, eds. *Disease and Distinctiveness in the American South*. Knoxville: University of Tennessee Press, 1988.

Scheiner, Seth. *Negro Mecca: A History of the Negro in New York City, 1865–1920*. New York: New York University Press, 1965.

Scott, James C. *Domination and the Arts of Resistance: Hidden Transcripts*. New Haven, CT: Yale University Press, 1990.

Secundy, Marian Gray, ed., with Lois La Civita Nixon, collaborator. *Trials, Tribulations, and Celebrations: African-American Perspectives on Health, Illness, Aging and Loss*. Yarmouth, ME: Intercultural Press, 1992.

Sernett, Milton C. *Bound for the Promised Land: African American Religion and the Great Migration*. Durham, NC: Duke University Press, 1997.

Serra, Ilaria. *The Value of Worthless Lives: Writing Italian American Immigrant Autobiographies*. New York: Fordham University Press, 2007.

Shah, Nayan. *Contagious Divides: Epidemics and Race in San Francisco's Chinatown*. Berkeley: University of California Press, 2001.

Skloot, Rebecca. *The Immortal Life of Henrietta Lacks*. Crown Publishers, 2010. New York: Broadway Paperbacks, 2011.

Sklar, Kathryn Kish. "Protestant Women and Social Justice Activism, 1890–1920." Conference keynote essay presented at the Women and Twentieth-Century Protestantism Conference, Chicago, April 23, 1998.

———. "The Historical Foundations of Women's Power in the Creation of the American Welfare State, 1830–1930." In *Mothers of a New World: Maternalist Politics and the Origins of Welfare States*, edited by Seth Koven and Sonya Michel. New York: Routledge, 1993.

Sleet, Jessie, R.N. "Tuberculosis Among Negroes." In *The Third Annual Report of the Committee on the Prevention of Tuberculosis of the Charity Organization Society of the City of New York, for the Year 1904–1905*. New York: Charity Organization Society of the City of New York, 1905. 28–32.

Springarn, Arthur B. *Laws Relating to Sex Morality in New York City*. New York: Century Company, Publications of the Bureau of Social Hygiene, 1915.

Smith, Susan L. *Sick and Tired of Being Sick and Tired: Black Women's Health Activism in America, 1890–1950*. Philadelphia: University of Pennsylvania Press, 1995.

Smith-Rosenberg, Carroll. *Disorderly Conduct: Vision of Gender in Victorian America.* New York: Oxford University Press, 1985.

Snow, John. *On the Mode of Communication of Cholera.* London: John Churchill, 1855.

Snowden, Frank M. *Naples in the Time of Cholera: 1884–1911.* Cambridge: Cambridge University Press, 1995.

Solomon, Harry Caesar. *Syphilis of the Innocent: A study of the Social Effects of Syphilis on the Family and Community.* Washington, DC: United States Interdepartmental Social Hygiene Board, 1922.

Stanley, Amy Dru. *From Bondage to Contract: Wage Labor, Marriage, and the Market in the Age of Slave Emancipation.* New York: Cambridge University Press, 1998.

Stansell, Christine. *American Bohemians: Bohemian New York and the Creation of a New Century.* New York: Metropolitan Books, 2000.

Stella, Antonio, M. D. *Some Aspects of Italian Immigration to the United States: Statistical Data and General Considerations Based Chiefly upon the United States Census and Other Official Publications.* New York: G. P. Putnam's Sons, 1924.

———. "Tuberculosis and the Italians in the United States." First published in *Charities* 12 (1904). In *The Italian in America: The Progressive View*, edited by Lydio F. Tomasi. New York: Center for Migration Studies, 1972.

Stepan, Nancy Leys. "Race and Gender: The Role of Analogy in Science." In *The "Racial" Economy of Science: Toward a Democratic Future*, edited by Sandra Harding. Bloomington: Indiana University Press, 1993.

Summers, Martin. *Manliness and its Discontents: The Black Middle Class and the Transformation of Masculinity, 1900–1930.* Chapel Hill: University of North Carolina Press, 2004.

Sutton, Constance R., and Elsa M. Chaney, eds. *Caribbean Life in New York City: Sociocultural Dimensions.* Center for Migration Studies, 1987. New York: Center for Migration Studies, 1994.

Sylvander, Carolyn Wedin. *Jessie Redmon Fauset: Black American Writer.* Troy, NY: Whitston, 1981.

Tandy, Elizabeth C. "Infant and Maternal Mortality Among Negroes." *Journal of Negro Education* 6, no. 3 (July 1937): 322–349.

Taylor, Clarence. *The Black Churches of Brooklyn.* New York: Columbia University Press, 1994.

Teller, Michael E. *The Tuberculosis Movement: A Public Health Campaign in the Progressive Era.* New York: Greenwood Press, 1988.

Terborg-Penn, Rosalyn. *African American Women in the Struggle for the Vote, 1850–1920.* Bloomington: Indiana University Press, 1998.

Terry, C. C. "Midwives: Their Influence on Early Infant Mortality." *American Journal of Public Health* 1914: 695–699.

Terry, C. E., M.D. "The Negro, a Public Health Problem." *Southern Medical Journal* 7, no. 6 (June 1914): 458–467.

Thompson, Loyd, M.D., and Lyle. B. Kingery, M.D. "Syphilis in the Negro." *American Journal of Syphilis* 3 (1919): 384–397.

Tilly, Louise A., and Joan W. Scott. *Women, Work, and Family*. New York: Holt, Rinehart, and Winston, 1978.

Tomasi, Lydio F., ed. *The Italian in America: The Progressive View*. New York: Center for Migration Studies, 1972.

Tomasi, Silvano M. *Piety and Power: The Role of the Italian Parishes in the New York Metropolitan Area, 1880–1930*. New York: Center for Migration Studies, 1975.

———, and Edward C. Stibili. *Italian Americans and Religion: An Annotated Bibliography*. 2nd ed., revised and enlarged. New York: Center for Migration Studies, 1992.

Tomes, Nancy. *The Gospel of Germs: Men, Women, and the Microbe in American Life*. Cambridge, MA: Harvard University Press, 1998.

de Toqueville, Alexis. *Democracy in America*. First translated from the French by Henry Reeve and published by Saunders and Otley, London, in 1835. An Electronic Series Publication http://www2.hn.psu.edu/faculty/jmanis/toqueville/dem-in-america1.pdf.Aaccessed February 25, 2014.

Trotter, Joe William, Jr. *The African American Experience*. New York: Houghton Mifflin, 2001.

———, ed. *The Great Migration in Historical Perspective: New Dimensions of Race, Class, and Gender*. Bloomington: Indiana University Press, 1991.

Tyndall, Rose Mary Murphy. "A History of the Bellevue School for Midwives: 1911–1936." PhD diss., Columbia University Teachers College, 1978.

Van Blarcom, Carolyn Conant, R.N. "Midwives in America." *American Journal of Public Health* 4, no. 3 (1914): 197–207.

Van Teijlingen, Edward, George W. Lowis, Peter G. McCaffery, and Maureen Porter, eds. *Midwifery and the Medicalization of Childbirth: Comparative Perspectives*. Huntington, NY: Nova Science Publishers, 2000.

Vecchio, Diane C. *Merchants, Midwives, and Laboring Women: Italian Migrants in Urban America*. Urbana: University of Illinois Press, 2006.

Vecoli, Rudolph J., and Suzanne M. Sinke, eds. *A Century of European Migrations, 1830–1930*. Urbana: University of Illinois Press, 1991.

Wailoo, Keith. *Dying in the City of the Blues: Sickle Cell Anemia and the Politics of Race and Health*. Chapel Hill: University of North Carolina Press, 2000.

———. *How Cancer Crossed the Color-Line*. New York: Oxford University Press, 2011.

Wald, Priscilla. *Contagious: Cultures, Carriers, and the Outbreak Narrative*. Durham, NC: Duke University Press, 2008.

Walkowitz, Daniel J. *Working with Class: Social Workers and the Politics of Middle-Class Identity*. Chapel Hill: University of North Carolina Press, 1999.

Wall, Cheryl. *Women of the Harlem Renaissance*. Bloomington: Indiana University Press, 1995.

Wallace, Helen M., M.D., Curtis L. Mendelson, M.D., Leona Baumgartner, M.D., and Ruth Rothmayer, R.N. "The Practice of Midwives in New York City." *New York State Journal of Medicine* (January 1948): 67–71.

Wallerstein, Immanuel. "The Construction of Peoplehood: Racism, Nationalism, Ethnicity." *Sociological Forum* 2, no. 2 (Spring 1987): 373–388.

Ward, Thomas J., Jr. *Black Physicians in the Jim Crow South*. Fayetteville: University of Arkansas Press, 2003.

Warner, John Harley. "From Specificity to Universalism in Medical Therapeutics: Transformation in the 19th Century United States." In *Sickness and Health in America: Readings in the History of Medicine*, edited by Judith Walzer Leavitt and Ronald L. Numbers. 3rd rev. ed. Madison: University of Wisconsin Press, 1997.

———. *The Therapeutic Perspective: Medical Practice, Knowledge, and Identity in America, 1820–1885*. Harvard University Press, 1986. Princeton, NJ: Princeton University Press, 1997.

———, and Janet A. Tighe, eds. *Major Problems in the History of American Medicine and Public Health*. Boston: Houghton Mifflin, 2001.

Washington, Harriet A. *Medical Apartheid: The Dark History of Medical Experimentation on Black Americans from Colonial Times to the Present*. New York: Harlem Moon, 2006.

Waters, Mary C. *Black Identities: West Indian Immigrant Dreams and American Realities*. Cambridge, MA: Harvard University Press, 2001.

Watkins-Owens, Irma. *Blood Relations: Caribbean Immigrants and the Harlem Community, 1900–1930*. Bloomington: Indiana University Press, 1996.

Watson, G. Llewellyn. *Jamaican Sayings: With Notes on Folklore, Aesthetics, and Social Control*. Tallahassee: Florida A & M University Press, 1991.

Watson, Steven. *The Harlem Renaissance: Hub of African-American Culture, 1920–1930*. New York: Pantheon Books, 1995.

Wechselmann, Wilhelm, M.D. "Reports of Salvarsan Fatalities." *Urologic and Cutaneous Review* 17 (1913): 649–651.

Wedin, Carolyn. *Inheritors of the Spirit: Mary White Ovington and the Founding of the NAACP*. With a foreword by David Levering Lewis. New York: John Wiley and Sons, 1998.

Weindling, Paul. *Health, Race and German Politics Between National Unification and Nazism, 1870–1945*. Cambridge: Cambridge University Press, 1989.

Weiner, Lynn. *From Working Girl to Working Mother: The Female Labor Force in the United States, 1820–1980*. Chapel Hill: University of North Carolina Press, 1985.

Weiss, Nancy. "Save the Children: the History of the Children's Bureau, 1903–1918." PhD diss., University of California, Los Angeles, 1974.

Wells-Barnett, Ida B. *On Lynchings, Southern Horrors, A Red Record, Mob Rule in New Orleans*. Reprint ed. Salem, NH: Ayer, 1991.

Welz, Walter E., M.D., and Alfred E. Van Nest, M.D. "Observations on the Treatment of Syphilis in Pregnancy in the Department of Health in Detroit." *American Journal of Obstetrics and Gynecology* 4 (1922): 174–182.

Wertz, Dorothy C. "What Birth Has Done for Doctors: A Historical View." In *The Medicalization of Obstetrics: Personnel, Practice, and Instruments*, edited by Philip K. Wilson. New York: Garland, 1996.

Wheeler, Leigh Ann. *Against Obscenity: Reform and the Politics of Womanhood in America, 1873–1935*. Baltimore: Johns Hopkins University Press, 2004.

White, Deborah Gray. *Ar'n't I a Woman? Female Slaves in the Plantation South.* New York: W. W. Norton, 1985.

——. *Too Heavy a Load: Black Women in Defense of Themselves, 1894–1994.* New York: W. W. Norton, 1999.

White, Newman Ivey. *American Negro Folk-Songs.* Cambridge, MA: Harvard University Press, 1928.

Whitney, Charles M., M.D. "The Impossibility of Curing Syphilis by Salvarsan Alone and the Dangers Arising From Insufficient Treatment." *Interstate Medical Journal* 23:80–88.

Wilkerson, Isabel. *The Warmth of Other Suns: The Epic Story of America's Great Migration.* New York: Vintage, 2011.

Williams, Phyllis H. *South Italian Folkways in Europe and America: A Handbook for Social Workers, Visiting Nurses, School Teachers, and Physicians.* New Haven, CT: Yale University Press, 1938.

Wilson, Harriet E., et al. *The Soul of a Woman.* London: X Press, 1998.

Wilson, Philip K., ed. *The Medicalization of Obstetrics: Personnel, Practice, and Instruments.* New York: Garland, 1996.

Winslow, C.-E. A., Dr. P. H. *The Evolution and Significance of the Modern Public Health Campaign.* New Haven, CT: Yale University Press, 1923.

——. *The Life of Herman M. Biggs, M.D., D. Sc., L.L.D.: Physician and Statesman of the Public Health.* Philadelphia: Lea and Febiger, 1929.

Wolcott, Roger T, and Dorita F. Bolger, compilers. *Church and Social Action: A Critical Assessment and Bibliographical Survey* Westport, CT: Greenwood Press, 1990.

Wolf, Stewart, and John G. Bruhn, with Brenda P. Egolf, Judith Lasker, and Billy U. Philips, collaborators. *The Power of Clan: The Influence of Human Relationships on Heart Disease.* New Brunswick, NJ: Transaction, 1993.

Wolters, Raymond. "Personal Connections and the Growth of the NAACP." Review of *James Weldon Johnson: Black Leader, Black Voice,* by Eugene Levy, and *J. E. Springarn and the Rise of the NAACP, 1911–1939,* by B. Joyce Ross. In *Reviews in American History* 2, no. 1 (March 1974), 138–145.

Woodson, Carter G. *A Century of Negro Migration.* Association for the Study of Negro Life and History, 1918. Mineola, NY: Dover Publications, 2002.

Woodward, C. Vann. *Origins of the New South, 1877–1913.* Baton Rouge: Louisiana State University Press, 1971.

Work, Monroe N., compiler. *A Bibliography of the Negro in Africa and America.* 1928. New York: H. W. Wilson Company, 1965.

Yans-McLaughlin, Virginia. *Family and Community: Italian Immigrants in Buffalo, 1880–1930.* 1971. Ithaca, NY: Cornell University Press, 1977.

Zuberi, Tukufu. *Thicker Than Blood: How Racial Statistics Lie.* Minneapolis: University of Minnesota Press, 2003.

——, and Eduardo Bonilla-Silva, eds. *White Logic, White Methods: Racism and Methodology.* New York: Rowman and Littlefield, 2008.

INDEX

Abolitionism, 8
Acculturation, 39, 69
Addams, Jane, 87
African Americans, 1–3, 157; ancestors of, 32–33; Baker and, 88; Blascoer and, 101–6; British West Indians and, 37–39; cultural artifacts of, 12; culture and, 110–30; diseases and, 155; as domestic workers, 28; education and, 5; environmental factors and, 6; Great Migration of, 6, 9, 26, 28, 30, 45, 147; health data and, 140–41; historiography of, 23–32; housing and, 94–95; immigrants, 11–12, 17–18, 19–35; infant mortality rate for, 6; marriage and, 44, 94; maternalism and, 71; men, 31, 41, 119–22; music and, 117–30; Negro question, 53–54, 67; nonnative-born, 41–42, 253n64; as nurses, 83–84; Ovington and, 96–101; poverty and, 245n3; racial discrimination against, 4–5; racialization of motherhood and, 111; sociological study on, 92–96; stereotypes of, 10, 44, 109, 123–24, 128, 134, 220; syphilis and, 2, 13, 15, 147–48, 152; tuberculosis and, 173–85. *See also* Columbus Hill
Afro-Caribbeans, 251n51; immigrants, 37, 41–43, 51; language of, 132–33
AICP. *See* Association for Improving the Condition of the Poor
Albuminuria, 214, 285n67
American Association for the Study and Prevention of Infant Mortality, 207

American Child Hygiene Association, 172, 210
American Civil War, 256n94
American Dream, 48
American Journal of Nursing, 181
American Journal of Public Health, 70
American Medical Association, 219
American Social Hygiene Association, 153
Ames, Jessie, 265n18
Anthropology, 53
Anti-Italian sentiments, 192, 193
Antimiscegenation laws, 39
Anti-tuberculosis campaigns, 10, 75
Arsphenamine, 170
Asian Americans, 248n4
Asian immigrants, 40
Assimilation, 252n57, 255n90
Association for Improving the Condition of the Poor (AICP), 103, 138–39, 150, 161–64, 171, 183; Columbus Hill and, 22–23, 151–58, 239–40; health demonstrations by, 2–3, 13, 16, 140, 151; housing and, 22; marriage and, 10; midwives and, 13–14, 204, 206–7, 223–26, 235, 286n5; Mulberry District and, 189, 190–91; prenatal care and, 219–21; *Protecting the Mother and Child*, 14, 218, 221–39; Southern Italians and, 192; "What Next in Mulberry Bend?," 239–43
Astral settlements, 97, 99
Atlanta University, 98
Autopsies, 76

315

Bacteria, 7, 142–43
Bacteriology, 149, 209, 282n24
Baetz, Walter, 159
Baker, Sara Josephine, 12, 85–86, 107, 205, 207–8; African Americans and, 88; Department of Health and, 85, 89; ethos of maternalism and, 86–91; immigrants and, 90; Southern Italians and, 90–91
Bananas, 252n54
Barbados, 45, 48, 130, 251n51
Barolini, Helen, 264n11
Barry, John M., 268n8
Beals, Alfred Tennyson, *224*
Beals, Jessie Tarbox, *181*
Beecher, Henry Ward, 96
Bell, Rosalie, 206
Bellevue Hospital, 205–6
Bellevue School of Midwifery, 206
Bertellini, Giorgio, 54
Bible, 130
Biculturalism, 132
Big Brothers, 103, 104
Big Sisters, 103, 104
Bilingualism, 132
Billings, John S., 145
Biogenetic engineering, 4
Biological determinism, 67
Bird of passage, 57, 195
Birth, as pathology, 204
Birth Registration Area, U.S., 228, 229–30, 233, 287n24
Black and White Sat Down Together: The Reminiscences of an NAACP Founder (Ovington), 98
Black Death, 141
"Black Mountain Blues" (Smith), 128–29
Blascoer, Frances, 10, 12, 64, 92, 101–6, 107
Blondes, 265n18
Bloomingdale Academy, 20
Blues music, 117–19, 121, 122–30, 266n24
Boards of health, 74
Bodnar, John, 254n89

Bond, Thomas, 77
Bourbon Democrats, 250n29
Breastfeeding, 147
Bright's disease, 199
Brindisi, Rocco, 258n102
Brisbane, Arthur, 20
British West Indians, 1, 2, 51, 251n51; African Americans and, 37–39; in Columbus Hill, 19–23, 43; cultural artifacts of, 12; cultural representations of, 130–36; environmental factors and, 6; Henrietta Industrial School and, 103; historiography of, 35–49; immigrants, 11–12, 19–23, 35–49; literacy and, 253n73; sociology and, 92; syphilis and, 13; as third-party population, 253n64; transportation links and, 252n54
Bronx, 146
Brooklyn, 97
Brooklyn Literary Society, 108
Brown Girl, Brownstones (Marshall), 45–49
Bruce, Robert, 96
Bruck, Carl, 158
Bubonic plague, 141–42
Bureau of Child Hygiene, 153, 205
Burgess, Ernest, 254n89
Burritt, Bailey B., 23, 138, 146–47, 162–65, 222, 275n1

Cadogan, William, 209
Calhoun, Katie, 35–37, 60, 62
Calhoun, Lester, 35
Cancer, 199
Carby, Hazel, 108, 124, 266n24
Caribbean, 9, 131. *See also* Afro-Caribbeans
Caroline Rest Home, 138
Cartwright, Samuel, 8, 174
Catholic Church, 202
Cavelleri, Rosa, 264n11
Central Africans, 17
Central Americans, 20

Chaddock, Robert, 140, 141, 144–46
Chemotherapy, 158
Chicago School, 29, 38, 254n89
Child-rearing methods, 3, 15
Children's Aid Society, 103
Children's Bureau, U.S., 71
Chinese Exclusion Act (1882), 40
Cholera, 7–8, 141–44, 148; infant, 208–9; *vibrio cholera*, 143, 269n16
City and Suburban Homes Company, 21, 95
Civil rights movement, 51
Civil War, 256n94
Climatization, 134–35
Colonialism, 51
"Colored Prenatal" report (AICP), 162
Color Struck (Hurston), 114–17
Columbia College of Physicians and Surgeons, 165, 168–70
Columbia University, 13, 140, 192
Columbia University School of Dental Hygiene, 223
Columbus Hill, 2–3, 11, 34–35, 48–49, 92, 107, 139, 150, 185–87, 249n9; AICP and, 22–23, 151–58, 239–40; Blascoer and, 101–6; British West Indians in, 19–23, 43; crime in, 95; health demonstrations in, 162–73; health work in, 12–13; housing in, 20–23, *21*; immigrants in, 19–23; marital status in, 10; neglect in, 64; nurses in, *82*; population by race in, *19*; prenatal care in, 220, 226, 238; results of demonstrations in, 171–73; sanitary districts in, 146–47; syphilis in, 162–73, 183–84, 226; truancy in, 64; tuberculosis in, 180–85
"Columbus Hill Health Center Album, Man on Sofa with Family" (Beals, J. T.), *181*
Committee of Dispensary Development, 194
Committee on the Hygiene of School Children, 101

Community Organization Society (COS), 11, 49, 97–98, 105, 180; Calhoun, K., and, 35–36; Simms, E., and, 24–25
Community Service Society of New York (CSSNY), 249n20
Community ties, 52
Congenital syphilis, 15, 156, 162–63, 170–71, 215, 272n47; infant mortality and, 184, 186, 216; racialization and, 111–12; sterility and, 154
Consumption. *See* Tuberculosis
Contadini (southern Italian townsfolk), 8, 191, 221
COS. *See* Community Organization Society
Coser, Rose Laub, 61
Creole dialects, 132–33
Crime, 95
Crosby, Alfred, 268n8
'Cruiter (Matheus), 32–35
CSSNY. *See* Community Service Society of New York
Cubanos, 43
Cultural artifacts, 136; of African Americans, 12; of British West Indians, 12; of Progressive Era, 113
Cultural capital, 43, 48, 132
Culture, 108–10; acculturation, 39, 69; African Americans and, 110–30; biculturalism, 132; British West Indians and, 130–36; conclusion to, 136–37; music and, 117–30; racialization of motherhood and, 110–17; transmission of, 16

Daniel, Annie Sturgess, 85, 88
Danzi, Angela D., 220
Darwinism, 53, 66, 70, 150
Davis, Angela, 117, 124
Day care centers, 72
De Lee, Thomas, 219
Dental care, 223
Department of Charities, 50
Department of Dermatology, 169, 170

Department of Health, 12, 151, 188–90, 195, 218, 238, 242–44; Baker and, 85, 89; midwives and, 204–6; mortality study by, 1, 158, 169; prenatal care and, 219, 221, 227–28; sanitary districts and, 2, 145–46; sore spots and, 15, 188; spitting and, 193
Department of Labor, 71
Department of Syphilology, 169, 170
Depression (1930s), 83, 201, 207, 243
DeWitt Clinton Park, 20
Diarrhea, 233–34; diseases, 162; infant mortality and, 208
Differentiation, 104
Discrimination: economic, 27; in housing, 29; racial, 4–5, 83, 106
Disease and difference, 7, 246n12
Diseases, 73, 111–13, 246n12; African Americans and, 155; Bright's disease, 199; diarrheal, 162; epidemic, 7–8, 74, 141–43; etiologies of, 7, 148–50; heart, 199; immigrants and, 73; infectious, 147; prevention of, 178–79; racialization of, 179; religion and, 7–8; respiratory, 2, 13, 147, 175–77; tropical, 174; venereal, 109, 128, 153, 157–58, 169. *See also specific diseases*
Dispensary Development Committee, 223
Dissemblance, 32
Division of Child Hygiene, 12, 85
Division of Child Welfare, 90
Division of Midwifery, 205
Division of Statistical Research, 188
Doctoresses, 203
Domestic violence, 121
Domestic workers, 28, 250n36
"Don't Fish in My Sea" (Rainey), 126
Double-shift women, 27
Dublin, Louis I., 172–73, 193, 197–201, 210, 213; MCA and, 214–15; stillbirths and, 211–12; syphilis and, 216
Du Bois, W. E. B., 12, 65, 90, 129, 252n54, 259n3; marriage statistics and, 44; Ovington and, 98; push/pull migration and, 29; sociological study by, 92–96
Duffy, John, 89
Duffy antigen, 174
Duster, Troy, 244
Dystocia, 216, 285n71

The East Side (Norris), 56–62
Eclampsia, 214–15, 285n67
Economic discrimination, 27
Education, 34, 75; African Americans and, 5; medicine and, 77
Effluvia, 7, 149
Ehrlich, Paul, 158–60, 166, 273n64
Elias, Lewis W., 274n67
Ellis Island, 8, 194, 281n21
Ellison, Ralph, 45
Emancipation, 27, 157, 173
Emerson, Haven, 138
Emerson, Helena Titus, 105
Empowerment movements, 51
English language, 42
"Enlightened Womanhood" (Harper), 108
Enteritis, 13, 15, 190, 233–34, 243
Environmental factors, 5–6, 67, 145; tuberculosis and, 177, 197, 200
Epidemic diseases, 7–8, 74, 141–43
Epidemiology, 149, 209
Episcopal Church, 103
Ethnic capital, 48
Ethnicity, 39
Ethnic purity, 71
Ethos of maternalism, 86–91
Eugenic theory, 39–40, 149
Eurocentrism, 18
European Jews, 199
European migration, 9, 50–51
Everett, Ray H., 153
Evil eye (*malocchio*), 194
Exodusters, 27
Exogamy, 39

Familial violence, 56–57
Families: matriarchal, 44, 253n74; sexuality and, 61
Fauset, Jessie Redmon, 266n26
Feldberg, Georgina D., 264n9
Feminism, 52, 284n52
Feminization, 256n94
First Peoples, 17
First-stage syphilis, 167
Five Points, 93
"Flame-Heart" (McKay), 131
Flexner, Abraham, 77, 80, 83
Forceps, 204
Fordyce, John A., 164
Foul air. *See* Miasmas
France, 70; midwifery and, 202–3
Franklin, J. L., 153
Frazier, E. Franklin, 29, 44
Free white persons, 248n4
Friedman-Kasaba, Kathie, 50–52, 255n90

Galen, 76
Galloping consumption, 176–77
Garrison, William Lloyd, 96
Gastrointestinal disorders, 208
Gebhart, John C., 153–54, 229, 238–40, 242, 272n43, 287n20
Gender class, 52
Germans, 6, 199, 250n36
German School, 142
Germ theory, 73–75, 148–50, 156, 209, 282n24; tubercle bacillus and, 142, 149; tuberculosis and, 178
Ghetto model, 29
Gilded Age, 109, 112
The Golden Door (Kessner), 254n89
Gonorrhea, 166, 194
Granny midwives, 203–4
Great Depression (1930s), 83, 201, 207, 243
Great Migration (1910s), 6, 26, 28, 30, 147; Barbadians and, 45; European migration and, 9
Greenwich House, 98–99

Griffin, Farah Jasmine, 30, 32
Guilfoy, William, 146–47, 184, 188–90, 223, 269n23
Gutman, Herbert, 10, 44

Hacker, Andrew, 39
Half a Man (Ovington), 100
Hall, Stuart, 245n3
Handlin, Oscar, 38, 254n89
Harding, Sandra, 52
Harlem, 23, 92, 102, 171, 256n93
Harlem Renaissance, 114, 124–25, 266n26
Harper, Frances Ellen Watkins, 12, 108–9, 129, 137
Harris, Abram, 10
Harris, Alice Kessler, 250n35
Hazen, Henry H., 160, 276n9, 276n11
Health data, racialization of, 140–50
Health Work for Mothers and Children in a Colored Community (AICP pamphlet), 14, 287n20
Hearst, William Randolph, 20
Heart disease, 199
Hell's Kitchen, 86–87
Henrietta Industrial School, 103
Henry, Florette, 29
Henry Street Settlement, 151, 153, 172, 213–16
Hereditarianism, 71, 111, 146, 148, 150, 173
Heritage, 259n4
Hidden transcripts, 9–10
Higham, John, 254n89
Hill, Robert, 266n24
Hine, Darlene Clark, 32, 83, 121
Historiography, 17–19; African American, 23–32; British West Indian, 35–49; Southern Italian, 49–62
Hoffman, Eric, 158
Hoffman, Frederick, 140
Holden, Arthur, 271n38
Holloway, Karla FC, 65, 107
Holmes, Norman, 21
Horsman, Reginald, 257n94

Hospitals, 76, 78; nurses and, 82; teaching, 168. *See also specific hospitals*
Housing: African Americans and, 94–95; AICP and, 22; in Columbus Hill, 20–23, *21*; discrimination in, 29; Tuskegee Apartments and, 98–99
Howells, William Dean, 97
Human capital models, 255n90
Humoralism, 73, 76, 142
Humors, 76
Hurricanes, 37–38
Hurston, Zora Neal, 114–17, 123, 137
Hygiene, 75; social, 109
Hyman, Paula E., 252n57

Illiteracy, 255n90
Illness as Metaphor (Sontag), 112
Illness censuses, 188–89
Immigrants: African American, 11–12, 17–18, 19–35; Afro-Caribbean, 37, 41–43, 51; Asian, 40; Baker and, 90; British West Indian, 11–12, 19–23, 35–49; conclusion to, 62–63; diseases and, 73; Japanese, 40; migration history and, 17–19; SCE, 5, 9, 40, 70, 110; Southern Italian, 8–9, 11–12, 49–62; stigma of, 7
Immigration Restriction Act (1924), 150
"The Impossibility of Curing Syphilis by Salvarsan Alone and the Dangers Arising From Insufficient Treatment" (Whitney), 166
In-betweenness, 226
Indoctrinization, 134–35
Infant cholera, 208–9
Infant diarrheal diseases, 162
Infant mortality, 69–70, 160, 275n1; African American, 6; Afro-Caribbean, 37; congenital syphilis and, 184, 186, 216; diarrhea and, 208; hot spots, 15, 72; movement, 71; in Mulberry District, 229, *229*, 230, *231*, 233; neonatal deaths and, 172, 213; racialism and, 110; rates of, 138–39, *139*, 141, 146, 153, 162, 229

Infectious diseases, 147
Infectious Fear (Roberts), 279n48
Influenza, 268n8
International Congress on Hygiene and Demography, 140
Interracial marriage, 39
Invisible Man (Ellison), 45
Iola Leroy (Harper), 108
Irish, 6, 149, 250n36; cholera epidemic and, 8; morbidity and, 199
"I Shall Return" (McKay), 132
Italians. *See* Southern Italians
""It Jus Be's Dat Way Sometime'" (Carby), 266n24

Jacobson, Matthew Frye, 53
Jamaica, 35–36, 38, 44, 130–35, 251n51
Japanese immigrants, 40
Jews, 50–51, 199–200, 258n102
Jim Crow segregation, 27, 30, 43, 150
Job Corps, 253n74
Johns Hopkins Hospital, 160, 216
Johns Hopkins School of Medicine, 79–80
Johnson, Lil, 127–28
Johnson-Reed Immigration Act (1924), 200
Jones, Jacqueline, 27, 253n73
Jones, James, 272n53

Kelley, Florence, 87
Kessner, Thomas, 254n89, 258n102
Kinship, 52
Kirkbride, Franklin B., 138–39, 145, 162, 275n1
Klevan, Mirian, 37
Koch, Robert, 73, 142–43, 148, 178, 269n16, 282n24
Koven, Seth, 68, 261n5
Kraut, Alan, 7, 8, 11, 73

Laboratory science, 77, 79
Laboratory testing, 281n20

Language: Afro-Caribbean, 132–33;
  English, 42
Lewin, Olive, 134–35
Lieberson, Stanley, 4–5
Lincoln Center complex, 3
Lincoln Day Nursery, 103
Lincoln House, 22, 48, 101, 146, 151
Literacy, 38, 40, 42, 241, 253n73, 255n90
Literacy Act, U.S., 38
Literary black migration, 30–31
Literature: social science, 45; transmigration, 254n89. *See also specific works*
Little Italy. *See* Mulberry District
Locke, Alain, 256n93
Lodgers, 95
Long Island Medical College, 160
Lowell, Josephine Shaw, 97
Lynching, 265n18

Malaria, 7, 143, 155, 174–76, 246n12
Malocchio (evil eye), 194
Mammy trope, 4, 32
Manhood, 108, 122
Marriage: African Americans and, 44, 94; AICP and, 10; interracial, 39; sex and, 128
Marshall, Paule, 45–49
Marxism, 51
Massini, Guilio, 57
Massini, Maria, 49, 50, 60, 62
Maternal Center Association, 172
Maternalism, 145, 261n5; ethos of, 86–91; movements, 12, 55; permutations of, 68–73; professionalization and, 66–73; religious beliefs and, 87–88; World War I and, 69–70
Maternal mortality rates, 15, 153, 230; eclampsia and, 215; maternalism and, 72–73; puerperal fever and, 232
Maternity Center Association (MCA), 213–16
Matheus, John F., 32–35
Matriarchal families, 44, 253n74

Mayo-Smith, Richmond, 192
MCA. *See* Maternity Center Association
McKay, Claude, 131–32
Meckel, Richard, 110, 263n7
Medical schools, 77, 79–80
Medicine: education and, 77; municipal, 12; professionalization of, 12, 75–80; rationalized, 79; tropical, 143
Meharry and Howard medical facilities, 83
Men: African American, 31, 41, 119–22; manhood, 108, 122; midwifery and, 203–4
Menard, Russell, 18
Mental health, 36
Mercury, 170, 274n71
Metropolitan Life Insurance Company, 172, 193, 210
Mexican Americans, 248n4
Miasmas (foul air), 7, 73–74, 143, 149
Michel, Sonya, 68, 261n5
Microbial agents, 73, 282n24
Midwifery, 183, 239, 242, 284n52; AICP and, 13–14, 204, 206–7, 223–26, 235, 286n5; French, 202–3; granny midwives, 203–4; licensing and, 205; men and, 203–4; in Mulberry District, 13–14, 202–17, 219–20, 223–26, 232, 235, 239, 242; schools for, 204–5; slavery and, 203; witchcraft and, 202
Migration: European, 9, 50–51; Great Migration, 6, 9, 26, 28, 30, 45, 147; history, 17–19; literary black, 30–31; post-migration identities, 1–2; push and pull, 17, 29, 33, 37, 51, 255n90; selective, 240; transmigration literature, 254n89; world-systems migration theory, 52. *See also* Immigrants
Milk stations, 74, 103, 210, 236; Strauss and, 141; venereal diseases and, 153
Miller, Herbert, 67, 259n4
Mink, Gwendolyn, 68
Minnie, Memphis, 118, 122, 124–26

Miscarriages, 171
Modern, 245n3
Monkkonen, Eric, 6
Morbidity, 73, 111, 198; data, 140; Irish and, 199; malaria and, 175; rates, 141; scrofula and, 177; sore spots and, 189; surveys, 223
Morrison, Toni, 32
Mortality: data, 140; tables, 198. *See also* Infant mortality; Maternal mortality rates
Motherhood, racialization of, 110–17
Mothers of a New World (Koven and Michel), 261n5
Moynihan, Daniel Patrick, 253n74
Mrs. W., 182, 185
Mulattos, 135–36
Mulberry District (Little Italy), 2–3, 11, 55, 107, 188–91, 218, 239–43; antituberculosis campaigns in, 10; birth rates for, 225; conclusion to, 243–44; health workers in, 91; infant mortality in, 229, 229, 230, 231, 233; midwives in, 13–14, 202–17, 219–20, 223–26, 232, 235, 239, 242; mortality rates in, 15; population by age group in, *241*; prenatal care in, 219–21; *Protecting the Mother and Child* and, 221–39; totally reported deliveries in, *236*; tuberculosis in, 191–201
Mulberry Health Center, 218, 233–34, 236, 238, 242–43, 289n54; health surveys by, 190; infant mortality and, *229*; prenatal care and, 220, 222–23; sanitary districts and, 228
"Mulberry Health Center Album, Prenatal Nurse with Family," *234*
"Mulberry Health Center Album, Visiting Nurse with Mother and Three Children" (Beals, A. T.), *224*
"Mulberry Health Center Album—Mothers and Kiddies Waiting for Care," *237*

Municipal medicine, 12
Music: blues, 117–19, 121, 122–30, 266n24; work songs, 119–22

NAACP. *See* National Association for the Advancement of Colored People
NACW. *See* National Association of Club Women
National Association for the Advancement of Colored People (NAACP), 12, 92, 101, 104
National Association of Club Women (NACW), 71
National Conference of the American Public Health Association, 156
National Congress of Mothers, 70
National League on Urban Condition Among Negroes, 104
Native Americans, 7, 141
Native-born African Americans, 41–42
Nativism, 7–8, 40, 179
Naturalization, 18, 39, 248n4
Needle trades, 56
Neglect, 64
Negro Consumption, 176
The Negro Immigrant: His Background, Characteristics, and Social Adjustment, 1899—1937 (Reid), 38–39
"Negro Poisoning," 176
Negro problem, 54, 92, 147, 256n93
Negro question, 67, 107
Neisser, Albert, 158
Neo-Marxism, 51–52
Neonatal deaths, 211–13, 215
Neosalvarsan, 160, 164, 166, 273n64
Nervous impulses, 66
Neurasthenic effect, 49
New Deal, 111
Newman, Louise, 69, 256n93
"The New Negro" (Locke), 256n93
New Negro Womanhood, 124
New York Diet Kitchen Station, 222, 236, 289n54

New York Free Kindergarten Association for Colored Children, 105
New York Hospital-Cornell Medical Center, 169
New York Infant Asylum, 169
New York Infirmary, 85
New York Medical Journal, 159
New York Nursery and Child's Hospital, 151–54, 162, 169, 185–86
New York Times, 60
Niagara Movement, 101
Nichols, Franklin O., 153
914 (neosalvarsan), 273n64
Nineteenth District, 93
Nonnative-born African Americans, 41–42, 253n64
Nordic European immigrants, 42
"The Normal Child" (course), 85
Norris, Zoe, 56–62, 257n97, 257n98
Norther, Emiliana P., 255n90
Northern Italians, 54–55
Nosology, 76, 148
"Nothing in Rambling" (Minnie), 124
Nott, Josiah, 8, 174, 256n94
Nursing: professionalization of, 80–84; standardized, 82

Obstetrics, 204, 209, 219
Office of the Registrar of Records, 204
Old World Origins, 18
"O Little Green Island far over the Sea" (Redcam), 131
Opportunity (magazine), 6, 114
O'Reilly, Leonora, 97
Orsi, Robert, 226
Out-of-wedlock births, 44
Overcrowding, 20–21, *21*
Ovington, Mary White, 12, 22, 92, 95, 96–101, 107
Owens, Katie. *See* Calhoun, Katie

Padrone, 221
Paesane, 239

Painter, Nell, 26
Pale spirochete (*spirochaeta pallida*), 158
Panama Canal Zone, 131, 159
Paris School, 78, 142
Park, Robert, 29, 67, 254n89, 259n4
Pasteur, Louis, 73, 142
Patriarchy, 50
Peasantry, 255n90
Pediatrics, 209
Pelvic measurement, 202
Phillips, Ethel, 152, 154
Phipps, Henry, 95, 98, 101
Phipps Houses, 21–22
Physiological method, 79
A Piece of the Pie: Blacks and White Immigrants Since 1880 (Lieberson), 4–5
Plasmodium falciparum, 174–75, 247n12
Plasmodium vivax, 174–75, 247n12
Pneumococcus, 142
Pneumonia, 13, 15, 179, 190, 199, 233–34; tuberculosis and, 183; virgin soil and, 177
Poetry, 131
Polio, 270n33
Political structures, 52
Population: by age group, *241*; growth of, 72; by race, *19*; third-party, 253n64
Post-migration identities, 1–2
Poverty, 96–97, 105, 141, 183, 245n3
Preeclampsia, 214–15, 285n67
Prenatal care, 87, 272n43; in Columbus Hill, 220, 226, 238; Department of Health and, 219, 221, 227–28; in Mulberry District, 219–21
Presbyterian Hospital, 168
Preschool public health, 14, 222
Price, Clara, 237, 269n25, 275n1
Private nurses, 83
Professionalization, 64–66; conclusion to, 84; maternalism and, 66–73; of medicine, 12, 75–80; of nursing, 80–84; of public health, 12, 74–75; of social work, 12

Progressive Era, 23, 65, 76, 109–12, 129–30, 137, 148, 164, 185; cultural artifacts of, 113; laboratory testing in, 281n20; maternalism and, 68–70, 71, 89; medical journal articles in, 272n53; music in, 117–18; poverty and, 245n3; religious beliefs and, 87; tuberculosis and, 178
Progressivism, 68
Proletarian model, 30
Prostitution, 100–101, 109, 166
Protecting the Mother and Child (AICP pamphlet), 14, 218, 221–39
Protestants, 202
Proverbs, Jamaican, 133–34
Prudential Life Insurance Company, 140
Public Health Service, U.S., 144, 194, 234
Public transcripts, 9–10
Puerperal maternal deaths, 172, 232
Push and pull migration, 17, 29, 33, 37, 51, 255n90

La questione meridionale (southern question), 53, 67, 107

Rabies, 142
Race relations model, 29
Race suicide, 39, 70, 157, 195
Racial discrimination, 4–5, 83, 106
Racial groups, 18, 38–39
Racism, 6, 67, 157, 244; infant mortality and, 110; tuberculosis and, 179
"Racism and Infant Death" (Meckel), 110
Racialization: of disease, 179; of health data, 140–50; of motherhood, 110–17; of science, 188
Racial uplift, 83
Radcliffe University, 97
Ragged Edge Klub, 60
Rainey, Gertrude "Ma," 118, 122, 126–27
Rape, 121

Rationalized medicine, 79
Reconstruction Era, 26–27, 108
Redcam, Tom, 131
Reid, Ira De Augustine, 38–39, 41, 45, 51
Religion: beliefs of, 87–88; diseases and, 7–8. *See also specific religions*
Resettlement centers, 72
Respectability, 123
Respiratory diseases, 2, 13, 147, 175–77. *See also specific diseases*
Risorgimento, of Italy, 53
Roberts, Samuel Kelton, Jr., 279n48
Rogers, Lina, 89
Roman Catholic Church, 202
Roosevelt, Theodore, 70, 249n9
Rosen, George, 73
Rosen, Isadore, 164–65, 170
Rosenberg, Charles, 66
Ross, E. A., 192
Russian Jews, 50–51, 199–200

Salvarsan, 158–60, 164, 166–68, 273n64, 274n67, 274n71
Sanitarianism, 8, 74–75, 142–44, 149, 209, 244
Sanitary districts, 6, 184, 188–89, 269n23, 279n53; in Columbus Hill, 146–47; Department of Health and, 2, 145–46; Mulberry Health Center and, 228
San Juan Hill. *See* Columbus Hill
Savitt, Todd, 175, 278n42
Scaffolding, 26, 65
SCE. *See* Southern, central, and eastern Europeans immigrants
Schaudinn, Fritz, 158
School for Midwives, 205
Scientific management, 81–82
Scott, James, 9
Scrofula, 177, 278n42
Seasoning, 175–76
Second-stage syphilis, 167
Selective migration, 240

Sexuality, 108–9, 265n18; family and, 61; music and, 117, 119, 123, 124, 127–28; slavery and, 135–36
Sheppard-Towner Act (1921), 210
Shippen, William, 203
Sickle-cell trait, 174–75
"The Silent Half: *Le Contadine del Sud* before the First World War" (Norther), 255n90
Silent Travelers: Germs and the Immigrant Menace (Kraut), 7
Simms, Ellen, 23–26, 60, 62
Simms, Thomas, 23
606 (salvarsan), 273n64
Skilled workers, 42
Sklar, Katherine Kish, 87, 261n5
Slavery, 8, 9, 27, 108, 132, 155; midwifery and, 203; out-of-wedlock births and, 44; sexuality and, 135–36; tuberculosis and, 173–74, 176–78, 180
Sleet, Jessie, 98, 180–83, 186, 197
Sloane Hospital, 150, 152, 168–69, 186
Smallpox, 177
Smith, Bessie, 118, 122, 128–29
Snow, John, 142
Social disorganization, 29
Social hygiene movement, 109
Social purity, 109
Social Reform Club (SRC), 97
Social science literature, 45
Social transmission, 16
Social welfare system, 71
Social work, 91–106; Blascoer and, 101–6; conclusion to, 107; Du Bois and, 92–96; Ovington and, 96–101; professionalization of, 12
Society for the Prevention of Cruelty to Children, 103
Socioeconomic factors, 1, 37
"Sociological Study" (Holmes), 21
Sociology, 92
"The Song of the Tubs" (Norris), 57
Sontag, Susan, 112

Sore spots, 15, 188–89
South Americans, 9, 20
Southern, central, and eastern Europeans immigrants (SCE), 5, 9, 40, 70, 110
Southern Italians, 1, 2; AICP and, 192; Baker and, 90–91; environmental factors and, 6; historiography of, 49–62; immigrants, 8–9, 11–12, 49–62; poverty and, 245n3; spitting and, 10–11, 194; stereotypes of, 54–55, 192, 221, 257n96; syphilis and, 281n17; tuberculosis and, 112, 179, 193, 195; writings by, 264n11. *See also* Mulberry District
Southern Italian townsfolk (*contadini*), 8, 191, 221
Southern problem, 256n93
Southern question (*la questione meridionale*), 53, 67, 107
Spanish-American War, 249n9
Spanish influenza, 139
Spanish Inquisition, 202
Specificity, 75–76, 78
Spirochaeta pallida (pale spirochete), 158
Spitting, 10–11, 75, 193–94
SRC. *See* Social Reform Club
Standardized nursing, 82
Staphylococcus, 142
Status quo, 17–18
Stay-at-home mothers, 106
St. Cyprian's Parish House and Chapel, 103
Stella, Antonio, 8, 193–97, 200–201, 258n102, 281n17
Stereotypes, 226, 255; of African Americans, 10, 44, 109, 123–24, 128, 134, 220; self-identification and, 136; of Southern Italians, 54–55, 192, 221, 257n96; tuberculosis and, 185; of womanhood, 266n23
Stillbirths, 171, 211–12, 215, 275n5
Strangers in the Land: Patterns of American Nativism (Higham), 254n89
Strauss, Nathan, 141

Streptococcus, 142
Stryker, Garrit Hopper, 20
Subfields, in history, 17
Sugar industry, 37
Surgeries, 78
Syphilis, 138, 140, 151–58, 185–86, 194, 226, 272n43, 272n47; African Americans and, 2, 13, 15, 147–48, 152; arsphenamine and, 170; British West Indians and, 13; in Columbus Hill, 162–73, 183–84, 226; MCA and, 215–16; mercury and, 170, 274n71; salvarsan and, 158–60, 164, 166–68, 273n64, 274n67, 274n71; Southern Italians and, 281n17; Wassermann tests and, 152, 159–60, 162–64, 184, 215–16, 269n25; World War I and, 169. *See also* Congenital syphilis

Talented Tenth, 94
Tammany Hall, 89
Teaching hospitals, 168
Tenderloin District, 93–95, 102
Tenement House Act (1901), 99, 144
Terry, C. E., 157
Therapeutic empiricism, 78
Tomes, Nancy, 244
Toqueville, Alexis de, 91, 262n11
Toxemia, 285n67
Tracy, Roger S., 146
Transmigration literature, 254n89
Transplantation, 255n90
The Transplanted: A History of Immigrants in Urban America (Bodnar), 254n89
Tropical diseases, 174
Tropical medicine, 143
Trotter, Joe William, Jr., 29
Truancy, 64
Tubercle bacillus, 112, 176, 179, 197, 264n9, 282n24; etiology and, 148–49; germ theory and, 142, 149; spitting and, 193
Tuberculosis, 15, 111–13, 142, 147–49, 186, 233, 264n9, 278n42, 279n48; African Americans and, 173–85; AICP and, 13; anti-tuberculosis campaigns, 10, 75; in Columbus Hill, 180–85; environmental factors and, 177, 197, 200; germ theory and, 178; mortality rates, 282n24; in Mulberry District, 191–201; racialism and, 179; slavery and, 173–74, 176–78, 180; Southern Italians and, 112, 179, 193, 195; stereotypes and, 185
"Tuberculosis among Negroes: A Report to the Committee on the Prevention of Tuberculosis" (Sleet), 182
Tuskegee Apartments, 95, 98–99, 101
Tuskegee Experiment, 274n66
Tuttle, William, 29

UCLA. *See* University of California, Los Angeles
Unification, of Italy, 53
University of California, Los Angeles (UCLA), 6, 266n24
University of Chicago, 29
University of Pennsylvania, 77
Unskilled workers, 38
The Uprooted (Handlin), 254n89
Uprooting, 255n90
Urbanization, 196
Urban League, 25, 64, 65, 104
Urban Studies, 6
Urine testing, 214

Vanderbilt Clinic, 13, 151, 153, 162–68, 170, 185–86
Van Ingen, Philip, 207, 208
Vedove bianche (white widows), 57
Venereal Disease Clinic, 153
Venereal diseases, 109, 128, 153, 157–58, 169. *See also* Syphilis
Vibrio cholerae, 143, 269n16
Violence, 128; domestic, 121; familial, 56–57; against women, 121–22
Virgin soil epidemics, 7, 177, 247n13
von Pettenkofer, Max, 142, 144, 269n16

Wald, Lillian, 87, 89
Walkowitz, Daniel, 91
Washington, Booker T., 97
Wassermann, August, 158
Wassermann tests, 152, 159–60, 162–64, 184, 215–16, 269n25
Wechselmann, Wilhelm, 159
Wedlock, births out of, 44
Welch, William H., 79
Wells-Barnett, Ida B., 265n18
West Africans, 17
Westchester Association, 139
West End Workers Association, 105
The West Indian Americans (Klevan), 37
West Indies, 9
West Virginia State College, 34
"What Next in Mulberry Bend?" (AICP), 239–43
White, Deborah Grey, 44
White ethnics, 192
Whiteness, 28, 114, 192, 248n4, 264n7; exogamy in, 39; gradations of, 250n35; naturalization and, 18
White widows (*vedove bianche*), 57
White witchcraft, 202
White Women's Rights (Newman), 69
Whitney, Charles M., 166, 167

Williams, J. Whitridge, 160, 216, 219, 272n47
Witchcraft, 202
Wolters, Raymond, 259n3
Womanhood, 108–9, 137; blues music and, 122–30; stereotypes of, 266n23
Woman problem, 256n93
Woman question, 53, 67, 107
Women's lore, 202
Women's Medical College, 85
Woodson, Carter G., 252n54
Woodward, C. Vann, 250n29
Worker's rights, 97
Work songs, 119–22
World-systems migration theory, 52
World War I, 29, 41, 45, 89, 241; maternalism and, 69–70; syphilis and, 169
World War II, 39, 41
Wright, Richard, 31
Writings, by Southern Italians, 264n11
Wynne, Shirley, 146–47, 184, 188–90, 223, 269n23

Yellow fever, 7, 155, 174
Yertsinia pestis, 141
"You'll Never Miss Your Jelly" (Johnson), 127–28

ABOUT THE AUTHOR

Tanya Hart is Associate Professor in the Department of History at Pepperdine University. Her areas of interest are U.S. women's history, African American studies, the histories of public health and medicine in the United States, and migration studies, all with an overarching emphasis on identity formation.